Sofie Bager-Charleson • Alistair McBeath
Editors

Supporting Research in Counselling and Psychotherapy

Qualitative, Quantitative, and Mixed Methods Research

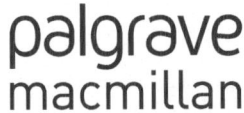

palgrave
macmillan

Editors
Sofie Bager-Charleson
Metanoia Institute
London, UK

Alistair McBeath
Metanoia Institute
London, UK

ISBN 978-3-031-13941-3   ISBN 978-3-031-13942-0   (eBook)
https://doi.org/10.1007/978-3-031-13942-0

Cover illustration: © Bernhard Fritz / getty images

This Palgrave Macmillan imprint is published by the registered company Springer Nature Switzerland AG.
The registered company address is: Gewerbestrasse 11, 6330 Cham, Switzerland

Contents

Notes on Contributors

Sofie Bager-Charleson is a UKCP and BACP registered psychotherapist. She works as Director of Studies for PhD at the Metanoia Institute, specialising in psychotherapy research and training, reflexivity and reflective practice. She chairs the Metanoia research group 'Therapists as Research-informed Practitioners (TRP)', aimed at supporting psychotherapists and counselling psychologists to become confident researchers. She is the co-founder of the annual Metanoia Institute Research Academy for practitioners and has had her work published widely in the field of research methodology and reflexivity, most recently as co-editor with Alistair McBeath of the book *Enjoying Research in Counselling and Psychotherapy*. sofie.bager-charleson@metanoia.ac.uk

Emily Banwell is a PhD researcher at the University of Manchester, where she is conducting a service evaluation on children and young people's mental health provision in the Greater Manchester city region. She also works as a researcher on a number of quantitative and qualitative-focussed studies alongside her doctoral research. These all focus upon the development and evaluation of mental health services, including the exploration of web-based therapy services. Banwell has contributed to postgraduate research methods modules at the University of Manchester, where she has facilitated SPSS workshops. She also holds an MSc in Mental Health Research from the University of Nottingham. In her free time, Emily is a keen world traveller, who likes getting 'off the beaten track'.

Clio Berry is Senior Lecturer in Healthcare Evaluation and Improvement at the Brighton and Sussex Medical School. Her research focuses on social and positive clinical psychology approaches to understanding and treating mental health problems, particularly in youth and student mental health and psychosis. She has a particular interest in the intersection between socio-occupational activities and mental health (problems), with specific focus on student and early career researcher, young people not in employment, education or training, and healthcare professional populations. Her teaching practice focuses on evidence-based practice in healthcare and applied research methods. Berry studied for her undergraduate degree in Psychology and Philosophy at the University of Reading 2004–2007, completed her PhD in Clinical Psychology at University of Sussex 2010–2014, and her PGCert in Higher Education at University of Sussex in 2021. Between 2013 and 2020, Berry held postdoc, research fellow and trial manager positions in observational and interventional studies in youth and complex mental health and student mental health, with the School of Psychology, University of Sussex and Sussex Partnership NHS Foundation Trust. More information about Berry's research and publications can be found here: https://profiles.sussex.ac.uk/p256671-clio-berry/publications

Virginia Braun is Professor in the School of Psychology at Waipapa Taumata Rau/The University of Auckland, Aotearoa New Zealand. She is a feminist and critical health psychologist and teaches gender and psychology and critical health psychology at undergraduate and graduate levels. Her research explores a wide range of topics across the intersecting areas of gender, bodies, sex/sexuality and health. Alongside this, she writes methodologically about qualitative research, with Victoria Clarke, and others including Nikki Hayfield and Gareth Terry. This includes work on thematic analysis—Braun and Clarke's highly cited *Using thematic analysis in psychology* was published in *Qualitative Research in Psychology* in 2006 (since translated into Turkish, and adapted into Brazilian Portuguese). Since then, they have written numerous papers, chapters, editorials, commentaries and encyclopaedia entries on thematic analysis, and the methods of qualitative surveys and story completion. They have written an award-winning and bestselling introductory qualitative textbook—*Successful Qualitative Research: A Practical Guide for Beginners* (2013)—translated into Hindi and Marathi—and most recently *Thematic Analysis: A Practical Guide* (2022). Their edited textbook—with Debra Gray—*Collecting Qualitative Data: A Practical Guide to Textual, Media and Virtual Techniques* (2017) has also been translated into (Brazilian) Portuguese. With Victoria Clarke, Ginny has developed websites on thematic analysis (www.thematicanalysis.net) and story completion (www.storycompletion.net). She can be followed on *Twitter* @ginnybraun.

Divine Charura is Professor of Counselling Psychology and the programme director for the Doctorate in Counselling Psychology at York St John University. He is a Chartered Psychologist, and Counselling Psychologist with the British Psychological Society. He is registered as a Practitioner Psychologist with the Health and Care Professions Council in England. Charura is also an Honorary Fellow of the United Kingdom Council for Psychotherapy (UKCP) and an adult psychotherapist. As a psychologist, psychotherapist and researcher, Charura's work focuses on the impact of trauma across the lifespan. His pedagogical research interests are in qualitative, mixed, relational, constructivist, duoethnographic and decolonial approaches. Charura has co-authored and edited numerous books in counselling, psychology and psychotherapy. These include *Love and Therapy: In relationship* [co-edited with Stephen Paul] and [co-edited with Colin Lago] the following books: *The Person-Centred Counselling* and *Psychotherapy Handbook:*

Origins, Developments and Current Applications (2016) and recently, *Black Identities + White Therapies: Race, Respect and Diversity* (2021).

For a complete list of Charura's publications, please see: https://ray.yorksj.ac.uk/profile/2104

Victoria Clarke is Associate Professor in Qualitative and Critical Psychology at the University of the West of England (UWE), Bristol, UK. Her research interests lie in the intersecting areas of gender and sexuality, family and relationships, and appearance and embodiment. With Virginia Braun, she has developed a widely used approach to thematic analysis, now called reflexive thematic analysis (see thematicanalysis.net), and has written extensively about this, including most recently, the book *Thematic Analysis: A Practical Guide* (2022). They have also co-authored an award-winning textbook on qualitative research: *Successful Qualitative Research: A Practical Guide for Beginners* (2013) and with *Debra Gray* co-edited *Collecting Qualitative Data: A Practical Guide to Textual, Media and Virtual Techniques* (2017). With Virginia Braun and others, Clarke has also written about the novel creative method of story completion (see storycompletion.net). She is also active on Twitter—mainly tweeting about thematic analysis and qualitative research @ drvicclarke.

Sally Rachel Cook obtained her PhD in Applied Linguistics in 2019 from Birkbeck College, University of London. She is an Associate Research Fellow there. She is committed to deepening knowledge and understanding of multilingualism in asylum seekers and refugees in the context of their rehabilitation. Through her work she aspires to open up new reflection and discussion on the best means of caring for such people. Cook's doctoral research explores the lived-experience of acquiring and using a second language in the healing journeys of survivors of torture within a unique London-based therapeutic community. To carry out the project she developed an innovative methodology integrating Interpretative Phenomenological Analysis with strategies from ethnography. She has disseminated her research through publications, workshops with health professionals working with refugees and at national and international Applied Linguistics conferences. She also took part in the interdisciplinary Oxford Talks, presenting her research findings in the seminar entitled 'Translating Distress'. Cook founded and directed for several years an English Theatre Workshop in Florence, Italy, and intends to use theatre as a means for her findings to reach a broader general audience. In 2020 she won the Harmonious Bilingual Network (HaBilNet) Travel Award to attend the Georgetown University Round table. Her publications can be found here: https://orcid.org/0000-0002-2656-802X

Beverley Costa is the founder of *Mothertongue* multi-ethnic counselling service (2000–2018) for multilingual clients. In 2009 she created a pool of mental health interpreters and in 2010 she established the national *Bilingual Therapist and Mental Health Interpreter Forum* and founded *The Pásalo Project* in 2017 https://www.pasaloproject.org/ to disseminate learning from Mothertongue. In 2013, she established *Colleagues Across Borders* offering support to refugee psychosocial workers and interpreters based mainly in the Middle East and Eastern Europe. She is a Senior Practitioner Fellow at Birkbeck, University of London and has written multiple papers and chapters. She shared the Equality and Diversity Research Award from the *British Association for Counselling and Psychotherapy* (2013) with Jean-Marc Dewaele. She created the online training resource on multilingualism and mental health in 2021/22 https://www.pasaloproject.org/multilingualism-mental-health-and-psychological-therapy---course-content.html

Her publications can be found here: https://orcid.org/0000-0002-3128-235X

Louise Davey is a counselling psychologist working in an NHS inpatient psychology service and in private practice. She also has many years of experience working with a Sexual Assault Referral Centre. Her work has shaped her interests in internal and social power dynamics, gender, appearance and embodiment, and the insights that critical and qualitative research can generate for applied psychology practice. This includes the ways that these approaches can produce knowledge to help practitioners understand the meanings available to their clients and the relational processes through which empowerment and healing can take place.

Maria Dempsey is a counselling psychologist and lecturer in the School of Applied Psychology, UCC. Her research interest is concerned with developing knowledge of individuals' understanding of self. While this has been realised in three primary areas, that is sexuality and parenting, mental health and reflective teaching and learning, the unifying cord through this work is methodology. She co-founded Ireland Network for Pluralism in Qualitative Research (2020) and views practice, research and teaching as being interwoven.

Jean-Marc Dewaele obtained his PhD from Free University of Brussels, in 1993 and he is Professor of Applied Linguistics and Multilingualism at Birkbeck, University of London. He has authored and edited 9 books, written over 300 papers and chapters on individual differences in psycholinguistic, sociolinguistic, pragmatic, psychological and emotional variables in Second Language Acquisition and Multilingualism. He is the author of the monograph *Emotions in Multiple Languages* published in 2010 (2nd ed in 2013). He is former president of the *European Second Language Association* (2007–2011) and the *International Association of Multilingualism* (2016–2018). He is the incoming President of the *International Association for the Psychology of Language* (2022–2024). He was General Editor of the *International Journal of Bilingual Education and Bilingualism* (2013–2019) before taking over as General Editor of the *Journal of Multilingual and Multicultural Development* (2019–). He won the Equality and Diversity Research Award from the *British Association for Counselling and Psychotherapy* (2013) with Beverley Costa, the Robert Gardner Award for Excellence in Second Language and Bilingualism Research (2016) from the *International Association of Language and Social Psychology* and the EUROSLA Distinguished Scholar Award (2022) from the

European Second Language Association. His publications can be found here: orcid. org/0000-0001-8480-0977.

Victoria S. Dixon is a doctoral student in Clinical & Counselling Psychology at the University of South Alabama. Prior to doctoral studies, she earned an MS in Clinical Mental Health Counselling at South Alabama in 2021, and a bachelor's in Psychology at South Alabama as well. Dixon's clinical experience includes counselling and assessment of children in an intensive, community health setting as well as adolescents in juvenile justice settings with an emphasis on trauma.

Broadly, Dixon's research interests revolve around child maltreatment. Specifically, she has focused on how adults, particularly those serving in the legal system, interact and impact children who have been sexually abused. Dixon has worked on several projects related to the intersection of psychology and law such as the Promise Initiative in Mobile, AL, a programme established to address the police department's sexual assault kits backlog, which was part of the Department of Justice's SAKI grant initiative, and helping conduct a programme evaluation of the Child Advocacy Center of Mobile, AL.

Sarah Foley is Lecturer in the School of Applied Psychology, University College Cork. Her research employs participatory and qualitative methods and focuses on experience relating to health and social care. She received her PhD in Applied Psychology in 2020, which examined the potential of technology to enhance social engagement in dementia care. She is a founding member of the Ireland Network for Pluralism in Qualitative Research (INPQR).

Nollaig Frost is Adjunct Professor at the School of Applied Psychology, University College Cork, Ireland. After many years as a psychodynamic counsellor in psychiatric and community settings, she pursued a PhD at Birkbeck, University of London, to research women's transitions to second-time motherhood within a psychosocial framework. Her interest in pluralistic research was piqued, and on completion of her PhD she began to work with a team of researchers to explore the benefits and tensions of combining methods. This project led to one of the first books about pluralistic research: Frost, N. (ed) (2011; 2021). *Qualitative Methods in Psychology: Combining Core Approaches*, Open University Press, now in its second edition. With colleagues, Frost established the Network for Pluralism in Qualitative Research (www.npqr.wordpress.com) and the Ireland Network for Pluralism in Qualitative Research, to provide resources, support and training to researchers and practitioners interested in pluralistic research. She has also written *Practising Research: why you are part of the research process even if you think you're not,* Palgrave Macmillan. Frost teaches research methods and provides doctoral research supervision to academic, clinical and counselling psychologists, and trainee counsellors and psychotherapists, at various universities and training institutions in the UK and Ireland.

Gilbert Garza is Associate Professor and graduate director of Psychology at the University of Dallas. He earned his PhD and Master's in Phenomenological

Psychology from Duquesne University and a Bachelor's degree in psychology from the University of Dallas. He teaches undergraduate and graduate students about the foundations of phenomenological psychology as well as qualitative and quantitative approaches to psychological research. His scholarly interests include qualitative and phenomenological research methodology, mixed methods research and the philosophical foundations of and the relationship between quantitative and qualitative research methodologies.

Terry Hanley is a Reader in Counselling Psychology at the University of Manchester. He is also a HCPC Registered Counselling Psychologist and a Fellow of both the BPS and the Higher Education Academy. Hanley works on a Doctorate in Counselling Psychology programme and has a particular interest in training therapists in humanistic approaches of therapy and research skills. He has edited 'The SAGE Handbook of Counselling and Psychotherapy', is a co-author of 'Introducing Counselling and Psychotherapy Research' and lead editor of text 'Adolescent Counselling Psychology'. He has worked as a therapist with young people and young adults for a number of third sector organisations, a football therapist with the organisation Freedom from Torture and a clinical supervisor for staff at Bury Involvement Group. He has been researching web-based therapy for over 20 years and has a growing interest in surfing therapy. Follow him on twitter @ drterryhanley.

Nikki Hayfield is an Associate Head of Department for Research and Knowledge Exchange in the Department of Social Sciences at the University of the West of England (UWE), Bristol. Hayfield is a keen qualitative researcher who uses a range of data collection methods, including interviews, focus groups, qualitative surveys and story-based methods. She has a particular interest in reflexive thematic analysis and has previously been a co-author on a number of papers and book chapters on research methods with Victoria Clarke, Virginia Braun and Gareth Terry—most recently publishing *Essentials of Thematic Analysis* with Gareth Terry as part of the American Psychological Association's *Essentials of Qualitative Methods* series. Her research interests are primarily in sexualities and marginalised identities, with a particular focus on how bisexual, pansexual and asexual identities are experienced and understood. She also has an interest in reproductive lives including the experiences of those who are childfree by choice. At UWE, Hayfield leads the *Identities, Subjectivities and Inequalities* theme which is part of the *Social Sciences Research Group*. Her first book entitled *Bisexual and Pansexual Identities: Exploring invisibility and invalidation* was published in 2020. You can see Hayfield's most recent research on their UWE staff page and on Google Scholar and ResearchGate.

Cassie Hazell is Lecturer in Clinical Psychology at the University of Surrey. She completed her PhD at the University of Sussex on the topic of guided self-help for people distressed by hearing voices. She has since completed postdoctoral positions at the University of Sussex, Sussex Partnership NHS Foundation Trust, Brighton and Sussex Medical School, and the University of Oxford all in the area of mental health and mostly working on clinical trials. Hazell is the co-founder and chair of the international Early Career Hallucinations Research (ECHR) group and current Early-Mid Career Research Representative on her institution's research council. Her research interests include implementation science, psychosis, hearing voices, cognitive behaviour therapy, increasing access to psychological therapies, well-being of mental health carers, mental health stigma, suicide and student mental health. More information about Hazell's research and publications can be found here: https://www.surrey.ac.uk/people/cassie-m-hazell.

Elizabeth Jenkinson is Senior Lecturer in Health Psychology and Research Methods at the University of the West of England, Bristol. She leads teaching and training for health psychologists at UWE and at NHS Health Education England. Liz conducts research in health psychology, appearance psychology, health promotion and well-being, and the design and evaluation of effective support for people with chronic and acute health conditions. She has authored over 70 peer-reviewed articles, policy documents, books and book chapters, and supervised over 100 research dissertations and theses. Liz is also a registered Health Psychologist, Practitioner Psychologist and Chartered Psychologist who has worked clinically in the NHS. As a result, her research takes an applied and pragmatic approach using both qualitative and quantitative methods, with a focus on the use of thematic analysis in health psychology. You can follow Liz on their UWE staff page, on Google Scholar and Twitter @DrLizJenkinson.

H. Burke Johnson is a retired professor in the Department of Counselling & Instructional Sciences at the University of South Alabama. His PhD is from the REMS (research, evaluation, measurement and statistics) programme in the College of Education at the University of Georgia. He also has graduate degrees in psychology, sociology and public administration, which have provided him with a multidisciplinary perspective on research methodology. He was guest editor for a special issue of Research in the Schools focusing on mixed research and completed a similar guest editorship for the American Behavioural Scientist. He was an associate editor of the *Journal of Mixed Methods Research*. Johnson is first author of *Educational Research: Quantitative, Qualitative, and Mixed Approaches* (2014); second author of *Research Methods, Design, and Analysis* (2014); co-editor (with Sharlene Hesse-Biber) of *The Oxford Handbook of Multimethod and Mixed Methods Research Inquiry* (2015); co-editor (with Paul Vogt) of *Correlation and Regression Analysis* (2012); and associate editor of *The SAGE Glossary of the Social and Behavioural Sciences* (2009).

Brittany Landrum is Assistant Professor of Psychology at the University of Dallas. She earned a PhD and a Master's in experimental psychology from Texas Christian University and a Bachelor's degree in phenomenological psychology from the University of Dallas. She teaches statistics, quantitative research methods, qualitative research as well as cognitive and social psychology electives. Her research interests include quantitative and qualitative research methodology, mixed methods, phenomenological psychology and philosophical foundations of research.

Alistair McBeath is a Chartered Psychologist and UKCP registered psychotherapist. Trained at Regents College and Guys Hospital, he is Director of Studies for the Doctorate by Public Works at the Metanoia Institute. He also works for an Edinburgh-based therapeutic consultancy. McBeath considers himself to be a researcher-practitioner and is keen to promote this identity within the psychotherapy profession. McBeath is a strong advocate of mixed methods research and has authored several research projects using this approach. McBeath favours a collaborative approach to research and has worked extensively with Sofie Bager-Charleson across a range of practitioner-relevant issues and they co-edited an earlier book *Enjoying Research in Counselling and Psychotherapy*. McBeath is a senior practitioner member on the BPS Register of Psychologists Specialising in Psychotherapy and co-editor of the *European Journal for Qualitative Research in Psychotherapy*.

Saira Gracie Razzaq is a Registered Chartered Psychologist accredited by the British Psychological Society, the Health Professional Council and a Registered member of the United Kingdom Council for Psychotherapists. She is an Associate Fellow of the British Psychological Society as a Registered Psychologist. Razzaq has been the Director of Psychotherapy and Well-being Services working with complex needs in the NHS for over 20 years and is a Clinical Supervisor. She has been a Primary Tutor and Lecturer on the Doctoral Programme for Counselling Psychology at Metanoia Institute and continues to act as a Research supervisor and Viva Examiner for the Programme. Razzaq's Doctoral research was an Autoethnographic account of Racist Trauma, where the concept of Autoethnographic Psychotherapeutic Research (APR) emerged. Razzaq is also a meditation and yoga teacher, and she is interested in how embodiment can be integrated within practice and research.

Louise Rolland obtained her PhD in Applied Linguistics at Birkbeck, University of London, in 2019. She is an Associate Research Fellow with research interests spanning the social and psychological aspects of multilingualism. She has studied how multilingual clients use their languages in psychotherapy to regulate emotion and access plural identities, highlighting the positive impact of therapists being open to multilingual practices. She has disseminated her interdisciplinary work through publications, workshops and seminars for psychotherapists and applied linguists. She also writes about the methodological aspects of researching multilingually, developing researcher awareness of the implications of participants' and researchers' language repertoires for the research. Her current research plans focus on bilingual language development and family language transmission. Alongside her research, she has lectured on the psycholinguistics of bilingualism and second language acquisition. Prior to academia, she enjoyed teaching English and French, and worked in a range of research management roles. Her publications can be found here: https://orcid.org/0000-0002-9814-2685.

Aaron Sefi is Chief Product Officer at Kooth, leading UK provider of digital mental health services for young people. He completed his Master's in Counselling at University of Manchester, is studying for a Doctorate in Clinical Research at the University of Exeter and specialises in the use of nomothetic and idiographic outcome measures for digital use. Sefi is driven by aligning user needs and wants an evidence base to ensure meaningful and valuable research and data is shared, understood and implemented, particularly in digital service provision. He lives in Cornwall and is actually (and proudly!) Cornish.

"Trés" Stefurak Trés is the Associate Dean and Professor of Counselling Psychology in the College of Education and Professional Studies at the University of South Alabama. He has served on the core-faculty of the Combined-Integrated Clinical & Counselling Psychology PhD programme here since its inception in 2009. Tres's scholarly works focuses on youth placed at-risk, particularly youth involved in the juvenile justice system, youth who have experienced trauma and the intersection between the two. More recently, his work has occurred within law enforcement agencies serving rape and child sexual abuse victims. In addition, Tres's writing has focused on mixed methods programme evaluation in these settings and scholarship focused on the use of philosophical pragmatism in research and evaluation as well as contributing to the development of the Dialectical Pluralism metaparadigm.

Keith Tudor is Professor of Psychotherapy at Auckland University of Technology, where he is also co-Lead of a Group for research in the Psychological Therapies. He is also a Visiting Associate Professor at the Univerza na Primorskem (University of Primorska), Slovenia, an Honorary Senior Research Fellow of the University of Roehampton, and a Fellow of The Critical Institute. He has had a long and varied career in the psychotherapy profession as a practitioner, teacher, supervisor and academic. He trained originally in gestalt therapy, and subsequently in transactional analysis and person-centred psychology, and is a Certified and Teaching and Supervising Transactional Analyst, accredited by the International Transactional Analysis Association. Tudor is a widely published author in the field of psychotherapy and counselling, and mental health, with over 250 peer-reviewed outputs, including 17 books. He is the series editor of 'Advancing Theory in Therapy', and the co-editor of *Psychotherapy and Politics International*. He works closely with heuristic research, having completed his own doctorate using heuristics, and, subsequently, supervised ten Master's dissertations/doctoral theses based on heuristic methodology and method.

Rachel Wicaksono is Associate Professor in TESOL and Applied Linguistics, and Head of the School of Education, Language and Psychology at York St John University. She was awarded a National Teaching Fellowship in 2013. Wicaksono is a member of the British Association of Applied Linguistics (BAAL) Executive Committee. As a teacher of, and researcher into, the uses of English(es) for (international) communication, Wicaksono's work focuses on the construction of meaning in contexts where difference (languages, cultures, educational traditions) are thought, by individuals and institutions, to be relevant. Her pedagogical research interests are in the practical/professional applications of thinking about ontology, and transformative research designs. Wicaksono has co-authored and edited books on applied linguistics and research methods. These include [with Christopher J. Hall and Patrick H. Smith] *Mapping Applied Linguistics: A Guide for Students and Practitioners* (2017,), [with Christopher J Hall] *Ontologies of English: Conceptualising the Language for Learning, Teaching and Assessment* (2020) and [with Dasha Zhurauskaya] *York's Hidden Stories: Interviews in Applied Linguistics* (Palgrave, 2020). For a complete list of Wicaksono's publications, please see: https://ray.yorksj.ac.uk/profile/1008

List of Figures

List of Tables

List of Boxes

Chapter 1
Introduction: Aim, Key Themes and an Overview of the Coming Chapters

Sofie Bager-Charleson and Alistair McBeath

Learning Goals

After reading this chapter you should have:

- familiarised yourself with some of the basic terminology and principles of qualitative, quantitative and mixed-methods research
- gained an overview of the different chapters and their contents
- started to reflect over your own relationship to research, including potential areas in need for support

Therapy is a multifaceted and ever-developing practice which frequently is described as both an art and a science. This book invites to discussions about therapist-researchers' 'epistemological home(s)'. Where do we as counsellors, psychotherapists and counselling psychologists 'belong' in terms of academic disciplines? What do we hold as 'true' and how do we generate knowledge about that?

Working within a practice referred to as an 'Art and/or Science' positions the researcher-practitioner often between a scientific, medical and a phenomenological and/or socially constructionist-based stance—with a rich variation both between and within the different approaches. For most therapists, their client sessions will be guided by both an evidence-based, scientific interest—focusing on generalisations and commonly held 'truths' which help us to 'know *about*' our client, and an aim to 'know *with*' guided by a focus on unique, individual experience and meaning makings. While evidence-based approaches favour a research focus on commonalities, certainties and objectivity, the social constructionist approaches view mental health and emotional well-being with biographical, socio-cultural, linguistic, gender-related and other context-dependent interests in mind. The latter include

S. Bager-Charleson (✉) • A. McBeath
Metanoia Institute, London, UK
e-mail: sofie.bager-charleson@metanoia.ac.uk; Alistair.mcbeath@metanoia.ac.uk

S. Bager-Charleson, A. McBeath (eds.), *Supporting Research in Counselling and Psychotherapy*, https://doi.org/10.1007/978-3-031-13942-0_1

recognising what McGinley (2015) defines as the value of 'embodied understanding', which includes the knower's 'moods, affect, and atmosphere' (p. 88) as sources of knowledge. This broad positioning can both be an opportunity and an obstacle. Our studies conducted under the umbrella of Therapists as Research-informed Practitioners (see more: https://metanoia.ac.uk/research/research-groups-events/therapists-as-research-informed-practitioners-trp/) highlighted a sense of 'homelessness' and lack of belonging for many therapists when it comes to research. One of the doctoral research students in our study into therapists' relationship to research said for instance:

> When I think of research, I associate it with feeling lonely, the largest upset is to not find research which reflects what I work with. Being a psychotherapist can feel like being a second-class citizen in the NHS. Cognitive, neuro, biological, outcome measures—there's a whole bunch of people I can contact and speak to. But I'm not working within those approaches … I struggle with the idea that emotions are measurable. (Bager-Charleson et al., 2018, p. 8)

The often-ignored conundrum for psychotherapy in terms of its disciplinarian 'homelessness' (Bager-Charleson et al., 2018, 2019; Bager-Charleson & McBeath, 2021a, 2021b) forms a focus for this book. Our aim has been to support therapists in inhabiting the space between art and science rather than feeling homeless.

'Mixing' methods is a contentious venture. Simply speaking, mixing methods involves typically the use of both qualitative and quantitative approaches and methods in a single study or sequentially in two or more studies (Frost & Bailey-Rodriguez, 2020). Each approach brings, however, a different paradigmatic viewpoint or 'worldview' and combining the two is for many regarded as inappropriate or even impossible. In this book, contributors expand on this conundrum from different angles and with a dialogue between 'scientific' and 'aesthetic'(or intuitive, embodied) means of generating knowledge in mind. In doing so, we resonate with other pluralistically inspired disciplines like DeLyser and Sui (2013) who within human geography refer to unhelpful 'divisiveness' when exploring multi-layered aspects of our existence. Sui and DeLyser suggest that for multifaceted disciplines 'to develop and survive [they need] move beyond the qualitative-quantitative [divisive] chasm between scientific and humanistic knowledge' (p. 111).

Scientifically Descriptive or Artfully Interpretive Research?

This book starts with examples of how the one method, namely thematic analysis, can be used either as a 'scientifically descriptive' and an 'artfully interpretive' mode of knowing, depending on research question and interest. In their chapter, Braun et al. describe the rich and multidisciplinary history of thematic analysis. They explain firstly what unites the different TA versions in terms of processes of coding and theme generation, whilst also reflecting over how 'the many ways versions of TA differ and can be imbued with quite different paradigmatic assumptions'. Building on a distinction suggested by Finlay (2021) in terms of a *scientifically descriptive* versus an *artfully interpretive* way of using thematic analysis, Braun et al. expand on 'reflexive TA' (Braun et al., 2022) as part of the latter. We will return to later example of more 'scientifically descriptive' uses of TA in this book, whilst focusing on 'artful interpretation' in context of qualitative research in this chapter. Qualitative research typically regards researcher subjectivity as a resource rather than a hindrance for research; that researcher subjectivity becomes in this sense something which shapes the research process and knowledge is regarded as inevitably partial, perspectival and contextually located. As the 'artfully interpretive TA' is embedded in these values, it 'moves beyond descriptions and summaries' towards a focus on 'how meanings might relate to the wider social contexts, and to what significance and implications this may have' as Braun et al. put it in their chapter.

Exploring Meaning Makings in Social Contexts

Questions around how meanings relate to wider socio-political, gender-related and cultural contexts form the core of the next chapter about arts-based decolonising research, by Charura and Wicaksono. They focus on arts and artful in context of the 'art of' decolonising research. Their research raises, for instance, questions about what objects, things, art are to different people; and to how they shift power. Charura and Wicaksono draw on a 'duo-ethnographic' process which includes their own questioning of meanings in their narratives and conceptualisations of what arts-based research and decolonizing research means to them. Their chapter highlights stages of where possibilities of decolonised approaches emerge in terms of opportunities to demonstrate a deep respect and valuing of participation/participants aiming for a *power-with* rather than *power-over*—the latter synonymous with 'colonising dynamics' where researchers focus on having their own research questions answered rather than engaging with the diversity of world views/experiences of the other as part of the research process. Decolonising research is, assert Charura and Wicaksono, a relational and a 'deeply reflexive process'. Special attention is paid to the themes of 'beginnings'—and to an active engagement thereafter with the unfolding research dynamics, referred by the authors to as the 'real inner drama', before 'endings' with space for debriefing and further reflections after the research interviews/encounters. Silence plays, further, an important role in the research interaction to secure space for material to emerge and/or to be held in reflection.

The Researcher's Critical Self-reflection: Bridging Tacit and Explicit Knowing

In Chap. 4 the focus turns specifically onto the researcher's critical self-reflection, with an interest into how the researcher's own meanings impact the findings. With the researcher's self-awareness in mind, Tudor expands on heuristic research as a 'disciplined and critical self-reflection and engagement in a process of discovery of self and others'. Again, art and intuitive knowing play a significant role. Tudor refers to intuition as a 'bridge' between the implicit, tacit knowledge and the explicit, observable and describable knowledge—with music, poetry and other forms of arts being drawn upon as part of the bridging. Like in previous chapter, Heuristics balances an 'autobiographic' focus with an interest into how personal meaning makings are of universal importance. With almost every question of personal importance, there is a social and often universal significance, asserts Tudor.

Chapter 5, by Dr. Saira Razzaq, offers another example of how key principles addressed in Chaps. 2, 3 and 4 can be incorporated in research. She explains turning to autoethnography from feeling constrained by the types of stories the dominant research discourses were made available. When starting her study into intergenerational trauma and racism, Razzaq wrestled with a 'daunting array of distancing academic texts and conceptually rigid frameworks' which contrasted the reflexive relationality of her psychotherapeutic training. Originating from the field of anthropology, ethnography (people and cultures with their customs, habits and differences) and sociology, authoethnography comes in many forms and overlapping styles, ranging from literary autoethnography, poetic autoethnography, meta-autoethnography, performance autoethnography to duoethnography and other collaborative forms as shown in Chap. 3. Autoethnography draws on a creative analytic practice which builds on novels, fiction, poems, prose, script, song, performance, art, photography, documentaries, images or performance narratives and ways of generating feelings *with* a story rather than being told *about* it—resonating with the distinction between *power-with* rather than *power-over* in research in Chap. 3.

Quantitative Research

In our next section of this book, our focus turns towards quantitative research. Our aim is to provide each research approach a platform to be 'heard' in the words of an expert in that approach, and this includes paying attention to different topics and focus but also to how different approaches convey and express different 'tones'/ voices across the chapters. For instance, when different contributors expand on what they regard as powerful research, Razzaq expands on turning to autoethnography after *feeling baffled by dominant discourses, distancing academic texts and conceptually rigid frameworks* whilst Hazell and Berry (in Chap. 7) describe feeling attracted by the tangible, writing *surveys are an incredibly powerful research tool; helpful in turning 'fuzzy' phenomena into something tangible and measurable, and allowing the collection of lots of data from lots of people in a short period of time.*

Activity 1.1 Ways of Speaking in Research

Our qualitative survey into Research Methods in Therapy Studies (McBeath & Bager-Charleson, 2022 in press) asked *what, if at all, might a research approach involving the use of both qualitative and quantitative methods offer to researchers in the field of counselling and psychotherapy?* The 3–5 minutes long survey included closed and open questions, ending with optional 'story completion question' for participants to expand on the theme of research methods in third person, as below:

> Kate is planning her research project for her psychotherapy doctorate. She is interested to explore the issue of compassion fatigue in therapists. She knows that she wants to explore the individual experience of compassion fatigue and so will use some form of qualitative research method. But she also wants to get an idea of how common compassion fatigue is across the profession.
>
> Kate is going to discuss how to progress her research with her supervisor (What could happen next?—feel free to add what might be seen as a story of what might happen).

We analysed the replies in pairs—first independently, then by comparing and agreeing on shared themes aligned with reflexive thematic analysis. Sofie's analysis was guided by an interest in 'narrative knowing' (Polkinghorne, 1991) focusing both on what people say and how they do it. When reading the story stem accounts, her attention turned to how some respondents chose to expand on the scene with Kate with reference to conundrums, uncertainties and different kind of 'feelings' in mind.

In the example below, the narrator expands on the researcher *as a person—* for instance by describing her as *a words person* who sometimes is *comfortable* and other times *fearful* and/or *excited*. Expressions like *not really knowing, exploring options* and *possibilities opening up* punctuate the account—incorporating shifting emotions and ambiguity in their account about what 'doing research' entail. The story starts, for instance, with Kate 'discusses options' and being 'comfortable' and finishes with 'excited by possibilities opening up' with references to 'fearful' and 'hopeful' in between.

"Kate discusses options with her supervisor and decides that she wants to capture both quantitative and qualitative data. She is a words person and so is comfortable with the qualitative side of things. She feels slightly fearful of number and not really knowing how to crunch them to make a story. She hopes from the discussion with her supervisor that there is a solution she can work with. She wants depth of insight but also breadth across the therapy profession. With help from her supervisor she begins to explore the option of an online survey, where the quantitative data are analysed by the survey platform. From the survey she can recruit participants for follow-on interviews. Kate starts to feel excited about the possibilities opening up for her" (127).

(continued)

(continued)

Others narrate in a more factual way, leaving emotional content out of their description, choosing expressions like *already established, already thought about* and *wants/needs to, will suit, demands establishing, can be measured* and *cross-check*—which to me imply choosing to focus on more practical, rational side of Kate as a researcher. The story starts with *having already established* and finishes with *cross-check and corroborate findings*.

"Kate has already established her research idea or research question, so she needs to identify which methodology will suit her question, she has already thought about employing qualitative methods, however, the research question also fits the quantitative methods since she wants to also have an idea of how common compassion fatigue is across the profession which demands establishing numerical figures/statistics that can be measured for her to explore their experiences and to potentially cross-check and corroborate findings" (79).

Whilst the accounts refer to actual obstacles and opportunities with MMR as a methods/technique, they also highlight how different researchers chose to punctuate their story and plot lines about doing research with different qualities, and with different 'valued' (Gergen & Gergen, 1988) starts and end points in mind. To use Polkinghorne's (1991) distinction, some emphasised 'paradigmatic' knowing by focusing on facts and events, whilst others organised events guided by 'narrative knowing' conveying experiences of the world in ways that integrate aspects like emotion, social context and time.

- Return to the vignette above and complete the story stem in your own words:

Kate is going to discuss how to progress her research with her supervisor. What could happen next—please add what might be seen as a story of what might happen.

- Compare your replies with the two 'types' referred to above. Reflect over your choice of words, and discuss, if possible, in pairs or with colleagues.

How Many, How Often, How Much…

In Chap. 6, Banwell, Hanley et al. begin our quantitative section by concluding that:

If the richness of your clients' unique experiences is something that you wish to capture, we must admit, a qualitative approach is probably the one you are looking for.

Quantitative research is typically, continue Banwell, Hanley et al., guided by questions about *how many; how often; what percentage of…; what is the difference between…; how are X and Y associated; what is the relationship between…?* They sum up these questions into descriptive, comparative and relationship-based categories of research questions. Many therapists might ask, continue the authors: 'how is my client represented in a quantitative study of their data?' and especially when compared to qualitative research, it is easy to see how concepts like 'variable', 'statistical test', 'p-value' seem slightly depersonalised. And so how then may the 'person' represented in quantitative work?

Banwell, Hanley et al. expand on how numerical or statistical data from our services can add knowledge into *what is working, and what is not working, including for whom, and why* to, in turn, help us see 'where time, effort, money, or further research attention might be needed'. Their chapter offers a substantial overview of both core principles of quantitative research and how they can be used to answer descriptive, comparative or relationship-based research questions. In their section titled 'humanising numbers' they assert that while quantitative research always may be reductive, collecting numerical information can 'place the individuals seeking support in the driving seat' of the study. Whilst this adds complexity to our understanding from such measures, the authors conclude that 'we believe that this can help to humanise the numbers being collected and has the potential to enhance the therapeutic work engaged in'. Following on from this, the authors discuss adventurous projects attempting to articulate a theory of change for online therapeutic services. The overarching mixed-methods design is described before going on to discuss the way that quantitative methods have been used to complement earlier qualitative research.

Online Surveys

Surveys are explored from different angles in this book. The following chapters expand on the use with mixture of qualitative and quantitative data in mind. In their chapter about dilemmas and decisions in quantitative-driven online survey, Hazzel and Berry share the different stages of their survey into doctoral researchers' mental health and need for support. The earlier mentioned large-scale survey in Chap. 7 by Hazell and Berry adds significant layers to our understanding of the obstacles and opportunities for doctoral researcher. It brings attention to not only aspects like shame, loneliness and exhaustion that are alarmingly common for doctoral researchers but also levels of mental health and suicide rate among doctoral researchers. The authors describe using both quantitative and qualitative data for an as nuanced understanding of contextual-dependent aspects surrounding doctoral students and their mental health.

The authors conclude that surveys predominantly are used as a quantitative method, but how they also can be used for qualitative and mixed-methods research. For reading about surveys in qualitative research, we refer the readers to Braun and Clarke's Chap. 2, but also recommend their earlier texts about qualitative research (Braun et al., 2017, 2021).

Surveys can be distributed in-person, via telephone or video calling, on paper and using digital technologies like computers and other mobile device. Online surveys offer participant anonymity and privacy in ways which can facilitate collection of data about more sensitive or potentially controversial topics—such as the topic of suicide in this study. Starting with practical aspects for setting up the survey, the chapter expands on how surveys can collect a combination of quantitative and qualitative data, in this chapter through incorporating a control group in the study, combined with questionnaires to measure 'latent constructs' such as the PHQ-9 to measure depression and with closed and open questions.

Reaching Out with the Research

A not insignificant benefit of quantitative research is its easy-to-present format. Hazell and Berry conclude that their decision to take a primarily *quantitative* mixed-methods approach was 'shaped by the traditional prominence of quantitative research in policy and practice' with opportunities to publish, presenting for stakeholders and generally be heard.

The use of online surveys is expanded upon further in Chap. 8, where McBeath concludes that survey is a powerful but often under-utilised research tool among counsellors and psychotherapists. Again, the significant point of reaching out is raised by McBeath's (2020) earlier studies into 'therapists and academic writing' which highlight how marginalised many therapists felt in academic writing.

McBeath also expands on benefits with online surveys both in terms of reaching participants who might not engage in less anonymous research methods allowing for more ethical focus on very personal and sensitive issues. He addresses significant advances in online survey use, for instance how they can act as effective *qualitative* research methods through a range of intuitive analysis tools—including the mentioned story completion method. His chapter also offers an introduction to 'survey logic' as the basis of so-called intelligent surveys. The chapter builds on and continues on McBeath's starter chapter about survey (McBeath, 2020) with information about how to construct a survey and what types of questions can be used.

Mixing...

In the next section, the focus turns to different theories for mixed-methods integration. Mixed-methods research is, as mentioned, a contested approach, with many theories around how to do it. The section in this book about mixed-methods integration ranges from pragmatism to dialectical method of dialog and synthesising—both guided by respectful and constructive ways of drawing on the strengths of quantitative and qualitative approaches.

Holding that 'good fences make good neighbours', Landrum and Garza instigate this section about mixed-methods integration. They expand both on the domains of quantitative and qualitative research and on traditional borders between them—with new bridging in mind. The chapter offers an overview of some different mixed-methods theories, with practical, step-by-step integrative examples of designing and conducting mixed-methods research into the relationship between social media use and anxiety during the pandemic. Chapter 10 makes, in turn, a case *for the pragmatic researcher*. McBeath expands on the issue of mixed-methods research in terms of traditional conflicts and new opportunities reach deeper and richer understandings of life experiences when combining and mixing approaches rather than keeping to qualitative or quantitative research methods on their own. The rationale and advantages of mixed methods are discussed, together with the importance of its underlying methodological pluralism that favours an inclusive logic of 'both/and' as opposed to the dichotomous logic of 'either/or'. The history of, and some fundamental design variants of, mixed-methods research is described in the chapter, with a special focus on the 'world view of pragmatism' which typically puts the research question to the forefront and advocates a choice of methods on the basis of 'what works' and brings us closer to an answer of the question rather than focusing on what is 'true' and 'real'.

The following Chap. 11 expands on a 'dialectic integration' of mixed methods. Stefurak, Dixon and Johnson discuss what relevance a dialectical dialogue may have on the progress of psychotherapy research often—as suggested earlier, characterised by polarities of evidence-based practice and manualised therapy versus more theoretically driven, intuitive, culturally responsive and non-directive forms of therapy. The authors use the term Dialectical Pluralism to capture an intentional and systematic process of listening to multiple paradigms, disciplines, values systems, inquiry methodologies, worldviews and cultures guided by aims of finding new, common ground. Dialectical Pluralism is *a process in which we work together to understand and solve problems, while thriving in our differences and intellectual tensions*, conclude Stefaruk et al. This involves 'carefully listening to multiple paradigms' guided by a *back-and-forth interaction* between what often might be regarded as conflicting or contradictory standpoints between for instance qual and quant research. This type of integration assumes, in turn, an openness for that both perspectives will alter through the dialogue. Johnson refers to dialectics as aback-and-forth examination following the logic of moving from thesis to antithesis with a synthesis and integration in mind (Johnson, 2017, p.157). The dialectical method of dialog and reasoning, assert the authors, is one of the oldest in history with roots both in the ancients West, through Socrates, Plato and Aristotle, and in the East via Hindu philosophy, Jain philosophy, Buddhism. The chapter expands on how dialectical thinking is being revised across many academic disciplines and areas to help deal with dualisms and contradictions and the changing nature of intersubjective and subjective reality and knowledge. This is, in turn, an area of interest for Frost et al. in Chap. 12, which offers theoretical and practical guidance for doing qualitatively driven mixed-methods research. Until recently qualitative method(s) were used with quantitative methods primarily to confirm and enrich results reached through quantitative methods, write Frost et al. Qualitative research was used to 'humanise' objective research or to act as a pilot to a larger quantitative study. *Qualitatively driven* mixed-methods research has emerged as a way of placing human experience to the forefront, with an interest in multiple realities—rather than a universal truth, in mind. Chapter 12 leads us back to the beginning of this book, using research to explore the multi-dimensionality of human experience often to uncover earlier subjugated or dominated (colonised) forms of knowledge. This chapter considers how to carry out research this way, and when and how it can be appropriate for conducting counselling and psychotherapy research. A range of study designs for this research approach are described. Ethics, quality criteria and some writing-up styles are discussed, and the chapter ends with consideration of some challenges and benefits in using this approach in counselling and psycho-therapy research. Our final Chap. 13 expands on the rich choices in mixed methods, ranging from qualitative- to quantitative-driven mixed-methods research with the interests raised earlier in terms of the emotionally and often political and socio-cultural challenging reality therapists engage with. Dr. Sally Cook explains stages within a qualitative mixed-methods approach combining Interpretative Phenomenological Analysis and Ethnography to explore the meaning survivors of torture ascribe to using a second language in their healing journey. Torture devas-tates and shatters a person's sense of self and trust in others, concludes Cook, as she expands on her 'ethnographic sensibility' allowed her 'to go beyond what face-to-face encounters and interview settings alone could have given me'. As part of her qualitative-driven mix of ethnography and IPA she writes about how it supported an emotional engagement with her participants to glean the meanings they attributed to their language experiences and to understand their meaning makings in the context of their everyday lives. Dr. Louise Rolland describes, in turn, how combining a web survey with interviews enabled her to unpack the initial, quantitative findings regarding multilingual clients' language use, revealing rich associations between languages, emotions and identity. Professor Dewaele and Dr. Costa add, finally, a meta-perspective on methodological choices—as earlier supervisors and mentors and based on their well-established authority in the field of multilingual therapy and mixed-methods research.

Supporting Therapists in Research

So, returning to the initial question about therapist-researchers' 'epistemological home(s)'. Where *do* counsellors, psychotherapists and counselling psychologists 'belong' in terms of academic disciplines? Well, we believe that the contributors convincingly show that for therapists the concept of 'truth' is a dynamic concept which follows the logic of psychotherapeutic practice where the multi-dimensionality of human experience is put to forefront. In clinical practice we move ongoingly between knowing 'with' and knowing 'about' our client. Borrowing a term from Chap. 11, we often move 'dialectically' between usually perceived as contrasting understandings (Bager-Charleson, 2003, 2020; Bager-Charleson et al., 2020) immersing ourselves on the one hand into world of the other whilst ongoingly 'checking in' with our therapeutic theory and modality. Research forms ideally an opportunity for us to systematically take note of this, ideally by engaging with others.

Research Supervision

Perhaps unsurprisingly, in our study (Bager-Charleson & McBeath, 2021a, 2021b) into therapist-researchers' experience of research supervision we found that supervisees rated the supervisor's capacity to engage in empathy almost as highly as research knowledge by the supervisees (Fig. 1.1).

Many supervisees also spoke about empathy aligned with clinical supervisors' ability to provide space for the supervisee to explore own reactions. In our earlier studies (Bager-Charleson et al., 2018, 2019) several therapists described becoming unwell during their data-analysis work with unexplained pain, hypertension, palpitations, chest pains, panic attacks and difficulty sleeping being some of the self-disclosed symptoms recorded where 'excessive immersion' whilst attempting to analyse their data. One therapist stated that 'I really did eat, sleep and breathe the research'. Many therapists described losing a sense of self. One therapist described 'I became stuck at the structural level of data analysis. I had played in the words so much I lost sight of the body'. Another therapist said 'My immersion in their stories [made it] difficult to 'let go'. I was overwhelmed by mixed emotions. I found myself laughing at some and crying at others'. The all-consuming nature of data analysis seemed disorientating different levels. One therapist said: 'It's been horrific, I've agonised so much, feeling like a fraud, so stupid … I've been feeling desperate, all the time thinking that I am doing this right with themes and codes and tables'. Another therapist expressed feeling unprepared for the lack of self-care in research, suggesting that 'the literature on qualitative research emphasises the importance of protecting the research participants. There is not much on protecting the researcher'.

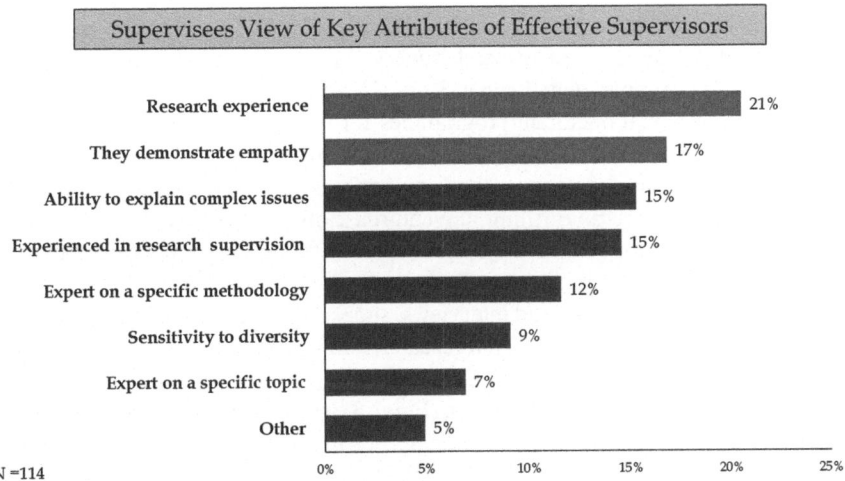

Fig. 1.1 Supervisees' view of effective supervision

Sailing instructor

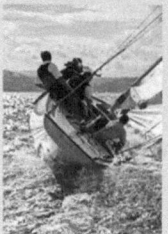

A helpful supervisor 'is in the boat with you, with a light hand on the tiller'

Like a Telescope

My supervisor is my telescope, navigating. I need freedom, but also the

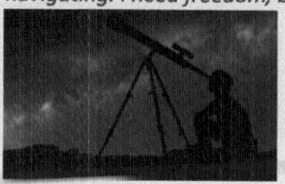

telescope; is it too far? Have I been looking in the wrong direction?

Seesaw

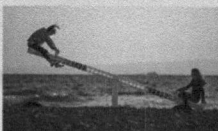

My supervisor was [knowledgeable], always there and slowly allowing me to even things out, reaching a point when I felt more in control. She'd still be there, but I could both hold my feet on the ground and be up in the air and trust my work.

Mountain leaders

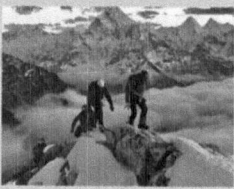

Supervisors can be like mountain leaders, guiding through challenging, complex uncharted landscapes – emotionally as well as socio-culturally, whilst supporting in 'not getting lost'.

Fig. 1.2 Supervisees describe doctoral research as thrilling, adventurous, often bordering on dangerous

Research supervisors play a critical role on different levels. In the mentioned study into the experience of research supervision (Bager-Charleson & McBeath, 2021a, 2021b) we approached supervisors (N=112) and supervisees (N=114) on PhD and professional doctorate programmes for psychotherapists and counselling psychologists with a survey using closed and open questions, and voluntary follow-up interviews. Figure 1.2 captures how supervisees expanded in the interviews on their doctoral research as thrilling, adventurous, often bordering on dangerous—with supervisors portrayed in ways that captured this through metaphors ranging from a sailing instructor to a mountain guide.

In the free text comments and interviews, supervisees stressed the value of empathy, containment and broad, updated research knowledge. In slight contrast, supervisors emphasised the importance of supervisee agency and self-direction.

One particularly illustrative example (Fig. 1.3) was how one supervisee described her supervisor as her 'telescope'—helping her to navigate and see far—whilst a supervisor chose a 'stethoscope' to describe how he regarded it his role to support

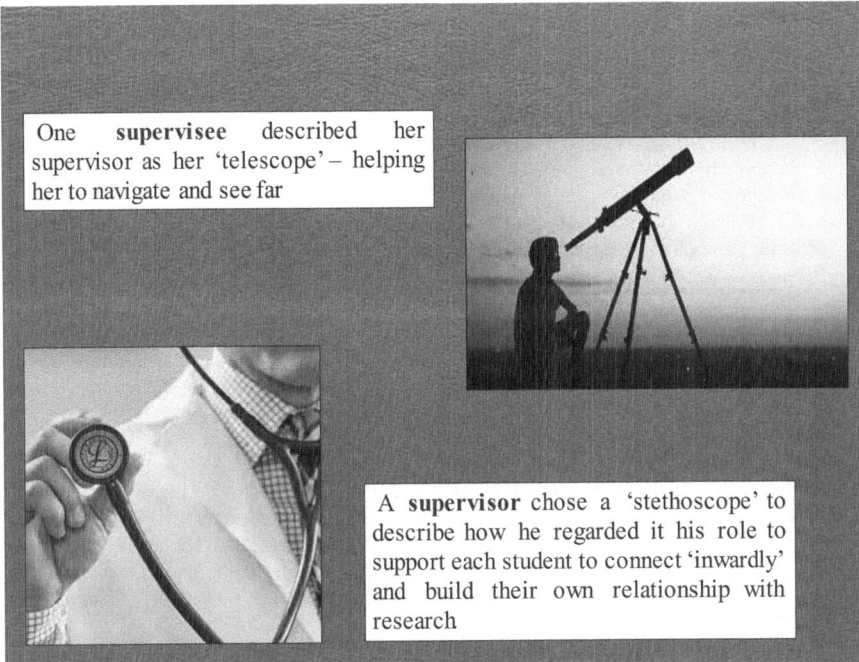

One **supervisee** described her supervisor as her 'telescope' – helping her to navigate and see far

A **supervisor** chose a 'stethoscope' to describe how he regarded it his role to support each student to connect 'inwardly' and build their own relationship with research

Fig. 1.3 The role of research supervision seen from different perspectives– seen from

each student to connect 'inwardly' and build their own relationship with research. We hope readers of this book will enjoy the opportunity of combining the two; travelling outwardly as well as inwardly in the amazing world of research.

perspectives.

Activity 1.1

- **Before reading this book: describe your relationship to research in one word.**

  In what areas, if any, might you benefit from support?
  To read more about others' experience of research and need for research support, please go to our 'relational research supervision guide' on this link:
  https://metanoia.ac.uk/research/relational-research-supervision-for-doctoral-psychotherapy-research/

References

Bager-Charleson, S. (2003). *The Parent's school? Narrative research about parental involvement in education.* Student Literature.

Bager-Charleson, S. (2020). *Reflective practice and personal development in counselling and psychotherapy* (2nd ed.). Sage.

Bager-Charleson, S., du Plock, S., & McBeath, A. (2018). "Therapists have a lot to add to the field of research, but many don't make it there". A narrative thematic inquiry into counsellors' and psychotherapists' embodied engagement with research. *Journal for Language and Psychoanalysis, 7*(1), 4–22. http://www.language-and-psychoanalysis.com/article/view/2603

Bager-Charleson, S., & McBeath, A. G. (2021a). What support do therapists need to do research? A review of studies into how therapists experience research. *Counselling and Psychotherapy Research, 21*(3), 555–569. https://doi.org/10.1002/capr.12432

Bager-Charleson, S., & McBeath, A. G. (2021b). Containment, compassion and clarity. Mixed methods research into supervision during doctoral research for psychotherapists and counselling psychologist. *Counselling and Psychotherapy Research, 22*(3), 689–707. https://doi.org/10.1002/capr.12498

Bager-Charleson, S., McBeath, A., & du Plock, G. (2019). The relationship between psychotherapy practice and research: A mixed-methods exploration of practitioners' views. *Counselling and Psychotherapy Research, 2019*(19), 195–205. https://doi.org/10.1002/capr.12196

Bager-Charleson, S., McBeath, A., & Vostanis, G. P. (2020). Guest editors: Special issue on mixed methods. *Research, for Counselling and Psychotherapy Research (CPR), 21*(1), 1. https://doi.org/10.1002/capr.12377

Braun, V., Clarke, V., Boulton, E., Davey, L., & McEvoy, C. (2021). The online survey as a qualitative research tool. *International Journal of Social Research Methodology, 24*(6), 641–654. https://doi.org/10.1080/13645579.2020.1805550

Braun, V., Clarke, V., Hayfield, N., Jenkinson, E., & Davey, L. (2022) Doing Reflexive Thematic Analysis. In S, Bager-Charleson & A.G McBeath, A.G. (Eds.) (2022) *Supporting Research in Counselling and Psychotherapy. Qualitative, Quantitative, and Mixed methods Research.* London: Palgrave Macmillan

Braun, V., Clarke, V., & Gray, D. (2017). *Collecting qualitative data: A practical guide to textual, media and virtual techniques.* Cambridge University Press. https://doi.org/10.1017/9781107295094

DeLyser, D., & Sui, D. (2013). Crossing the qualitative- quantitative divide II: Inventive approaches to big data, mobile methods, and rhythmanalysis. *Progress in Human Geography., 37*(2), 293–305. https://doi.org/10.1177/0309132512444063

Finlay, L. (2021). Thematic analysis: The 'good', the 'bad' and the 'ugly'. *European Journal for Qualitative Research in Psychotherapy, 11*, 103–116.

Frost, N., & Bailey-Rodriguez, D. (2020). Doing qualitatively driven mixed methods and pluralistic qualitative research. In S. Bager-Charleson & A. McBeath (Eds.), *Enjoying research in counselling and psychotherapy.* Palgrave Macmillan.

Gergen, K. J., & Gergen, M. M. (1988). Narrative And The Self As Relationship. *Social Psychological Studies Of The Self: Perspectives And Programs, 21*, 17–56. https://works.swarthmore.edu/facpsychology/965

Johnson, R. B. (2017). Dialectical pluralism: A metaparadigm whose time has come. *Journal of Mixed Methods Research, 11*(2), 156–173.

McBeath, A. G. (2020). Doing quantitative research with a survey. In S. Bager-Charleson & A. G. McBeath (Eds.), *Enjoying research in counselling and psychotherapy.* Palgrave Macmillan.

McBeath, A. G. & Bager-Charleson, S. (2022). Views about mixed methods research (MMR) from counselling and psychotherapy research students and supervisors. (manuscript in preparation). Metanoia Institute.

McBeath, A. G., Bager-Charleson, S., & Abarbanel, A. (2019). Therapists and academic writing: "Once upon a time psychotherapy practitioners and researchers were the same people". *European Journal for Qualitative Research in Psychotherapy, 19*, 103–116.

McGinley, P. (2015). *A phenomenological exploration of crying.* Ph.D. Dissertation. Regent's School of Psychotherapy and Psychology, Regent's University London.

Polkinghorne, D. (1991). Narrative and self-concept. *Journal of Narrative and Life History, 2*, 135–153.

36 of 296

Part I
Qualitative Research

Chapter 2
Doing Reflexive Thematic Analysis

Virginia Braun, Victoria Clarke, Nikki Hayfield, Louise Davey, and Elizabeth Jenkinson

Learning Goals

After reading this chapter, you should understand:

- The key characteristics of the thematic analysis (TA) family of methods, including reflexive TA—the main focus of this chapter.
- The wide scope of reflexive TA, related both to research design and conceptual issues.
- What data coding involves and how to go about developing codes using reflexive TA.
- What constitutes a (good-quality) theme and the practice of theme development in reflexive TA.
- Common problems to avoid when doing reflexive TA.

V. Braun (✉)
School of Psychology, Waipapa Taumata Rau/The University of Auckland,
Auckland, New Zealand
e-mail: V.Braun@auckland.ac.nz

V. Clarke • N. Hayfield • E. Jenkinson
School of Social Sciences, University of the West of England (UWE), Bristol, UK
e-mail: Victoria.Clarke@uwe.ac.uk; Nikki2.Hayfield@uwe.ac.uk;
Elizabeth2.Jenkinson@uwe.ac.uk

L. Davey
Lewisham and Greenwich NHS Trust, London, UK
e-mail: louisedavey@louisedavey.com

© The Author(s), under exclusive license to Springer Nature
Switzerland AG 2022
S. Bager-Charleson, A. McBeath (eds.), *Supporting Research in Counselling and Psychotherapy*, https://doi.org/10.1007/978-3-031-13942-0_2

Introducing Thematic Analysis

Thematic analysis (TA) is often presented as a singular method, but in actuality refers to a *family* of methods. TA has a long, if opaque, history, across multiple disciplines, although it most likely developed from (qualitative) content analysis. Like any method with a long history, different versions of TA have developed over time (for a detailed overview, see Braun & Clarke, 2021e). What—broadly—unites different versions is the use of processes of coding and theme generation for analysing qualitative data, and the production of a set of analytic 'themes'—with a theme capturing a pattern of meaning across the dataset. But there are many ways versions of TA differ, and approaches can be imbued with quite different paradigmatic assumptions (the values and principles that provide the foundation for research). A distinction we like comes from psychotherapy researcher Linda Finlay (2021) who differentiates TA approaches that are *scientifically descriptive* and those that are *artfully interpretive*. (NB: as Finlay notes, this is not a pure division, some approaches combine elements of both, e.g., Guest et al., 2012.)

Scientifically descriptive approaches to TA are characterised by the postpositivist research values of mainstream scientific research, typically drawing on realist philosophies and essentialist theoretical frameworks (e.g., Boyatzis, 1998). The postpositivist researcher strives to produce objective and reliable knowledge about the world, aiming to accurately describe and summarise data. Procedures for TA are designed to keep the understood-as-distorting effects of researcher subjectivity in check, and ensure the reliability of data coding. Because of this emphasis, we describe these approaches as *coding reliability TA* (Braun & Clarke, 2021e). If you have only been trained in scientific/quantitative approaches, this may sound reassuringly familiar, not radically different from what you are used to. But the broad domain of qualitative research encompasses so much more than what can effectively be a qualitative version of quantitative research. Finlay's (2021) artfully interpretive approaches to TA are part of the rich *qualitative* research tradition, combining qualitative data and techniques with qualitative research *values*. Defining qualitative research values is not simple, but many would agree with the following: 1) valuing researcher subjectivity as a resource for research (Gough & Madill, 2012); 2) that researcher subjectivity inevitably shapes the research process in various ways; and 3) that knowledge is always partial, perspectival and contextually located. Embedded in such values, artfully interpretive TA goes beyond description and summary, to ask questions about how particular patterned meaning might relate to the wider social context, and about the significance and implications of the patterned meanings.

The 'artfully interpretive' approach offered by reflexive TA (e.g., Braun & Clarke, 2021e) forms the main focus of this chapter. Since Ginny and Victoria's original paper on this approach (Braun & Clarke, 2006), reflexive TA has become widely used in many disciplines and research fields, including counselling and psychotherapy. In this chapter, we will introduce you to the defining characteristics and conceptual foundations of reflexive TA, and describe the six phases of the analytic process, illustrated with an example study from Louise's counselling and psychotherapy research (see Box 2.1). To make the most of this journey, we invite you to put aside any white-coated inner-scientist you may harbour, and (try to) embrace your inner creative storyteller—and embrace reflexivity!

Box 2.1 Introduction to the Example Study: Living with Alopecia Areata

Louise explored the subjectivities and lived experience of people living with alopecia areata (AA) for her Professional Doctorate in Counselling Psychology, supervised by Victoria and Liz (see Davey et al., 2019; Davey, 2020). AA is an autoimmune condition that results in hair loss. The hair loss is unpredictable; treatments have limited efficacy and potentially serious side effects, and hair loss resumes once treatment ends. People with AA experience high levels of depression and anxiety and lower quality-of-life. Louise aimed to explore how meanings associated with hair and hair loss shape the experience of living with AA, and—as a trainee counselling psychologist— how this might inform healthcare professionals to better support people living with AA. Louise collected data from 95 people living with AA—mostly White women. She used an online qualitative survey (see Braun et al., 2021) to ask a series of open-ended questions focused on experiences of living with AA and seeking psychological support. Responses were analysed using reflexive TA within a broadly critical realist framework, which attends to the social and cultural context of subjective meaning making. Louise developed four themes, which together captured the way participants' distress was contextualised by sociocultural meanings associated with hair loss:

(1) *It's (not) only hair* captured the extremely distressing nature of hair loss alongside a sense of not feeling entitled to distress or sympathy because hair loss was not life-threatening or a signifier of a life-threatening illness.
(2) *A restricted life* captured people's struggles with or avoidance of everyday activities because of anxiety around their hair loss being noticed or revealed.
(3) *Abandon hope all ye who lose their hair* explored the emotional rollercoaster of hopes raised and dashed because of the unpredictability of the condition and ineffective or only temporarily effective treatments; feelings of hopelessness were reinforced by encounters with non-empathic and insensitive health care professionals.
(4) *Seeking support in a 'highly personalised journey'* explored the social support from friends and family members, and contact with others with AA, that helped people to cope, alongside the difficulty of accessing cosmetic and psychological support.

Louise concluded that health professionals can better support people with AA with empathic and sensitive communication and signposting to alopecia support groups and psychological support.

Reflexivity for Reflexive Thematic Analysis

Reflexivity is an *essential* component of doing reflexive TA. But what is reflexivity? Simplifying somewhat, reflexivity captures the process of a researcher critically reflecting on their values, assumptions, expectations, choices and actions throughout the research process, and considering what these might enable, exclude and close off (see Finlay & Gough, 2003). It contains the acknowledgement that knowledge is never free of researcher influence, that our assumptions and choices *inevitably* shape the knowledge we create (create, rather than 'discover'). Reflexivity offers a form of quality control, through making space to question how we might be delimiting our analysis, and through articulating for readers the assumptions and values that contextualise the knowledge we have produced (Braun & Clarke, 2021a). To prepare yourself for learning about reflexive TA, we encourage you to try the reflexivity activity in Box 2.2.

Box 2.2 Flex Your Reflexivity Muscles!

We invite you to reflect on your perspectives on, and any personal experiences of, alopecia or unpredictable hair loss. The questions will prompt you to reflect on your personal positioning in relation to unpredictable hair loss, and to consider how your positioning might shape research on this topic.

How am I positioned in relation to this topic? Reflect on your experiences, perspectives and knowledge of hair loss:

- Am I an 'insider' (see Hayfield & Huxley, 2015) with personal experience of (unpredictable) hair loss?
- Do I know others with lived experience?
- Is my experience or knowledge specific to alopecia?
- What immediate responses and feelings do I have to the idea of hair loss, and specifically *unpredictable* hair loss?

How might my positioning shape my project design and analysis? Consider how your responses might impact if you were conducting a study with people who have lived experience of alopecia:

- How might having (or not having) insider knowledge, or a personal interest, inform my study design and research materials?
- How might I go about developing data collection questions in light of my professional and/or personal knowledge of the topic (or absence thereof)?
- In what ways could my positioning as insider/outsider impact on recruiting participants?
- In what ways could my positioning impact on data collection (particularly if this involved meeting your participants in person)?
- What might my positioning bring to the data analysis; how might it shape its development?

The activity in Box 2.2 highlights another aspect of reflexivity—how our positioning informs how we *design* and *do* our research. Thematic analysis offers much flexibility in regard to research design—indeed design and conceptual flexibility are distinguishing characteristics that set TA apart from most other analytic approaches (e.g., narrative analysis, interpretive phenomenological analysis) (Braun & Clarke, 2021b), which can be considered not methods but 'ready-made' *methodologies* (Chamberlain, 2012). Methodologies provide researchers with a theoretically informed framework for an entire research project, not just an analytic method. TA is closer to just an analytic method, although specific versions of TA reflect and are underpinned by particular research values (e.g., embracing or seeking to contain researcher subjectivity). The status of TA as method(ish) means a thoughtfully reflexive researcher, attuned to conceptual and design thinking, making considered and coherent choices, is essential for high-quality reflexive TA (Braun & Clarke, 2021c).

Designing a Reflexive Thematic Analysis Study

What we describe as 'design thinking' (Braun & Clarke, 2021c) covers diverse aspects of research, from the research questions we explore through to the size and constitution of the dataset or participant group; it's deeply connected to 'conceptual thinking' so read these processes (and sections) as interwoven. The design scope—flexibility—of TA is broad.

Research questions are a good place to begin. Broadly, qualitative researchers are often interested in people's lived experiences of a particular phenomenon (such as everyday experiences of living with alopecia), people's perceptions, understandings, views, needs or motivations in relation to a particular phenomenon (such as views on treatment options for alopecia, or social support needs), or people's behaviours or practices in relation to a particular phenomenon (such as wearing a wig in social situations and/or the workplace to conceal hair loss). Some seek to understand the social context of individual experience, and ask questions about the social factors or processes that influence particular phenomenon (such as what factors shape seeking the support of a therapist for alopecia-related distress), or the implicit rules or norms that govern particular phenomena (such as what values underpin the organisation of alopecia support groups). Some ask questions about the context of meaning, including a focus on representation or the social construction of meaning and consequent shared realities or truths (such as whether and how head, face and body hair are constructed in *gendered* ways in online alopecia support groups). TA offers an analytic tool to address this very wide range of questions (but not what we term 'language practice' questions, focused on the particulars of language use and function, or those oriented to narrative structures [Braun & Clarke, 2013], although researchers *are* blending methods, see Palomäki et al., 2013; Terry & Braun, 2016). To help determine whether a research question is appropriate for TA, reflect on whether it aligns with these broad forms (see more discussion in Braun & Clarke, 2021c).

What about *data*? Different data collection methods produce different data types, and—to use the language of a TV dating show—TA hasn't yet met a data type it's not compatible with! TA works with established methods like interviews and focus groups, and more novel ones (as well as in mixed method research, e.g., Rosen et al., 2012). This gives much design flexibility regarding data and TA, and we encourage creatively thinking 'beyond the interview' (Braun et al., 2017) for TA data. In counselling and psychotherapy research alone, TA has been used to analyse qualitative survey data (see Box 2.3), 'naturalistic' and pre-existing data sources such as psychotherapy sessions (e.g., Willcox et al., 2019) and data generated by *creative methods* such as story completion (e.g., Moller et al., 2021; Shah-Beckley et al., 2020).

Another key data design consideration is from whom/where and how many 'data instances' are collected—the latter is often referred to as 'sample size'. TA again offers valuable flexibility regarding the constitution and size of a dataset. Although it has been used in case of study research (e.g., Cedervall & Åberg, 2010), the method typically requires multiple data items, as it explores patterns of meaning (themes) *across* these. Beyond that, datasets can be larger or smaller in size, and homogenous or heterogeneous in constitution. It is impossible to precisely specify how many data instances will provide adequate data for a reflexive TA, as so many factors intersect in that question (see Braun & Clarke, 2021d). For a student in counselling and psychotherapy, our pragmatic lower limit recommendations for a rich, in-depth *interview* study would be: 5–6 interviews for a small diploma project; 6–12 for a medium-sized master's project; and 12–20 for a larger professional doctorate project (for a wider range of suggestions, see Braun & Clarke, 2013). Collecting the 'perfect' dataset is a myth, but how do we know ours is adequate in size and scope, and how do we explain that it provided good enough data to address our research question and support our claims? Researchers often resort to claims of 'saturation'—a widely (mis)used criterion for qualitative dataset size—sometimes supported by experimental claims to have determined the number of interviews needed for a TA to reach saturation (e.g., Guest et al., 2006). Saturation is also known as 'information redundancy' and amounts to the researcher's judgement—usually before analysis has started—that further data collection would generate 'no new information'. We do *not* recommend saturation, for several reasons, including—crucially—that it is very difficult to make definitive judgements about our data *before* we have analysed them, and meaning isn't fixed within data, so there is always scope for new information or interpretations (to read our full critique, see Braun & Clarke, 2021d). A looser concept called 'information power' (Malterud et al., 2016), which involves the researcher making subjective judgements about whether their data provide a sufficient basis for the proposed analysis, aligns conceptually with the values of reflexive TA.

A word of caution regarding design: our emphasis on flexibility in design for TA does *not* mean 'anything goes'. Holding onto a key principle of good qualitative design practice—variously known as 'fit' (Willig, 2013), design coherence or 'methodological integrity' (Levitt et al., 2017)—is crucial. You need to carefully consider your design choices, ensure the various elements of the research

Box 2.3 Why I Used Qualitative Surveys: Reflections by Louise
My study aimed to inform practice by increasing therapists' and healthcare professionals' understanding of lived experience of AA. With little existing research on the topic, I considered it important to collect data from lots of people. Qualitative surveys aligned well with these research objectives, as, unusually amongst qualitative methods, they allow for both breadth *and* depth of data (Braun et al., 2021). For therapist-researchers, they also offer the advantage of avoiding role conflicts—between researcher-self and therapist-self—that can arise in interactive methods, a particularly important consideration when collecting data on sensitive experiences (Davey, 2020). For participants, qualitative surveys offer a high degree of anonymity and the flexibility to respond at a time and location of choice. This can enable people who might not otherwise be present in qualitative research to participate—those constrained by work or caring commitments, or who struggle with face-to-face interactions. These advantages were apparent in my data—accounts were deeply intimate, high in emotional content and included descriptions of intense social anxiety and fear of revealing hair loss to others. Many were also submitted late at night or early in the morning. The qualitative survey therefore centres the needs of the client group being studied, making it an ideal fit for counselling and psychotherapy research.

design—including philosophical assumptions and theoretical frameworks discussed next—are coherent and align with each other; you also need to articulate a compelling rationale for these choices in your research report. Louise reflects on her reasons for using qualitative surveys for her alopecia study in Box 2.3.

Conceptual Understanding for Good Reflexive Thematic Analysis

Reflexive TA can be understood as a *fully* qualitative approach—involving the use of qualitative research *techniques*, underpinned by qualitative research *values*. As a researcher you are like a storyteller; the stories you tell about your data are inevitably shaped by your personal positioning, lived experience, assumptions and expectations about the topic. A base conceptual understanding for (good) reflexive TA is that you're not seeking to be a neutral, unbiased observer and reporter. From this conceptual base, reflexive TA gives you choices—the 'many questions of TA' (Braun & Clarke, 2006—in how you approach the artfully interpretative task of analysis. The broader domain of *fully* qualitative research is like the court of a mediaeval monarch, made up of various different—at times hostile—factions. Even though fully qualitative researchers share some common values, their research can be founded in quite *different* understandings of the world, and what it is we seek to know (referred to as ontologies, or theories of reality), and with quite different ideas on how (best) to do research (encapsulated in epistemologies, or theories of knowledge). We do not have space to detail the different 'ologies in this chapter, but want to signal that it's important to recognise that there are quite different ways to imagine these, and you need to consider and discuss this in conceptualising, designing and doing reflexive TA (see Braun & Clarke, 2021c, 2021e).

Ontological and epistemological issues connect to whether your reflexive TA is *experientially* or *critically* oriented. There are various ways of demarcating different qualitative factions—such as a fuzzy set of clusters of methods (Madill & Gough, 2008), or qualitative paradigms (Grant & Giddings, 2002). We like the analogy of two camps—an experiential camp and a critical camp (Reicher, 2000). Experiential TA encompasses approaches that take a broadly empathetic approach to interpretating meaning, centring participants' sense making, and aiming to stay close to how participants make sense of their worlds—such as in our example living with alopecia study. Experiential TA is used to address research questions about participants' lived experiences, views, perspectives and behaviours. Questions about influencing factors, norms and values may also be broadly experientially oriented. Experiential approaches constitute the vast majority of qualitative research in counselling and psychotherapy, with data often collected using interviews, focus groups and diaries. In critically oriented TA—which is a minority pursuit in counselling and psychotherapy (and indeed elsewhere)—a more interrogative approach is taken in interpreting meaning, with questions asked about what meanings exist, and are possible, and what their effects and implications may be (for an example, see Shah-Beckley et al., 2020).

Reflexive TA can also vary in relation to how meaning is explored in data: more semantically or more latently; more inductively or more deductively. Semantic/ latent refers to a continuum in how you go about reading the *content* of your data. Analysis at the more semantic level stays closer to the surface of the data, where meanings are explicitly stated; more latent analysis requires a dive 'under the surface', to focus on meaning that isn't so explicitly stated or 'visible' (latent isn't used in the psychoanalytic sense of unconscious, although it can encompass unconscious meaning in a psychoanalytically informed TA). In the alopecia study, the examples in Table 2.2 are of semantic codes, which dominated the analysis, as the aim was to stay close to participants' sense making. Looking at the ideas expressed in the familiarisation notes in Box 2.4, a more latent code would centre on participants' distress around being perceived as inauthentic (being assumed to be a cancer patient or the 'fakery' of wig wearing or drawn on eyebrows) and the underlying shared value of individual authenticity. A possible code label would be 'it's important to be authentic'.

The inductive/deductive continuum in reflexive TA captures whether analytic meaning exploration is more grounded in, and driven by, the data content, or more by existing/theoretical ideas the researcher is interested in exploring, using the dataset to do so. (NB these uses of induction/deduction are a bit different to the theory-generating and -testing meanings in scientific/quantitative research.) Induction in reflexive TA is not intended to be 'pure'—devoid of any outside influence; the researcher will influence!—but rather seeks to allocate interpretative *primacy* to the experiences, perspectives and so on expressed within the dataset. The alopecia example study exemplifies an inductive orientation. Deduction in reflexive TA is similarly not the application or testing of theory via the dataset, but rather using a theoretically informed analytic lens with the data, to offer new insights—and potentially develop theoretical understanding (e.g., Willcox et al., 2019). The researcher aims to hold existing theory 'lightly', as offering a way of opening up new ways of thinking about the data. Reflexive TA can combine elements of both—analysis is (initially) grounded in the data, but existing theoretical concepts and literature deepen the analytic interpretation (e.g., Shah-Beckley et al., 2020).

There is another crucial thing to understand to do conceptually coherent reflexive TA: what a theme is, and how themes are developed. In reflexive TA, themes are *not* conceptualised as real things, that reside within data, to be 'identified' during analysis—such ideas fit better with how themes are conceptualised in scientifically descriptive types of TA (see Braun & Clarke, 2021e). Instead, themes capture patterns only developed in *later* phases of analysis, after considerable analytic work to explore diversity and possible patterns of meaning. Themes in reflexive TA do more than cluster together the data related to a certain topic or issue (a 'topic summary'); they capture patterns of shared meaning, clustered around a central concept or idea, and tell stories about what such patterns mean and why they matter. A topic summary is *not* a theme in reflexive TA, though it is in some other approaches to TA, so it's crucial to understand the distinction to do reflexive TA well. A topic summary might be something like *barriers to accessing counselling for physically disabled adults*. Imagining a pre-pandemic world of face-to-face counselling, this 'theme' would overview all the *different* barriers the participants identified, such as inaccessible premises, lack of disabled parking, no accessible transport. What unites the observations is the topic of barriers, and the 'theme' maps the diversity of experience, rather than telling a shared-meaning-based story grounded in the experiences recounted. Taking a reflexive TA approach, you are interested in what unites, rather than diversity. Considering the data a bit more deeply (more latently, perhaps more deductively), you might start to notice all the barriers mentioned relate to ableism (Friedman & Owen, 2017). You might develop a shared-meaning-based, story-oriented theme on *the ableism of the built environment as a barrier to accessing counselling*. Researchers new to reflexive TA often fall into the trap of developing topic summaries—especially if data collection has asked particular questions where responses can simply be clustered. Developing shared-meaning-based, story-oriented themes can take more work, so, if your initial themes are topic summaries, there will be more work to do!

Getting Started with Analysis

Reflexive TA involves six phases that guide your analytic process (outlined in Table 2.1). The phases represent different types of engagement with your data, to develop analytic insights that help you to tell an interesting and important story about your data that addresses your research question.

Table 2.1 The six phases of reflexive thematic analysis

Phase	Process
1) Familiarisation	The starting point of 'getting to know' the data involves reading and re-reading textual data (and listening to audio data, viewing images, etc.). The researcher makes notes of things that strike them as interesting, and to be explored further.
2) Coding	The researcher reads their data closely, and tags all the data that capture interesting features relevant to the research question with code labels.
3) Initial theme generation	The researcher clusters and re-clusters similar codes to explore potential patterns of shared meaning, united around a core concept. These initial clusterings only have to be 'good enough' at this point.
4) Reviewing and developing themes	Starting from their initial themes, the researcher reviews, develops or radically changes them, to ensure they work to capture meaningful patterns in relation to the coded collated data, and the entire dataset. They consider the *story* each theme tells, as well as the developing overall analytic story.
5) Refining, defining and naming themes	Themes are further refined through writing short theme definitions—of up to a few hundred words—that capture the scope and core concept of each theme. The researcher settles on a name for each theme, based on its interpretative story.
6) Producing the report	The final phase finalises the analysis through writing. The analysis coherently weaves together data extracts and the researcher's analytic commentary, to tell the story of each theme. The overall analytic story is contextualised in relation to existing knowledge, and methodological processes are reflexively described.

Phase 1) familiarisation—which is separate to any 'familiarisation' gained during data collection—provides the foundations of your analysis! Although it involves a somewhat looser and freer-flowing engagement with the data than later phases, it is important, so do not skip over or rush this phase. During familiarisation, which involves reading and re-reading the data (and/or listening or viewing depending on data type), you should start to notice aspects of the data, perhaps those that feel most familiar or conversely strike you as quite unfamiliar. In this phase, it is common to initially (or indeed only) notice ideas that are at the surface of the data, or particularly common. As you immerse yourself more in the data, you might start to observe less immediately obvious features (Victoria's note in Box 2.4 illustrates this). Although it can be hard not to leap ahead, at this point you are *not* trying to notice particular patterns or develop themes, but rather intimately 'get to know' the data.

Louise, Victoria and Liz's analysis for the living with alopecia project was produced specifically in response to a call for papers for a special issue of the *British Journal of Dermatology* focused on skin conditions. It had to be produced in a fairly tight timeframe, and was more collaborative than Louise's main—more critically oriented—analysis for her thesis. Louise, Victoria and Liz familiarised themselves with the survey data by reading and re-reading them and making familiarisation notes in a way that suited them. The software used for the survey compiled the responses to each question, so this is how the data were read (while being mindful of the trap of summarising the responses to each question and presenting these topic summaries as 'themes'). To give an example of the familiarisation process, Victoria printed the data and read through the hard copy several times. She highlighted particularly vivid data extracts with a highlighter, and scribbled notes in the margins. She made overall familiarisation notes and observations on separate blank pages (Box 2.4 provides a brief excerpt from these). Louise, Liz and Victoria then met to discuss their initial impressions of the data and consider how to progress the analysis. They aimed to bounce ideas around, consider different 'takes' on the data and open up new ways of thinking about them, rather than reach some consensus. Another important function of the meetings was sharing emotional reactions to participants' accounts, supporting each other in working with a dataset that conveyed a huge amount of distress. After this first meeting, Louise and Victoria worked on coding the data and developing initial themes.

Box 2.4   A Brief Excerpt from Victoria's Overall Familiarisation Notes
I am really struck by the complexity of people's feelings—on the one hand, hair loss is profoundly significant, it's devastating, and the participants use various analogies to powerfully convey this: losing hair is like losing a limb, for women it's like having a mastectomy, it's like a bereavement, and they feel deeply frustrated, angry and hurt when GPs and others minimise the significance of hair and trivialise their hair loss, they don't feel seen, they don't feel listened to, so they feel entitled to their distress. But in other ways they don't feel entitled to their distress—because the hair loss is not physically painful, it's not life-threatening. Instances of being mistaken for a cancer patient provide really vivid examples of this—because they don't have cancer, because they're not at risk of dying, they don't feel entitled to people's sympathy, they feel fraudulent. If we were going deeper into the data, authenticity would be important to explore…

In *phase 2) coding*, you undertake a systematic, thorough approach to your data engagement, exploring and parsing out all the different meanings relevant to your research question. Coding involves closely reading the data, considering what is interesting and important, and then assigning a code label that captures your understanding of the meaning of a segment of the data. The size of any coded segment of data can vary, as can the number of codes applied to a segment. Parts of a dataset can be 'rich' with detailed content that invites or requires you to develop lots of codes to capture that detail; for some segments you will find yourself assigning fewer codes, or even none, if there is less or no relevant meaning. A code is a tool you create, that captures and briefly describes how/why you think some data are interesting and relevant—Table 2.2 provides examples of code labels and associated data from the alopecia study. Codes are not predetermined ahead of analysis; they can and should evolve as your understanding deepens—the boundaries of a code can be redrawn, the coding label tweaked, two or more codes can be collapsed

Table 2.2 Codes and example data extracts (from Davey et al., 2019)

Code label	Example extracts tagged with this code
Hair loss is like a bereavement	'it must be treated like grief. The psychological impact is all encompassing and never seems to diminish... It is extremely lonely and isolating'. (P84, female) 'losing hair is a grieving process and the emotions felt mirror those experienced by those suffering a bereavement'. (P2, female)
Hair loss is like losing a limb, a breast or part of the self	'It's like losing a piece of you. Nothing makes sense and you cannot recognise yourself'. (P34, female) 'it's a deeply personal feeling, and at times akin to women who have had a mastectomy and feel that something that made them a woman has been taken away from them'. (P49, female)
Feeling or looking monstrous or alien	'Also having to draw on eyebrows and eyeliner or face looking like an alien'. (P75, female) 'I get quite upset when I see myself bald. There is a reason monsters are portrayed bald. In Lord of the Rings when Gollum was a Hobbit he had hair when he turned evil—bald. Then of course there is Nosferatu, Voldemort, Trolls and Orcs'. (P61, female)
Feeling ugly and unfeminine	'having no eyebrows or eye lashes makes me feel like I'm no longer a woman as I don't have the womanly face anymore, it's just a blank canvas with no features at all now'. (P55, female) 'I have particularly low self-esteem when I consider the way I look, especially as a woman. I feel rather ugly when I'm not wearing my wig and it makes it difficult for me to feel that men would find me attractive (even with my wig on)'. (P17, female)

together, a code can be split into several more focused codes... Key is working systematically to *consistently* engage with the data throughout, going back through the coded data to recode when needed. You end this phase when you have coded the full dataset thoroughly, and then collated the data segments related to each code, to work with in the next phase. At this point, we encourage you to have a go at familiarisation and coding using the extracts presented in Table 2.3.

Developing and Completing Analysis

By now, you may be itching to develop themes, having felt constrained during familiarisation and coding. This is your moment! In *phase 3) initial theme generation* you develop your collated codes into possible themes. But: it is *very* easy to get attached to your first group of themes, so try to think of these as a 'first draft'. The terminology of *initial* themes is a useful reminder that you are still *early* in your analysis and everything is provisional, your analysis *will* shift and change—sometimes dramatically—from where you get to in this phase. Your aim is to develop *meaningful* patterns, rather than just organise data into categories. This means you need to actively explore your codes—which form the building blocks of themes— and how they might cluster together to tell a coherent story about a pattern of meaning. The most common process for generating themes is by combining codes that

Table 2.3 Have a go at familiarisation and coding!

What is it like to live with alopecia? Using this selection of data extracts from the alopecia study, engage with this question. First have a go at familiarisation. Read the extracts a few times; make notes on what strikes you as interesting and worthy of further exploration. Second, try coding, including developing more semantic and more latent codes. We encourage leaving a few days between familiarisation and coding, to allow your ideas to 'ferment'.

Data extracts	Familiarisation notes	Codes
'My family and I tried buying hair products and shampoos to help but they didn't and were a waste of money. I went to 4 wig shops within 40 miles of me and all made me feel worse because the products were not very good/ fit and colour etc. I then went all the way from [north of England] to [south of England] to see someone who had alopecia and was recommended and I felt better and bought an expensive wig'.		
'At first I wore acrylic wigs but since I've started wearing vacuum ones it's been much easier to cope. They are very expensive (£1900) and I need a new one every 3 or so years so it's a significant financial burden but since I wear it every day it's one I save for. I've also had temporary tattoos regularly for my eyebrows and eyeliner. The latter I gave up because it didn't last very long and it was really unpleasant as well as expensive. I've also tried microblading'.		
'The counsellor asked me what was the worst thing about it and I said that it was people staring at me. She stared at me for two sessions and it totally freaked me out. So she did exactly the things which I had told her was the worst thing. The counsellor had told me that she had never come across anyone with alopecia'.		
'In terms of psychological help, there was none. I had general counselling, but none of the counsellors knew what alopecia was nor did they understand the impact that alopecia can have on someone's life. I was never offered counselling, my parents had to look for counselling help on their own'.		

you consider fit together well. Less commonly, a rich and complex code might form the basis of a theme, with a few other codes potentially clustered around it. This process is active and interpretative—informed by your knowledge of the topic and your reflexive positions. Ultimately, each theme will contribute to you telling an overall story about the data to address the research question.

Not all codes need to fit into your initial theme mapping (or indeed the final story)—set aside but don't discard unused codes, and return to them at all development and review points. In this phase, it's good to consider a few different possible mappings, but when have you done enough to move on to the next phase? Your initial themes just need to be 'good enough'—remembering this is an *initial* set of themes might be helpful!—as the next phases involve considerable further analytic development work. It's also good to understand that moving through the phases is not like travelling down a one-way road. While we endorse initially engaging in the first three phases sequentially to build a robust foundation for your analysis, your subsequent analysis will likely be recursive, with developing insights requiring you to return to some or all of the earlier phases.

In *phase 4) reviewing and developing your themes* you explore how effectively your initial themes work to tell the story of your data. There are multiple processes for review: reconsidering your whole list of codes and coded data, including what has not been included in the initial thematic code clusters; re-reading your whole dataset to make sure your themes have not departed too far from it, and tell a good story of it; checking whether you have a clear core concept for each theme—that your story is built upon; evaluating how meaningful your interpretation of the data is in relation to your research question. Insight cannot be forced, so having breaks during theme development can be helpful to allow ideas to develop (Braun & Clarke, 2021e). Once you feel your developed themes capture well what you judge to be the, or an, important story of the dataset, you can shift towards the refining and then finishing phases.

The processes in *phase 5) refining, defining and naming themes* offer tools to further assess how well your themes are working, and move you towards finalising through writing up. Writing theme definitions is an important part of this phase. Start by simply writing what the theme is about to capture as its core concept. Themes are multifaceted (in contrast, codes are single-faceted), so will include various expressions of the core concept. Writing definitions offers opportunities for further refinement: you can work out the flow of theme content; ascertain whether a theme has too much happening, and might need separating into two or more themes, or the use of subthemes for clarification; you may find you have very little to say, so themes need to be further developed, by merging themes or revisiting coding and theme generation, or perhaps even discarded. Thorough work in the earlier phases usually means that refinement, rather than drastic action, is required here (though sometimes it is!).

Collectively, theme definitions may help you determine the best order to present your themes in your final report. They can provide the foundation for your analytic narrative, although the specific way they do so will depend on the structure of the final analysis. Box 2.5 provides an excerpt of a theme definition from the living with alopecia study, written for a medical journal. Such journals typically present qualitative research in a quite particular way, with analytic commentary/description of the theme in the main text, and data quotations in a separate table/box. Data quotations are generally used to illustrate broader observations, rather than more specific points, which they can do when embedded in the main text. Because of the tight word count for the main text of the paper, the theme descriptions were essentially polished versions of the initial theme definitions.

Box 2.5   Original Theme Definition for 'A Restrictive Life' [excerpt]
Many spoke about the things they avoided doing, or found difficult to do, because of their hair loss, fears and anxieties around being hyper-visible in public spaces and stared at by strangers, anxieties about managing their wig and their baldness/lack of hair being exposed in public if their wig should slip, or being exposed as a 'fake'. Many avoided activities like sport and

---

(continued)

Box 2.5 (continued)

exercise—particularly swimming and 'working out' in the gym. They also reported worrying about the weather—hot weather makes wigs feel uncomfortable; wind raises the potential of losing their wig. They related fears around making friends and forming partner relationships, and socialising generally, because of their feelings of self-consciousness. Many participants were grateful to have a long-term partner, but expressed concern for those who were younger/single. Some reported taking time off work or school when they were younger until they had a way of concealing their (often sudden) baldness or patchy hair loss (e.g., waiting for a wig), or because of depression and other mental health difficulties resulting from the hair loss. A few even avoided leaving the house altogether, such was their distress…

This phase also involves deciding final theme names—often developed from the working titles we use along the way. Key is ensuring theme names capture the central concept, and convey this clearly to the reader. The theme name *a restricted life* from the alopecia study (in Box 2.5) evocatively indicates to the reader the scope of this theme—how hair loss brought an element of often profound restriction to participants' lives. Including brief, evocative data extracts in the theme name can entice the reader, but the name still needs to convey the focus of the theme. Whilst some data offers 'gold'—such as an amazing quotation from an eloquent participant—don't be drawn by a snappy quotation that doesn't convey the core idea of the theme.

Phase 6) producing the report is not about simply writing up an already formed analysis; it also serves as final refinement of your themes, and assessing how well they tell the story of your overall analysis. Considering only the analytic section, your writing process will depend on how much you've already written as you've developed your analysis. The analysis needs to include data extracts, as well as *your* analytic narrative, the story you want to tell. Typically, you will introduce the core concept of each theme, then make a series of analytic claims—telling the story of the theme—with data that demonstrate the claims you are making about the data; narrative and extracts are often interwoven. Ensuring you include extracts from a range of data items, and that you *tell the story* of the data, rather than relying on the data to 'speak for themselves', will give credibility to your themes. Writing can be an engaging process, and another space for being reflexive, as Louise discusses in Box 2.6.

Box 2.6 Reflection on Writing Up: By Louise

The theoretical flexibility of TA allowed for quite different analyses: one critical-realist-based experiential analysis in which the story of the data was relevant and accessible to medical readers (the example study here; Davey et al., 2019), and another using a critical constructionist philosophical

(continued)

Box 2.6 (continued)

approach, where the coding and themes explored the depth, complexity and nuance of participants' subjectivities that are more the domain of counselling and psychotherapy (see Davey, 2020). As I reflected during the ongoing analytic process of writing my thesis (Braun & Clarke, 2021e), I realised the first analysis also enriched the second, deepening my engagement with the data and prompting insights about parallels between the therapy and research processes.

The patterns I developed from the data differed depending on the analytic lens I used (experiential or critical). Yet the two approaches spoke to each other in my reflexive process, challenging me to remain open and curious, even as I committed to codes, themes and the stories I was telling. I realised parallels with my role as therapist—as therapists we similarly continuously make choices about what information or patterns of experience to privilege as we respond to our clients, while simultaneously seeking to hold space for their meaning-making. The research process, like therapy, often felt confusing and messy, but my developing reflexivity helped me tolerate this, guiding my reflections and interpretations. Therapist capacity to tolerate messiness and uncertainty is a key quality in relational therapy, as is the ability to enable some structure to take shape so that a therapeutic process can unfold. This calls for a reflexivity through which the therapist can maintain ongoing awareness of their subjective responses to what the client brings. Reflexive TA allowed me to acknowledge and value my subjectivity in the research process, and along the way nurtured my understanding of reflexivity in the therapy process.

Avoiding Common Problems in TA

Unfortunately, problems in research using TA, including published studies, are all too common, and we briefly signal five easy ones to avoid (for a detailed discussion, see Braun & Clarke, 2021a, 2021e). Many of these seem to fall under the banner of what we might call *unknowing practice*, where researchers appear unaware of the diversity within TA, and blend together aspects or processes from different approaches, without any acknowledgement of, or justification for, this (for a counselling example of this, see Rosen et al., 2012).

1. We wish we were joking, but 'do your reading' is our first piece of advice. Too often we find examples where people use TA, citing methodological authors— including us—who advise different and sometimes diametrically opposed practices to what is reported as their research practice.
2. Don't unknowingly 'mash up' different versions of TA. Do demonstrate you understand that there are *different* approaches to TA, underpinned by different

research values and philosophical assumptions, and with very different conceptualisations of core constructs (such as themes) and procedures for coding and theme development/identification.

3. Don't implicitly treat TA as if it is atheoretical, rather than theoretically flexible. Specify the research values and theoretical assumptions that inform your use of TA. This provides the foundation for validity of your analytic claims—it determines what sorts of analytic processes or claims make sense, and what do not.

4. Don't present topic summaries as 'themes'—a theme is centred around a shared meaning; it tells your interpreted data story of *that* core idea or meaning.

5. Don't rush into themes! New to TA researchers often want to—or do—rush ahead to develop themes. Not only does a quick jump to themes risk analytic *foreclosure* (Connelly & Peltzer, 2016), the practice implicitly treats themes as real and 'identifiable' things, waiting to be discovered, or—gasp—emerge from the data. In reflexive TA, themes are produced at the intersection of the data, and your subjectivity and skill as researcher, and all that you bring to the analysis in terms of your values, assumptions and so on. The analytic insight needed for developing a rich, interpretative *story* about the data and topic comes from a combination of reflexive exploration and openness, and time for ideas to percolate (Braun & Clarke, 2021e).

What these common problems signal is the need to be a *knowing* practitioner of TA—demonstrating you understand the research values that underpin your chosen approach to TA, and how these give rise to particular conceptualisations of codes/ coding and themes, to particular coding and theme development procedures, and to quite different responses to researcher subjectivity. Doing TA well is less about following procedures exactly as specified, and more about understanding the values that shape those procedures. By understanding the values—and how they validate and invalidate different research processes—you can engage in analytic process in the way that works best for you and your project, yet remains conceptually coherent.

Chapter Summary

We have presented the essentials of conceptualising, designing and doing *reflexive* TA, in counselling and psychotherapy. We contextualised the TA family of methods, and introduced quite radically different approaches—from scientifically descriptive to artfully interpretative. We discussed the value of researcher subjectivity and practicing reflexivity, and encouraged a thoughtful, engaged, knowing researcher for quality reflexive TA. After outlining key design and conceptual considerations for TA research, we described the practice of reflexive TA, detailing a six-phase approach, illustrated with reference to our example study of living with alopecia. We concluded by signalling five all-too-common problems in (reflexive TA) research, problems which are easily avoidable even by a new researcher, by reading widely and becoming a *knowing* practitioner of TA.

References

Boyatzis, R. E. (1998). *Transforming qualitative information: Thematic analysis and code development*. Sage.

Braun, V., & Clarke, V. (2006). Using thematic analysis in psychology. *Qualitative Research in Psychology, 3*(2), 77–101. https://doi.org/10.1191/1478088706qp063oa

Braun, V., & Clarke, V. (2021a). One size fits all? What counts as quality practice in (reflexive) thematic analysis? *Qualitative Research in Psychology, 18*(3), 328–352. https://doi.org/10.1080/14780887.2020.1769238

Braun, V., & Clarke, V. (2021b). Can I use TA? Should I use TA? Should I not use TA? Comparing reflexive thematic analysis and other pattern-based qualitative analytic approaches. *Counselling and Psychotherapy Research, 21*(1), 37–47. https://doi.org/10.1002/capr.12360

Braun, V., & Clarke, V. (2021c). Conceptual and design thinking for thematic analysis. *Qualitative Psychology, 9*(1), 3–26. Advance online publication. https://doi.org/10.1037/qup0000196

Braun, V., & Clarke, V. (2021d). To saturate or not to saturate? Questioning data saturation as a useful concept for thematic analysis and sample-size rationales. *Qualitative Research in Sport, Exercise & Health, 13*(2), 201–216. https://doi.org/10.1080/2159676X.2019.1704846

Braun, V., & Clarke, V. (2021e). The ebbs and flows of qualitative research: Time, change and the slow wheel of interpretation. In B. C. Clift, J. Gore, S. Gustafsson, S. Bekker, I. C. Batlle, & J. Hatchard (Eds.), *Temporality in Qualitative Inquiry: Theories, Methods and Practices* (pp. 22–38). Routledge.

Braun, V., Clarke, V., Boulton, E., Davey, L., & McEvoy, C. (2021). The online survey as a qualitative research tool. *International Journal of Social Research Methodology, 24*(6), 641–654. https://doi.org/10.1080/13645579.2020.1805550

Braun, V., Clarke, V., & Gray, D. (Eds.). (2017). *Collecting qualitative data: A practical guide to textual, media and virtual techniques*. Cambridge University Press. https://doi.org/10.1017/9781107295094

Braun, V., & Clarke, V. (2013). *Successful qualitative research: A practical guide for beginners*. Sage.

Cedervall, Y., & Åberg, A. C. (2010). Physical activity and implications on well-being in mild Alzheimer's disease: A qualitative case study on two men with dementia and their spouses. *Physiotherapy Theory and Practice, 26*(4), 226–239.

Chamberlain, K. (2012). Do you really need a methodology? *Qualitative Methods in Psychology Bulletin, 13*, 59–63.

Connelly, L. M., & Peltzer, J. N. (2016). Underdeveloped themes in qualitative research: Relationship with interviews and analysis. *Clinical Nurse Specialist, 30*(1), 52–57. https://doi.org/10.1097/nur.0000000000000173

Davey, L. (2020). *Exploring the subjectivities of people with alopecia areata - a critical qualitative study to inform applied psychology practice*. Unpublished doctoral thesis, University of the West of England. https://uwe-repository.worktribe.com/output/3236744

Davey, L., Clarke, V., & Jenkinson, E. (2019). Living with alopecia areata: An online qualitative survey study. *British Journal of Dermatology, 180*(6), 1377–1389. https://doi.org/10.1111/bjd.17463

Finlay, L. (2021). Thematic analysis: The 'good', the 'bad' and the 'ugly'. *European Journal for Qualitative Research in Psychotherapy, 11*, 103–116.

Finlay, L., & Gough, B. (Eds.), (2003). Reflexivity: A practical guide for researchers in health and social sciences. .

Friedman, C., & Owen, A. L. (2017). Defining disability: Understandings of and attitudes towards ableism and disability. *Disability Studies Quarterly, 37*(1), 301. http://dsqsds.org/article/view/5061/4545

Gough, B., & Madill, A. (2012). Subjectivity in psychological research: From problem to prospect. *Psychological Methods, 17*(3), 374–384. https://doi.org/10.1037/a0029313

Grant, B. M., & Giddings, L. S. (2002). Making sense of methodologies: A paradigm framework for the novice researcher. *Contemporary Nurse, 13*(1), 10–28.

Guest, G., Bunce, A., & Johnson, L. (2006). How many interviews are enough? An experiment with data saturation and variability. *Field Methods, 18*(1), 59–82. https://doi.org/10.1177/1525822X05279903

Guest, G., MacQueen, K. M., & Namey, E. E. (2012). *Applied thematic analysis.* Sage. https://doi.org/10.4135/9781483384436

Hayfield, N., & Huxley, C. (2015). Insider and outsider perspectives: Reflections on researcher identities in research with lesbian and bisexual women. *Qualitative Research in Psychology, 12*(2), 91–106.

Levitt, H. M., Motulsky, S. L., Wertz, F. J., Morrow, S. L., & Ponterotto, J. G. (2017). Recommendations for designing and reviewing qualitative research in psychology: Promoting methodological integrity. *Qualitative Psychology, 4*(1), 2–22. https://doi.org/10.1037/qup0000082

Madill, A., & Gough, B. (2008). Qualitative research and its place in psychological science. *Psychological Methods, 13*(3), 254–271. https://doi.org/10.1037/a0013220

Malterud, K., Siersma, V. K., & Guassora, A. D. (2016). Sample size in qualitative interview studies: Guided by information power. *Qualitative Health Research, 26*(13), 1753–1760. https://doi.org/10.1177/1049732315617444

Moller, N., Clarke, V., Braun, V., Tischner, I., & Vossler, A. (2021). Qualitative story completion for counseling psychology research: A creative method to interrogate dominant discourses. *Journal of Counseling Psychology, 68*(3), 286–298. https://doi.org/10.1037/cou0000538

Palomäki, J., Laakasuo, M., & Salmela, M. (2013). "This is just so unfair!": A qualitative analysis of loss-induced emotions and tilting in on-line poker. *International Gambling Studies, 13*(2), 255–270.

Reicher, S. (2000). Against methodolatry: Some comments on Elliott, Fischer, and Rennie. *British Journal of Clinical Psychology, 39*(1), 1–6.

Rosen, D. C., Miller, A. B., Nakash, O., Halpern, L., & Alegría, M. (2012). Interpersonal complementarity in the mental health intake: A mixed-methods study. *Journal of Counseling Psychology, 59*(2), 185–196. https://doi.org/10.1037/a0027045

Shah-Beckley, I., Clarke, V., & Thomas, Z. (2020). Therapists' and nontherapists' constructions of heterosex: A qualitative story completion study. *Psychology and Psychotherapy: Theory, Research and Practice, 93*, 189–206. https://doi.org/10.1111/papt.12203

Terry, G., & Braun, V. (2016). "I think gorilla-like back effusions of hair are rather a turnoff": "Excessive hair" and male body hair (removal) discourse. *Body Image, 17*, 14–24.

Willcox, R., Moller, N., & Clarke, V. (2019). Exploring attachment incoherence in bereaved families' therapy narratives: An attachment theory-informed thematic analysis. *The Family Journal: Counseling and Therapy for Couples and Families, 27*(3), 339–347. https://doi.org/10.1177/1066480719853006

Willig, C. (2013). *Introducing qualitative research in psychology* (3rd ed.). Open University Press.

Further Reading

Ginny and Victoria's book—supported by an extensive open access companion website (https://uk.sagepub.com/en-gb/eur/thematic-analysis/book248481)—provides the definitive guide to doing reflexive TA: Braun, V., & Clarke, V. (2022). Thematic analysis: *A practical guide.* Sage Their website www.thematicanalysis.net includes FAQs, annotated reading lists, links to YouTube lectures and more.

Nikki and Gareth Terry's book provides a succinct accessible guide to reflexive TA: Terry, G., & Hayfield, N. (2021). Essentials of thematic analysis. American Psychological Association.

For more on research design in reflexive TA, see: Braun, V., & Clarke, V. (2022). Conceptual and design thinking for thematic analysis. *Qualitative Psychology, 9*(1), 3–26. https://doi.org/10.1037/qup0000196

For a detailed discussion of quality in reflexive TA, including common problems to avoid, see: Braun, V., & Clarke, V. (2021). One size fits all? What counts as quality practice in (reflexive) thematic analysis? Qualitative Research in Psychology, 18(3), 328–352.

Finally, for a detailed discussion of the (mis)use of the saturation concept in TA research, see: Braun, V., & Clarke, V. (2021). To saturate or not to saturate? Questioning data saturation as a useful concept for thematic analysis and sample-size rationales. Qualitative Research in Sport, Exercise & Health, 13(2), 201–216. https://doi.org/10.1080/2159676X.2019.1704846

Chapter 3
Doing Arts-based Decolonising Research

Divine Charura and Rachel Wicaksono

> As 'ontological colonizers', we must learn to let go of our
> profound desires to control, if not the course of History itself,
> the metaphysical meanings we attribute to the experience of
> historical temporality'.
>
> *(Malette, 2012: 381)*

This chapter outlines some conceptual issues in doing arts-based decolonised research. In this chapter, we take a broad view of 'art', one that includes the 'art of' (decolonising) research, and we highlight examples from our own research that show (1) how we have used objects ('arti-facts'?) to create data and (2) linking to psychotherapy and research, how the 'art of communication' (the delicate mechanisms of interaction and the way that we, as researchers, choose to report them) has created our data.

We approached this chapter using a duoethnographic research approach, in which we consider the meanings of our individual narratives and our conceptualisations of the different perspectives we were exploring (Breault, 2016; Norris & Sawyer, 2012). We began with two key questions: 'what "is" arts-based research?' and 'what does decolonizing research "mean"?'. In this chapter, we highlight the importance of seeing research as a relational and deeply reflexive process; we pay attention to the themes which we conceptualised as part of our analysis of the duo-ethnographic process. These themes are: 'beginnings'; active engagement with the research dynamics that unfold thereafter (which we have called the 'real inner drama'); and, finally, 'endings'. Through each of these themes, we explore the possibility of a decolonised approach which demonstrates a deep respect, and valuing, of participation/participants. This respect can be primarily demonstrated by

D. Charura (✉) • R. Wicaksono
York St John University, York, UK
e-mail: d.charura@yorksj.ac.uk; r.wicaksono@yorksj.ac.uk

© The Author(s), under exclusive license to Springer Nature
Switzerland AG 2022
S. Bager-Charleson, A. McBeath (eds.), *Supporting Research in Counselling and Psychotherapy*, https://doi.org/10.1007/978-3-031-13942-0_3

engagement with reflexivity and evidence of how we, as researchers and co-authors of this chapter, have tried to manage 'power-with' rather than 'power-over'. We show how the latter, being synonymous with colonising dynamics, plays out in practices in which, for example, researchers focus on having their research questions answered, rather than on engaging with the diversity of world views/experiences that participants bring to the research process. In ending research interviews/ encounters, leaving space for reflection and debriefing is important. Where artifacts, or other creative methodologies, are employed, respecting the participant and their objects/creations involves a discussion of what happens to them next, or how the participant would like to end their participation. Furthermore, dialogue about returning to the transcript to check with the participant about the representation of their narrative, as well as discussions about how they will be represented, or not, in the dissemination, is all part of the ending process. To demonstrate these themes we offer examples from our own arts-based decolonising research.

Central to our chapter are the following questions:

- What are objects, things, art, and how do they shift power?
- How are these issues relevant to counselling and psychotherapy research and practice?
- What are some of the dilemmas we have faced in doing arts-based decolonising research?

To end this chapter, we reflect on silence as a useful part of the research interaction; for example, in the provision of a space for material to emerge, or to be held, in reflection. We recommend increased awareness of our own and our research participants' multiple and changing understandings of 'things', both material and conceptual; whilst at the same time remaining committed to the process of searching for our own truths, and to the maintenance of ethical research and professional practice.

Origins of our Duoethnographical, Decolonised Approach and Writing Process

Given that we are from different fields and professions, with one of the authors (DC) being a practitioner psychologist, and Director of the Doctorate in Counselling Psychology at York St John University, and one (RW) being an applied linguist, we agreed that in writing this chapter we would engage in duoethnographic dialogue. This process began with discussion about our lived experiences: as people with some similar pedagogical interests; as researchers, academics; and by exploring our individual/personal experiences of being in the world (our epistemologies and ontologies). In addition, we focused on our understandings of what doing arts-based decolonising research meant to us and what our experiences of engaging in decolonised research were. This approach was important to us as we were also interested in engaging in a decolonised approach to collaboration in the writing of this chapter.

Such an approach enabled our multiple diversities and lived experiences (autoethnographies, autobiographies, life histories, and more) to become equal knowledge-generating partners in dialogue. It also meant that psychological theory/research perspectives did not have pre-eminence over applied linguistic research, or vice versa. And furthermore, it allowed us to attempt to illuminate our process for the readers of this chapter, thereby offering an example of an approach for future researchers to consider in creating their own collaborative encounters/research.

Our duoethnographic approach as an evolving form of inquiry draws on the work of Norris and Sawyer (2012, p. 12), who suggested that duoethnographies can be thought of as a kind of 'collaborative field testing' (Breault, 2016; Norris & Sawyer, 2012). The material for this chapter thus arose over a period, of about a year, which began with a workshop on *'Ontologies' in the context of doing research* with trainees on the Doctorate in Counselling Psychology programme, facilitated by one of the authors (RW). In this workshop, the trainees were invited to explore their perspectives on 'what different things are'. The facilitator invited the trainees to respond to different photographs of objects/things or people. After a few moments of silent reflection, the trainees were then invited to think about and share with other group members, 'what they thought, perceived or felt about what they had seen'. These reflections led to a class discussion about ontology as a questioning of 'the nature of reality' and one's own experience of 'being in the world' (Charura & Lago, 2021; Pring, 2004; Wicaksono & Hall, 2020); and epistemology as a questioning of how theories/bodies of knowledge, and the research methods that underpin them, inform our understanding of social reality, including our fundamental assumptions about human beings/research participants (Charura & Lago, 2021; Grix, 2001). Following this workshop, we were both moved by the trainees' diversity of perspectives on, and changes in, their understanding of why it is important for researchers in counselling, psychotherapy, and psychology to engage critically with their own ontological and epistemological positions. Some quotes from our post-workshop dialogue include DC's initial response to RW:

> As we all engaged in the process, Rachel, I was surprised and excited at the shifts in understanding, in myself as well as the trainees. It was particularly interesting when you showed the picture of hair in a sink and the responses of some participants in the workshop were "oh that is disgusting". Then when you asked about why it becomes "disgusting" in the sink and not when on one's head, the reflections about the importance of considering a diversity of personal/cultural perspectives on hair, and other things, demonstrated a shift in openness to the worldviews of others. This openness to continually develop a reflexive awareness of one's assumptions when engaging in research highlighted for me how the researchers' ontological and epistemological positions of 'what things are' can easily result in colonizing dynamics when faced with a different world-or-knowledge view.

In response to this RW responded,

> Thank you Divine... this is important in designing our own research. What are the possible definitions, understandings, categorizations, experiences of a thing? When comparing findings between studies. What was the researchers' conceptualization of the thing? .... I am trying to understand the work of the quantum physicist Karen Barad (2007) who asks us to think about how what we 'know' about things makes them into what they 'are'; and how these objects of knowledge are also agents in the production of knowledge.

We continued in dialogue in person and, at times, online, each month, and emailed thoughts and responses to each other in relation to doing arts-based decolonising research. Halfway through the writing process, one of the authors (DC) was hospitalised with critical COVID-19 complications for about a month, thus there was a break and pause in our process. We explored what this break meant for us as collaborating authors; including, how what we 'know' about things/people/states of health makes them into what they 'are', and how changing viewpoints about, for example, what it means to be a 'person', or a 'healthy person' determine those people's pasts and futures, and the entangled relationships between ontologies (being), epistemologies (knowing), and ethics (doing, in this case, writing).

Upon return to work, we continued to analyse our experiences, further interweaving our co-constructed narratives into key themes, which then cumulated in the co-authoring of this paper. As noted by Norris and Sawyer, we juxtaposed our personal voices with the voice of another, so that, through co-reflections, neither position could 'claim dominance or universal truth' (2012, p. 15). We also tried to notice how our naming of things (including, for example: 'real', 'research', 'co-author', 'health') interacts with those things, and, more broadly, how material objects, classes (including of people), ideas/concepts, institutions, practices, and ourselves come into being and, perhaps, fade away. We offer this aspect of our process, an unforeseen break and then a return to work, as possible example of the potential challenges/unforeseen circumstances that can emerge in any research process; what we refer to, later in the chapter, as 'the real inner drama'.

What Are Some Conceptual Issues in Doing Arts-based Decolonising Research that We Address Here?

Arts-based Research

In our chapter, we have taken a view of 'art' that includes the 'art of' (decolonising) any kind of research. Our own examples in this chapter show how we have used (1) objects and (2) the 'art of communication' (the delicate mechanisms of interaction and the way that, as researchers, we choose to report them) to create our data. Our view of art is a version of a definition of 'art therapy', which, according to the American Art Therapy Association (2018), is a process that takes place in the presence of a (disciplinary-sanctioned) certified/qualified art therapist (Regev & Cohen-Yatziv, 2018). Our 'arts-based' research is described as such in the context of our creation of common ground between our two disciplines. In creating this common ground, we named our examples, presented later in this chapter, as 'arts-based' for the purposes of exploring the art of decolonising (our) research. Our joint agreement to name/describe our process brought our territory into being into a way that avoided the dominance of one discipline over the other. For the, possibly temporary, purposes of this chapter, we are doing arts-based research, a definition which makes the chapter possible, in the context of this book.

Decolonising Research

> Making explicit our metaphysical assumptions in order to negotiate their formulations and implications openly with holders of different worldviews who may not share these assumptions could be a good first step to move beyond the grip of a colonial ontology. By doing so, we could minimize the risk of epistemic violence and subtle modes of domination working through our understanding of reality at a fundamental level. (Malette, 2012: 381)

We started this chapter with a quote from Sebastien Malette, and here we return to his work with another quote. These quotes for us embody the perspectives we raise in this chapter, in relation to an invitation to the reader/researcher to carefully examine and critique worldviews, and the meanings we attribute to things, knowledge and research. In line with Malette's (2012) call to move beyond colonial ontologies, and in order to shift towards a postcolonial ethos, we highlight the importance of challenging the power one holds as a researcher in the fields of counselling, psychotherapy, and psychology. Malette (2012, p. 369) advocates disrupting modes of domination by freeing *ourselves from ourselves* and shifts us to openness to that *which has not always been, that it could be otherwise.* As researchers, we have tried to learn to let go of our individual, profound desires to control the course of (this duo-ethnographic) research. We have used our different disciplinary perspectives to challenge our ontological and epistemological assumptions, and to co-create our new common ground. And we have tried to reflect on how what we have learned in participating in this duoethnographic process relates to the way we have related to our research participants in the past, and how we might name and categorise our research 'participants' of the future in ways which evidence a process of 'power-with' participants rather than 'power-over' them.

3.1 Researcher Reflection Point 1

1. What could be the connections between these types of questions/concerns and the issue of how you decolonise your own research?
2. Could you begin/continue to decolonise your research by asking these types of questions about what both material and conceptual things 'are'?

With specific reference to decolonising research, we suggest that researchers might need to:

- Endeavour to avoid assuming what freedom (and de/colonisation) is.
- Explore the various ways in which decolonising research can be achieved, with what consequences, for whom.
- Keep open to the possible meanings of things, concepts, participants' responses, or worldviews.
- Be reflexive about the ways in which they keep their practices open.

Doing Arts-based Decolonising Research: Themes Emerging from our Duoethnography Process and Research Examples

While we claim the importance of seeing research as a relational and deeply reflexive process, we also note the, 'risk of personal/autobiographical accounts becoming self-absorbed, and self-indulgent [….] without offering fresh insight into the phenomenon of concern' (Finlay, 2020 p. 335). In the hope of being able to provide some fresh insight into decolonising research, we will provide some examples from our research in the sections of this chapter that follow. In doing this, rather than showing 'straightforward, unreflective absorption in the objects of experience', as cautioned against by Finlay (2020 p. 335), we attempt to go 'beyond the personal' perspectives and experiences of our research (Toombs, 1993 p. xii; Finlay, 2020). Our approach is in line with the view that duoethnography uncovers different subjectivities, generates new meanings, and creates 'hybrid identities' (Asher, 2007 p. 68) instead of 'binary opposites' (p. 3). Here, a 'hybrid identity' is formulated through our combining of applied linguistics and psychotherapy research, in order to create fresh insights into the objects of experience and in the hope of going beyond our individual experiences of research.

In direct reference to decolonial practice, and in an effort to 'unpack' the cultural underpinnings of their thinking about teaching for equity and diversity, Sawyer and Liggett (2012) use a duoethnography process to explore their own history and the curriculum of colonialism (as schoolteachers in the U.S.). They use personal photographs of themselves as children, a school report, and lesson plans they designed, to compare their lives, their educational histories, and some critical educational incidents; reflecting on issues of representation, self-reflexivity, and trustworthiness.

In response to engaging with our reading and dialogue about what we had read, RW stated:

> After reading their [Sawyer and Liggett's] account of their process and reflecting on their learning, I was left wanting to try and spend more of my time talking/writing about what I see/hear/sense around myself, and less time saying what I think it 'means'. More time on what exploring perspectives on what people think 'it' 'is'. To stay longer with 'things' and spend less time with reasons, more description and less analysis (including more acknowledgement that description = analysis).

> This is something that I have also thought about as a transcriber of spoken interaction for research that explored the construction of 'stories' elicited as part of a community project. As part of our data analysis, we tried to pay careful attention to how we translated our audio recordings into written documents, mindful that transcription constructs what the data 'is'.

The importance of lingering over description, and the equal importance of recognising that description is also analysis, resonated with both of us. In thinking about decolonised counselling and psychotherapy research, DC responded:

> Doing arts-based decolonising research values the different uses of 'things', of objects/art-i-facts or research encounters, to express the lived experience. That which we may term arts-based research differs in each research encounter, but perhaps the central/common themes are the researcher's approach to power, knowledge, and curiosity. That, for example,

the researcher uses questions, or an approach, which offer(s) opportunities for the participant to employ any form of art/way of being to illuminate the phenomena in question. This could be responses to questions such as: Who are you? What is your lived experience or worldview? What happened to/in you? (rather than: What is wrong with you?). Having an openness to different participant worldviews may take the research interview/encounter in a direction that was not preconceived....and indeed it may require time to stay longer with 'things', the research design/process or the analysis.

In engaging with the question of what doing arts-based decolonising research is, from our different perspectives, we observed the following three themes:

1. Beginnings—welcoming the participant and their narrative/experience.
2. Active engagement with the research dynamics that unfold thereafter (which we have called 'the real inner drama').
3. Endings—reflecting on what feelings researchers may experience in letting go of power and how they can search their own truth whilst maintaining an ethical stance throughout the process.
4. In addition, we focused on the importance of paying attention to the use of language and use of silence when engaging in research encounter/dialogue. Towards the end of this chapter, we also consider some of the consequences of cleaning and interpreting things, including research data.

To illuminate these themes, we offer examples from our practice and research.

Beginnings

The research, and the writing, process has to start somewhere. The following are examples of questions which helped us to begin the duoethnographic research we describe here:

- How do we want to approach this research?
- What are the questions we want to ask?
- How do we want to present our experience in a way that is useful to us, and which allows us to explore how our conceptualisation of our research experience is brought into being through dialogue.

We then discussed the importance of welcome in the research process, and here we ask you to reflect on and respond to the following questions.

3.2 Researcher Reflection Point 2

1. How do you welcome participants in your arts-based research?
2. How do you begin entering dialogue about the phenomena being researched?
3. How does your welcome communicate how you will use your power and how you will respect the participant's worldviews that may emerge?

In one example of our research on trauma, loss, grief, and growth in asylum seekers and refugees (Taylor et al., 2020), participants were invited to bring an artifact that they felt represented their lived experience, in order to begin a dialogue in a way that was the participant's choice. Examples included: a patchwork quilt, shoes, inspirational songs, poems, photographs, a dress, a Bible (that the participant had carried from her home country), a bag, and an African percussion instrument (Mbira). The researchers acknowledged that some participants might not bring a physical object, given that many of their narratives included having lost all things as a result of forced migration. In our own process, following a break in our work due to one of the authors being (DC) having been on sick leave, we attempted to re-begin our duoethnographic process, and RW said:

> I had been thinking of you…. I did not want to carry on with the project without you. I wanted to respect your thinking, and your life as it was happening, your illness and trauma at the time, in a situation in which you were trying to recover, it made me want to be careful and not rush… our project is interdisciplinary and that also made me want to be careful, and not to assume that we would agree with each other… also, I had very much enjoyed the process of working together and don't want it to end. I have learnt so much from our dialogue.

In psychotherapy/counselling research, and in psychotherapy encounters, the beginnings of the process set the tone of how, and whether, one can begin to share a narrative/experience. An experience of autonomy in the beginning creates facilitative and conducive conditions for a successful and rich encounter. In re-beginning our duoethnography, we tried to keep the process open by, firstly, not assuming that it had (re-)begun, and then by allowing the other to introduce resources of their choice: an academic discipline, a story about trauma, an opportunity to learn/teach, or nothing. This account of (our) beginnings is an example of our next theme, the importance of showing 'the real inner drama' of research.

The 'Real Inner Drama'

> In an attempt to assert objectivity and rationality, scientists often report their work through a simplified pattern of (1) problem, (2) literature review, (3) methodology, and so on. This pattern suggests that their ideas developed solely along such a linear time-line and involved an exclusively logical progression of events. Through such highly standardized reporting practices, scientists inadvertently hide from view the real inner drama of their work, with its intuitive base, its halting time-line, and its extensive recycling of concepts and perspectives. (Bargar & Duncan, 1982, p. 2)

In our acknowledgement of the disruptions and uncertainties in our research, we aim to avoid presenting a linear pattern that hides how our thinking and writing was brought into being, and that runs the risk of one of us over-powering/colonising the process of the other.

As part of our duoethnography dialogue in relation to power, one of us (DC) stated:

Rachel, I like what you said about how power and responsibility can become placed in the frame of reference of the participant. One participant I interviewed brought a pair of shoes. It felt clear to me that, although he had been extremely disempowered by the asylum-seeking process, at least in this interview, he was feeling he had the resources and power to share whatever he wanted about his experience, journey and trauma. He also shared how psychotherapy had made a positive impact on his trauma symptoms.

In the example of the research in which participants brought artifacts/objects (Taylor et al., 2020) there are several common themes. These include:

1. Participants commented on how they appreciated the opportunity to use creative methodologies such as art, photo elicitation, and objects, and to choose what resources they would bring (including none).
2. Arts-based decolonising research that acknowledged the disruptions and uncertainties that are part of the research process enabled 'power with' the participants, by giving them control about how, and how much, they shared about their experiences.

An excerpt from our dialogue reflects the dynamics of re-constructing the lived experiences of participants, in the 'inner drama' of the process. RW stated:

I was struck with the idea that the stories, which were created in dialogue with the objects and their owners, are a re-counted, a re-constructed, past—the only past we have.

DC responded:

Rachel what you said in relation to the use of artifacts and objects, responds beautifully to the Bargar and Duncan quote which we used earlier to highlight how researchers can 'inadvertently hide from view the real inner drama of their work'. In engaging with dialogue, arts, objects and artifacts, I could not hide behind the mask of being a researcher. I was faced with narratives of trauma, loss, death, and difference that refugees and asylum seekers face. I had to quietly reflect on my privilege and power as a person and as a researcher. I was fully present and was being so careful not to 'colonise' the process/participant through conveying a desire to get my research questions answered or to bring my own worldview/interpretation of what the object/artifact represented. Through dialogue with each participant and open questions such as 'what would you like to share with me about this object/photograph?... their use or introduction of each object, photograph, or artifact led to an open sharing of their presenting past... in the here and now of our research interview. This way of being resulted in interviews that interweaved narratives of trauma, and loss, but also hope, meaning and post traumatic growth.

In the next stage of our dialogue we continued to talk about how, when researchers need answers to questions they may be particularly likely assert 'objectivity' and 'rationality', and to lose sight of 'the real inner drama' of how answers are achieved through interaction between the researcher and the research participants. To illustrate some of the ways in which this happens, we discussed data from a recent study conducted by Wicaksono and Zhurauskaya (2020) that explored the telling of migration stories. The study reported the experience of working with a community group based in York, a small city of approximately 220,000 residents in which, according to the 2011 government census, 90.2 per cent of residents identify as 'White British'. The community group created a project together with fifteen participants who had been born outside of the UK and, at some point, moved to York.

The community group leaders worked with the project participants on a number of awareness-raising activities, and also interviewed each of the participants about their migration experiences. It was these fifteen, one-hour long, audio-recorded, interviews which provided the data for the study.

Here we present one extract from the transcripts of these fifteen audio recordings. The transcript is a way of making the audio recorded interviews accessible in written form, and a key to the symbols used is available at the end of this chapter. Transcribers decide which aspects of the data to try and represent in writing and which to ignore; these are analytical choices that effect the responses of subsequent readers of the research, as well as any next steps that the researcher may take and are similar to a 'data cleaning' process. What the researcher decides is unnecessary or unimportant in the data is 'cleaned' away and is no longer visible to the readers of the transcript. The extract we present here is the result of this process of selection, and we know that we are implicated in these choices about what to preserve and what to ignore/hide/clean away, and that our choices are invisible to our readers.

In the extract, that follows below, the interviewer is asking the interviewee questions about their 'values' and 'treasures', before moving on to a new topic. The extract begins with the interviewer summarising what they have already heard the interviewee say, before beginning, what the interviewee treats as, a question in line 6.

After two small pauses (.) and a hesitation sound 'er', the interviewer begins to summarise the interviewee's previous answers: in lines 1–4 (you treasure your dad, who you left behind) and 6–8 (you treasure the opportunities available in the UK). After each of these summaries, the interviewee says 'yeah' (in lines 5 and 9). A pause follows, in line 10, providing a moment in which either speaker could self-select to talk. It is the interviewer who speaks, again, in lines 11–12, offering a further question 'I mean is there anything else that you treasure about the UK then?'

Several different types of interviewer contributions can be observed in the extract. One example is in lines 11–12, when the interviewer has a second attempt at asking about 'treasures' in the UK, having received only a minimal, ambiguous, response to the suggestions that 'opportunities' are to be treasured. Another example is in lines 16–17, after the second attempt at 'treasures' is unsuccessful, when the interviewer rephrases the question by narrowing its scope, asking about York instead of the UK, and changing 'anything' (line 11) to 'something' (line 16). A further example can be seen in line 30, where what might be an attempt to help the interviewee to find the right word actually constrains their subsequent answer and helps to project the kind of information the interviewer appears to want to hear more about.

If we assume that, in research interviews, answers follow questions, the only possible answer to the question of what this interviewee treasures in the UK is the interaction in line 9, where they say 'yeah', in response to the interviewer's assumption that *opportunities* are what they treasure. Conceptualising the interviewing process as an art and as a way of thinking about the 'real' experiences of a research participant relies on an idea of meaning as held by individuals, rather than in interaction with each other (the interviewer contributes, even controls, given their 'right' to ask questions, to the answers) or in interaction with the research methods (answers follow questions).

This extract shows some of the ways in which a research project which uses interviews, or focus groups or questionnaires, can be seen to 'discover' what residents of York miss about the country of their birth: amongst other things, the opportunities that the UK provides to migrants and the music of the country in which they were born. A close look at the interaction, however, shows how the research method and the researcher are as much a part of the findings as the research participants, and cannot be separated from them. We noted that, in the transcript, what seemed like a rather 'leading' set of interview questions helped us to see how answers are always a result of questions, and how 'thematic' analysis of these answers risks tidying up the data to such an extent that the analysis can no longer claim to represent a 'discovery', except in the specific context of the interview.

Offering a decolonising approach requires an awareness of how the act of interviewing underpinned a complex relationship between: interviewer and interviewee; the researcher/researched and the research methods; and the researcher/researched/research methods and the material/social context in which the research takes place. Charura and Lago (2021) in their writing on decolonising psychotherapy and counselling research note the importance of researchers' reflections on their power, as well as how they can actively challenge unequal power relations with disadvantaged, marginalised groups and communities. They further note the importance of acknowledging multiple realities and knowledge bases of participants. Figure 3.1 shows how the 'findings' of research are inextricably linked to the research method, most obviously when there is 'power over' rather than 'power with' the participants. Where the 'real inner drama' of the research is cleaned away, and the opportunities provided by halting time-lines and silence are not recognised, findings become the projections of the powerful researcher, and not an acknowledged result of collaboration and interaction between all parties, the methods, and the context.

In our duoethnographic dialogues, we went on to discuss the typology of silence, the place of silence in research, and the importance of the researcher seeing silence as part of the interaction. We noted the illocutionary force of silence and the question we ask the reader when faced with silence in an interaction with a participant is: what kind of silence is presenting? How does the researcher engage with the silence? Given our argument here that silence is functioning, do you, as the researcher, need to use silence more?

3.3 Researcher Refection Point 3

1. How do you respond to the material your participants share in interviews?
2. How do you begin the transcription and analysis process?
4. How do you use silence and ensure you are not rushing to 'suggest themes'?
5. How do you engage with reflexivity and use your developing insights to address power and ensure a decolonised approach to your research?

IR: Interviewer
IE: Interviewee

```
01 IR: so you (.) er (.) when you describe [country] then
02 (.) obviously (1.0) the thing tha:t (.) you treasure
03 most is >obviously< your dad that you left behind
04 [the:re]
05 IE: [yeah]
06 IR: when you think of thi:s country then (2.0) am
07 I getting an inkling that you treasure the
08 opportunities
09 IE: yeah
10 (1.0)
11 IR: I mean is there anything else that you
12 treasure about the UK then
13 (.)
14 IE: ((lip-smack)).hh erm (2.0) ((lip-smack)) what
15 do I treasure about the UK?=
16 IR: =or even York perhaps (.) is there something
17 about living in York=
18 IE: =Yes (.) I actually (.) really love (.) living
19 in York now (.) again when I first came to York
20 I thou:ght it was one of the most bo:ring cities
21 ((laughter))
22 IE: a:nd=
23 IR: =so what age where you when you came to York
24 then
25 IE: I wa:s (.) round about (.) thirteen fourteen
26 IR: ok
27 IE: (.) yes a:nd (.) one of the first things that
28 you notice of somebody of colour erm (.) is
29 (.) of course=
30 IR: =a rarity
31 IE: yeah (.) [and]
32 IR: [yeah]
33 IE: here wasn't much hehe
34 IR: okay
35 IE: e:m (.) so: it was another (.) moment of (1.0)
36 ((sigh)) hh just (.) being kind of (.) on your
37 own again (.) you know (.) e:rm (.) a::nd (.)
38 >it was a struggle< but ((lip-smack)) I think
39 those experiences sort of made me
40 (1.0) e:rm (1.0) what's the word (1.0) stronger
41 in a lot of ways
42 IR: so, they give you character
43 IE: erm (0.5) it did
```

Fig. 3.1 Transcription example

In responding to these questions, we now invite you to consider endings in research. How can we avoid trying to hide ourselves and our thinking (because doing so presents us, the researcher, as 'objective' and our research participants as 'subjective'/ subjects who are 'discovered' by the researcher)? How can we describe our process in a way that avoids 'cleaning it all up'? How can we stay with the process as researchers, without rushing to findings and in a way that enables the research encounters to be opportunities to hear the voice of those with lived experience, whilst at the same time furthering the stimulus of our thinking?

Endings can mean a number of things, including ending the interview, debriefing, ending the analysis, ending a research project, and dissemination of findings. In the section that follows we discuss our final theme of 'endings'.

Endings

> The past in its historical actuality, is gone: the reconstructed, that is, recounted past, the interpreted past, is all we have [....] That is, out of ongoing growth and integration of life experiences, individuals progressively create the found world [...] We create the world we live in by the lived interpretation we make about ourselves and about others. (Gargiulo, 2016 p. 14)

We start this section on 'endings' with a quote from Gargiulo's work on quantum psychoanalysis. His reminder that the reconstructed, recounted, interpreted past is all we have encouraged us to renew our commitment to the value of relational, decolonised research. If we believe that, in counselling and psychotherapy practice and in research, the participants are equal knowledge generating partners, and that their conceptualisations of what things matter, then our approach/research design should show (not hide) this.

In relation to endings, our dialogue focused on the importance of letting go, searching for our own truths, and continually being ethical in our research practice. DC stated:

> From our discussions last time we met, I drew the conclusion that if we insist on what we think things/or objects are, or if we rush to conclude or interpret what we think the meaning of the participant's lived experience is, we risk unethical practice and colonizing the other! That is because we will miss their experience or cultural perspective. I am also reminded of our contemporary understanding of quantum models that see the micro world as a 'mist of infinite possibilities', and 'a jittery foam of probabilities' (Gargiulo, 2016; Wheeler et al., 1973). This could be synonymous with the idea that we have repeatedly ended up with; that the things/artefacts or narratives and the experiences of participants we engage with, have multiple possibilities of meaning.

In the same discussion on the importance of letting go, searching for our own truths, and continually being ethical in our research practice. RW, responded, stating:

> We risk misunderstanding the other and devaluing their perspectives if we take the view that 'I know what it is!'. Stories are also things! We should try to be open to different uses of things. As we have agreed, we can perhaps begin to approach knowing what things are for others through curiosity and listening, and through giving space for others to name things from their frame of reference. In terms of endings, perhaps all we have is that 'mist of infinite possibilities'!

We noted the importance of referring back to the ethical guidelines of our professional body/institution. In relation to endings, the British Psychological Society [BPS] (2021) Code of Human Research Ethics states that when the research data is completed, 'It is important to provide an appropriate debriefing for participants' (p.26). The Code acknowledges that some participants may choose not to take up the offer of debriefing, but states that it should be offered when appropriate. We agree that giving research participants the space to have the last word is one way to increase the possibilities of the research, to open up the closing down stages of a project, and to keep the inner drama out in the open.

3.4   Researcher Refection Point 4

1. As a researcher committed to decolonised ethical research, how will you now approach your arts-based research, design, and analysis?
2. How will you respond to the material/objects (internal/physical artifacts) that participants share through the research process?

We conclude this chapter with some points of reflection on objects/subjects and how the creation of these can be related to a colonising process of fixing meaning as a way of getting power over things (objects, people, data, etc.). We aim to show our learning from our duoethnographic process, and the insights that have transformed us and our practice as decolonising researchers. We re-iterate the benefits of remaining curious, of not assuming knowledge of things, of engaging in dialogue, and the importance of watchful waiting/not rushing the encounter/participant in order to chase themes. We assert as researchers that it is important to:

1. Reflect on the work of beginnings, the real inner drama, and endings, in arts-based, decolonising research.
2. Reflect on the perspective that research participants are not *only* 'themselves', and don't *only* exist in relation to each other and with the researcher, but that they also 'intra-act' with material things that they may bring to the research context, as well as with the tools/methods of the research, including inorganic objects (such as a recording device) and technologies (such as a transcription code).
3. Pay attention to the potential relationships between research and the process of othering/division in the selection and description/categorisation of 'participants'. We can get power over participants when we position them as 'our participants', even when we are engaged in work that aims to re-dress this balance of power in their favour.
4. Take account not only of our relationships with participants, but also of the political, social, economic context of the research in which these colonising dynamics of power take place.
5. Avoid claiming knowledge about what others 'are' and avoid using naming practices that are not relevant or welcomed by the participants.

6. Consider cultural factors/humility when designing research, in the selection/ translation of instruments/toolkits/resources or artifacts, as well as in data analysis and interpretation of data.
7. Engage with literature that uses theory and reports research which demonstrates a decolonised, culturally sensitive/informed approach. Critique literature or practice that does not.
8. Notice when your question or reflection, in response to what your participant is saying, has narrowed the flow of the dialogue, or shifted the power dynamic negatively. Consider following up with a more general question such as 'I noticed you seem to have paused/held back, is there something else you want to say?' or 'Do you have some more comments in response to what I have asked/reflected?'
9. If the participant does not respond within a few seconds of a question, it is worth letting the silence be. Silences have different meanings for people and respecting pauses can allow time for the participant and researcher to reflect or to think of more detailed answers.
10. Question and reflect on your power as a researcher. This can be in relation to critiquing the dominance of Eurocentric perspectives that exclude the multiple realities and knowledge bases of your participants. It can also be in relation to challenging unequal power relations with disadvantaged, marginalised groups and communities.
11. Research is a site of creative struggle, of innovation and destruction, and a mist of infinite possibilities. We can demonstrate the delicate mechanisms through which this struggle takes place by paying attention to the effects of repetition, silence, overlap, and so on.
12. In designing research, we need to pay attention to, and include in our analysis: pre- and post-data collection talk with participants; moments of sampling, recruitment, and consent; the preparation of, and adjustments to, data collection instruments 'in the moment' of their use.

We concur with Marshall and Rossman (1999) who argue that researchers should try to be sensitive to the need for change and flexibility as it emerges in their research encounters. Although we had to finish the construction of this chapter in order to meet our deadline, we tried not to rush to the closing down of the process. And we expect to continue to develop, craft, and further refine what has yet to emerge in our writing.

Summary

We have found it useful to think about what things 'are' in de-colonising research; partly because this ontological thinking emphasises that the beginning of our research journey, the drama we experienced and the decisions we made along the way, and our reasons for finishing, are all part of a mist of infinite possibilities. Our research (methods) was/were not inevitable, but emerged in dialogue, and in a range of changing contexts. We have tried to show how the incorporation, through detailed exploration, of obstacles has been part of our own research experience. And we have tried to remain open to the multiple meanings of our dialogue, ourselves, and of each other. We are aware that there is much more work to do.

References

American Art Therapy Association. (2018). *About art therapy.* Accessed May 10, 2022, from https://arttherapy.org/about-art-therapy/

Asher, N. (2007). Made in the (multicultural) U.S.A.: Unpacking tensions of race, culture, gender, and sexuality in education. *Educational Researcher, 36*(2), 65–74.

Barad, K. (2007). *Meeting the universe halfway: Quantum physics and the entanglement of matter and meaning.* Duke University Press.

Bargar, R.R. & Duncan, J.K. (1982). Cultivating creative endeavor in doctoral research. *The Journal of Higher Education, 53*(1), 1–31.

Breault, R. A. (2016). Emerging issues in duoethnography. *International Journal of Qualitative Studies in Education, 6,* 777.

British Psychological Society. (2021). *Code of human research ethics.* Leicester.

Charura, D., & Allan J. (2017). Spiritual development, meaning-making, resilience and potential for post-traumatic growth among asylum-seekers and refugees: An interpretative phenomenological analysis. In *Qualitative methods in psychology (QMiP) conference, Aberystwyth University, Aberystwyth, Wales,* 5–7 July 2017.

Charura, D., & Lago, C. (2021). Towards a decolonised psychotherapy research and practice. In D. Charura & C. Lago (Eds.), *Black identities and white therapies: Race, respect and diversity.* PCCS Books.

Finlay, L. (2020). COVID-19 took my breath away: A personal narrative. *The Humanistic Psychologist, 48*(4), 321–339. https://doi.org/10.1037/hum0000200

Gargiulo, G. J. (2016). *Quantum Psychoanalysis: Essays on Physics, Mind, and Analysis Today.* International Psychoanalytic Books.

Grix, J. (2001). *De-mystifying postgraduate research: From MA to PhD.* University of Birmingham Press.

Jaworski, G., Mountain, C., Coan, S., Charura, D., & Fransman, K. (2020). *Home truths: Housing experiences of UK migrants.* PsyCen.

Malette, S. (2012). De-colonizing Foucault's historical ontology: Toward a postcolonial ethos. *Postcolonial Studies, 15*(3), 369–387.

Marshall, C., & Rossman, G. B. (1999). The "what of the study": Building the conceptual framework. In C. Marshall & G. B. Rossman (Eds.), *Designing qualitative research* (3rd ed., pp. 21–54). Sage Publications.

Norris, J., & Sawyer, R. D. (2012). Toward a dialogic methodology. In J. Norris, R. D. Sawyer, & D. Lund (Eds.), *Duoethnography: Dialogic methods for social, health and educational research* (pp. 9–40). Left Coast Press.

Pring, R. (2004). *Philosophy of educational research* (2nd ed.). Continuum.

Regev, D., & Cohen-Yatziv, L. (2018). Effectiveness of art therapy with adult clients in 2018—what progress has been made? *Frontiers in Psychology, 9.* https://doi.org/10.3389/fpsyg.2018.01531

Sawyer, R. D., & Liggett, T. (2012). Shifting positionalities: A critical discussion of a duoethnographic inquiry of a personal curriculum of post-colonialism. *International Journal of Qualitative Methods, 11*(5), 628–651.

Taylor, S., Charura, D., Williams, G., Shaw, M., Allan, J., Cohen, E., Meth, F., & O'Dwyer, L. (2020). Loss, grief, and growth: An interpretative phenomenological analysis of experiences of trauma in asylum seekers and refugees. *Traumatology.* Advance online publication. https://doi.org/10.1037/trm0000250

Toombs, S. K. (1993). *The meaning of illness: A phenomenological account of the different perspectives of physician and patient*. Kluwer Academic.

Wheeler, J., et al. (1973). *Gravitation*. McMillan.

Wicaksono, R., & Hall, C. J. (2020). Using ontologies of English. In C. J. Hall & R. Wicaksono (Eds.), *Ontologies of English: Conceptualising the language for learning, teaching, and assessment* (pp. 368–376). Cambridge University Press.

Wicaksono, R., & Zhurauskaya, D. (2020). *York's hidden stories: Interviews in applied linguistics*. Palgrave Macmillan UK.

Further Reading

Charura, D., & Lago, C. (Eds.). (2021). *Black identities and white therapies: Race, respect and diversity*. PCCS Books.

Kara, H. (2015). *Creative research methods in the social sciences: A practical guide*. Policy Press.

Wicaksono, R., & Zhurauskaya, D. (2020). *York's hidden stories. Interviews in applied linguistics*. Palgrave Macmillan.

Chapter 4
Supporting Critical Self-enquiry: Doing Heuristic Research

Keith Tudor

> There is no more urgent topic to research than the human realm
> of experience, action, and expression, especially the significant
> and exciting life events and the extraordinary experiences these
> can entail.
> —(Hiles, 2001, p. 1)

> [T]here is a terra incognita that may be far more available for
> human inquiry than any of these [external] places. This final
> frontier, I propose, is the interiority of our experience, where
> feeling, which may previously not have been noticed as
> significant, is not just a core component of the terrain but the
> dominant one.
> —(Sela-Smith, 2002, p. 54)

Introduction

Requiring disciplined and critical self-reflection and engagement in a process of discovery—of self and others—heuristic research is, arguably, the method of psychological research closest to the practice of therapy (a referent for all forms of psychological therapies). Indeed, Moustakas (1990) himself applies heuristic methodology to psychotherapy, and Merry (2004) does so with regard to supervision. Drawing on the pioneering work of Moustakas (1967, 1990) as well as other heuristic researchers, notably Sela-Smith (2002), this chapter summarises the key concepts of the heuristic method with illustrations from the literature, my own heuristic

K. Tudor (✉)
Auckland University of Technology, Auckland, New Zealand
e-mail: keith.tudor@aut.ac.nz

© The Author(s), under exclusive license to Springer Nature
Switzerland AG 2022
S. Bager-Charleson, A. McBeath (eds.), *Supporting Research in Counselling
and Psychotherapy*, https://doi.org/10.1007/978-3-031-13942-0_4

research, and some of the research students with whom I've worked. Written in a direct style, this chapter discusses key concepts of heurism which acknowledge its methodology and philosophical roots, and takes you (the reader/student/researcher) through the various stages or processes of heuristic research. In doing so, I offer some pauses and points for reflection, as well as some experiential activities designed to stimulate your identification and engagement with possible areas of enquiry and research, and three key issues with regard to heuristic research. Finally, in writing about doing heuristic research, I also hope to dispel some myths about heurism and this method of research and research methodology.

Ancestors of the Mind: Clark Moustakas and Sandy Sela-Smith

> There is no theory that is not a fragment, carefully prepared, of some autobiography.
> (Valéry, 1957)

For a long time, I have been interested in the autobiographical nature of theory, and of research, or, at least, the—or an—interest in a specific area of research. This is certainly true of Clark Moustakas (1923–2012), the founder of heuristic research, so this is where we're going to begin.

Clark Moustakas was an educational and clinical psychologist, whose publication, *The Self: Explorations in personal growth* in 1956, helped forge the humanistic psychology movement. As a result of a personal, family crisis, Moustakas went through a period of great loneliness, about which he subsequently wrote a book titled *Loneliness* (Moustakas, 1961). Reflecting on this experience, and the process of the experience, led to him defining and refining heuristics—from the Greek εὑρίσκειν, meaning to find, to find out, to discover—as a method of research (Douglass & Moustakas, 1985; Moustakas, 1967, 1990, 1994, 2000). Moustakas was an integral part of the humanistic psychology movement, helping to establish the American Association for Humanistic Psychology in 1961 (from 1963, the Association for Humanistic Psychology) and the *Journal of Humanistic Psychology*, which he edited for a time. Heuristic research was influenced by humanistic psychology, as Moustakas himself acknowledged (see Box 4.1).

Box 4.1   Influences of Humanistic Psychology on Heuristic Research

- Regarding delineations of subjective–objective truth (Bridgman, 1950).
- Regarding self-actualising persons (Maslow, 1956, 1966, 1971).
- Regarding explorations of dialogue and mutuality (Buber, 1958, 1961, 1965).
- Regarding the analysis of the meaning of experience (Gendlin, 1978).
- Regarding indwelling and personal knowledge (Polanyi, 1962), and the tacit dimension of knowing (Polanyi, 1964, 1966, 1969).
- Regarding self-disclosure (Jourard, 1968, 1971).
- Regarding human science (Rogers', 1969, 1985).

After Moustakas, the key person in the field of heuristic research is Sandy Sela-Smith (1944–2021) who was a teacher and counsellor before returning to study at the age of 51, graduating from Saybrook Graduate School, San Francisco, California, where she subsequently joined the faculty as an adjunct professor. Her own heuristic self-study encompassed childhood sexual abuse (Sela-Smith, 1998), transition, transformation, and heuristic theory itself (Sela-Smith, 2001), which doctoral research led to a clarification of Moustakas' method. As she puts it: 'Moustakas's research focus shifted from the self's *experience of the experience* to focusing on the *idea of the experience*' (Sela-Smith, 2002, p. 53; my emphasis), a shift that she attributes to Moustakas' own resistance to experiencing unbearable pain. Based on her re-reading of Moustakas and the experience of her own heuristic self-inquiry, Sela-Smith (2002) identifies six components in heuristic research, that is, self-experience, inward reach (for tacit awareness and knowledge), surrender, self-dialogue, self-search, and transformation. Using these components as factors, she then conducted a review of 28 research documents whose authors claimed to have followed Moustakas' research method, of which she considered only three to have fulfilled the method successfully (further details of which I discuss later in this chapter). Stimulated by this discrepancy, Sela-Smith then took another look at Moustakas' (1990) book and discovered what she describes as an ambivalence in his method, with regard:

- To the study of external situations, rather than the self.
- To the inclusion of co-participants as a distraction from the internal process of the researcher (see below, pp. **xx-yy**).
- To a confusion of language which is epitomised in the shift from the use of the word experience as a noun that is connected to observations, rather than experience as a verb that is connected to the internal self-search.
- To the observation of experience of self and others, rather than experience and self-search.

As a result of this, Sela-Smith clarifies her approach to heuristic research as "heuristic self-search inquiry" (HSSI), the implications of which I discuss throughout the chapter.

So, having introduced the parents—by now, grandparents—of heuristic research, I turn to considering methodology and method, key aspects of research that all researchers need to address, and many confuse and/or conflate (examples of which I also note in the chapter and in Table 4.1).

Heuristic Methodology

Heuristic research is generally viewed as drawing on a number of philosophical and psychological traditions, specifically heuristics, existentialism, and phenomenology, and humanistic and experiential psychology. Different researchers and authors emphasise different traditions (as may be seen in Table 4.1). For an example of how

Table 4.1 Heuristic research studies: methodologies and methods

Author(s)	Research subject	Methodology	Method
Shantall (1999)	The experience of meaning amongst holocaust survivors	Not discussed	Heuristic inquiry
Sela-Smith (2001)	Subjectivity, knowledge, and heuristic research	Experiential, autobiographical, narrative	Heuristic self-search inquiry (HSSI)
Atkins and Loewenthal (2004)	Lived experiences of psychotherapists working with older clients	Not discussed	Heuristic (based on Moustakas', 1990, six phases)
Ferendo (2004)	Ken Wilber and personal transformation	Heuristic hermeneutic, transpersonal psychology	Heuristic hermeneutic HSSI
Casterline (2006)	The experience of the act of praying	Heuristic, phenomenological	Heuristic (based on Moustakas' six phases)
Meents (2006)	Intuition	HSSI (based on Ferendo, 2004; Sela-Smith, 2001; and Wilber's work)	HSSI
Djuraskovic and Arthur (2010)	Acculturation and identity construction	Heuristic	Heuristic
Tudor (2010, 2017)	The fight for health	Heuristics, phenomenology	Heuristic *enquiry*
Grennell (2014)	Being Māori and Pākehā (cultural hybridity)	Kaupapa (Māori) research theory (K[M]RT), phenomenology	Heuristic (in terms of Moustakas' six phases)
Haertl (2014)	The power of the written word	Phenomenology (Husserl, 1919/1983; Moustakas, 1994)	Heuristic inquiry (using Douglass & Moustakas', 1985 three-phase approach)
Schulz (2015)	Existential psychotherapy	Constructionism, phenomenology	Heuristic inquiry and case study
Wiorkowski (2015)	The experiences of students with autism spectrum disorders	Heuristic (not elaborated)	Heuristic (not elaborated)
Hammond (2016)	Therapists' experience of working with shame	Heuristic (defined in terms of Moustakas' (1990) concepts	Heuristic (elaborated in terms of Moustakas' six phases)
Alleyne, 2017	A psychotherapist's experience of grief	Heuristic, based on phenomenology	HSSI
Ozertugnul (2015, 2017b)	Obsessive compulsive disorder	Holistic	HSSI
Kumar (2017)	Healing through writing a dissertation	Unclear	Heuristic
Harrison (2018)	Physical activity and psychotherapy	Heuristic, based on phenomenology	Heuristic (elaborated in terms of Moustakas' six phases)

(continued)

Table 4.1 (continued)

Author(s)	Research subject	Methodology	Method
Yeh (2018)	Leadership practices of female faculty in higher education	Heuristic (phenomenological) (not elaborated)	Heuristic (not elaborated)
Sherwood (2019)	Psychological infanticide	Heuristic inquiry	Heuristic inquiry, imaginal psychology, and transformational writing
Shelburne et al. (2020)	Problematic eating	Heuristic (not elaborated)	Heuristic (not elaborated)
Williams (2020)	The experience of people of colour engaging in an asynchronous, smartphone application	Qualitative, imaginative, creative (not specified), heuristic	Heuristic (from case study)
Chue (2021)	Abrupt endings	Heuristic (not elaborated)	HSSI
Ciurlionis (2021)	Humour in psychotherapy	Phenomenology, heuristic	Heuristic (not elaborated)
Lyons (2021)	Ambivalence in psychotherapy	Heuristic	HSSI (elaborated in terms of Moustakas' six phases)

different qualitative approaches can be negotiated, see the chapter in this book by Frost et al. (2022). The issue here is not about who's right and who's wrong but, rather, what traditions you as a researcher draw on and what connections you make between your heuristic research, including the methods you're employing or considering employing, and the underlying methodology or methodologies on which they rest. Thus, some people claim that heuristics are both a methodology and a method and, indeed, this has a long and honourable history (see Hertwig & Panchur, 2015).

Describing heuristics as a conceptual framework, Douglass and Moustakas (1985) describe its objective as one of discovery—of "the nature of problem or phenomenon *as it exists in human experience*" (p. 42; my emphasis). They follow this by stating that: "This orientation makes palpable a theoretical marriage of existential philosophy and perceptual psychology" (p. 42).

Later, Moustakas (1990) distinguishes heuristics from phenomenology:

> Whereas phenomenology encourages a kind of detachment from the phenomenon being investigated, heuristics emphasizes connectedness and relationship … phenomenology loses the persons in the process of descriptive analysis, in heuristics the research participants remain visible.… Phenomenology ends with the essence of experience; heuristics retains the essence of the person in experience. (p. 43)

For further discussion of the differences between phenomenology and heuristic enquiry, see Patton (2002). Ozertugrul (2017a) also puts this well: "Contrary to phenomenological inquiry, heuristic research does not involve definitive descriptions or universal structures; rather, it entails depictions of the felt and thought experience of an individual" (p. 240).

From this we can see that the philosophical and psychological traditions on which Moustakas draws are more experiential (see Box 4.1).

However, as I note above, Sela-Smith (2002) criticises Moustakas (1990) for confusing this issue by promoting (in the later chapters of the same book) a more phenomenological focus and, therefore, inquiry. Moreover, in their original article, Douglass and Moustakas (1985) state that *"heuristics offers an attitude with which to approach research, but does not prescribe a methodology"* (p. 42; my emphasis). This statement represents possibly the most important and radical contribution of heuristic research, one that challenges you, the researcher, to discover your methodology.

In his work, Moustakas (1990) identifies a number of key concepts or processes, which I think of as offering portals to his—and/or your—philosophy, that is, identifying with the focus of inquiry; self-dialogue; tacit knowing; intuition; indwelling; focusing; and the internal frame of reference.

Activity 4.1

1. Read what Moustakas (1990) and Sela-Smith (2002) write about these concepts.
2. Read what other authors have to say about these and how they have applied them in their thinking about heuristics and other methodologies.
3. As you read this section, reflect on what these concepts mean to you.

Here, I offer some thoughts about these and pointers for further reading.

Identifying with the Focus of Enquiry

As Moustakas (1990) puts it:

Heuristic inquiry is a process that begins with a question or problem which the researcher seeks to illuminate or answer. The question is one that has been a personal challenge and puzzlement in the search to understand one's self and the world in which one lives. (p. 15)

This is crucial to any understanding of heuristic research: it's personal and subjective, even if your data is a text or involves co-researchers/participants. If you're struggling to find a question, problem, or topic, try the following exercise.

Activity 4.2   Identifying with the Focus of Enquiry

Write a stream of consciousness.

I did this some years ago and wrote the following:

1955 Born and raised in Leamington Spa, the Midlands (of England) • Midland Oak • Keith, name, family, extended family • Unitarianism • Warwickshire, Shakespeare • 1965 Sheffield, Sheffield Wednesday, Steel City, Socialist Republic of South Yorkshire • 1969 Burford, upset, school, sport, Maggie • 1973 Oxford, philosophy and theology, theatre, prison seminars • 1976 temporary probation office, radicalised • 1977 University of Kent at Canterbury, radical social work • friendships • 1979 London (Hammersmith, Shepherd's Bush), unemployed, community and political activism • Big Flame • 1981 collective house I, youth counsellor, personal therapy • 1983 collective house II, group therapy • training, Gestalt • Sue • 1985 Italy (Montercorice, Milano), lo straniero • 1987 London, psychiatric social worker, 1988 Louise • 1990 training position with Louise • 1992 Move to Sheffield ...

Reflecting on this then, I discovered and identified a focus on friendships, love, and loss—which could constitute the focus of a heuristic research enquiry.

Doing this exercise again as I was writing this chapter, I wrote:

Here I stand. Where I stand ... Kei te whenua o Te Kawerau a Maki taku kāinga nainei | My house stands on the lands of Te Kawerau a Maki [the local iwi or tribe in West Auckland]. What is my standing? What is my understanding. What is under my standing? Leaves. Soil. Rock. Mountain. Sea....

Reflecting on this now takes me to a sense of ground and place, belonging and not belonging, knowing and not knowing—and uncertainty—and would constitute another and a different heuristic research enquiry.

From this perspective, I would say that the heuristic researcher needs to have experienced what they are researching. Douglass and Moustakas (1985) write about heuristics as "a passionate and discerning personal involvement in problem solving, an effort to know the essence of some aspect of life through the internal pathways of the self" (p. 39); and Sela-Smith (2002) suggests that there is—and needs to be— some "intense or passionate concern that causes the investigator to reach inward" (p. 69).

As people who are educated/trained to reflect, therapists are in a good position to identify subjects of personal enquiry. My own heuristic doctoral research was into mental health which I framed as "The fight for health" (Tudor, 2010, 2017), a phrase which my examiners picked up on and asked me to self-search further in my subsequent required amendments to my thesis (see Tudor, 2017). Subsequently, the heuristic research I have had the good fortune to supervise includes cultural and personal identity (Grennell, 2014; Grennell-Hawke & Tudor, 2018; Hill, 2022); therapists' experience of working with shame (Hammond, 2016); a psychotherapist's experience of grief (Alleyne, 2017); a psychotherapist's experience of exercise (Harrison,

2018; Harrison & Tudor, 2020); psychological infanticide (Sherwood, 2019); ambivalence in psychotherapy (Lyons, 2021); humour in psychotherapy (Ciurlionis, 2021); abrupt endings (Chue, 2021); and racial microaggressions (McCann, 2022; McCann & Tudor, 2022)—all of which represent quite a range of enquiry.

Self-dialogue

> In addition to the significance of becoming one with what one is seeking to know, one may enter into dialogue with the phenomenon, allowing the phenomenon to speak directly to one's own experience, to be questioned by it. In this way, one is able to encounter and examine it, to engage in a rhythmic flow with it—back and forth, again and again—until one has uncovered its multiple meanings. (Moustakas, 1990, p. 16)

For Sela-Smith (2002) one of the components intrinsic to heuristic inquiry is that "Self-dialogue, [is] not simply a one-way reporting of thoughts or feelings, is evidenced. To report a feeling is not the same as dialoguing with the feeling" (p. 69). In his research, Ozertugrul (2017b) embodies this in real-time self-to-self conversations in which he was both "I–Researcher" and "I–Participant", explaining that "My goal in using self-dialogue in this context was to add to the existing research in terms of what really takes place inside the mind, and how that relates to the world outside" (p. 218). He also links this to methodology and, specifically, ontology and epistemology when he states that "I used dialectics because it is inherent in the self's experience; the self wants to make sense of experience through the array of voices that exist within, including epistemic role playing" (p. 218).

Many students who undertake heuristic research keep some form of diary or journal and, whilst this can be useful as an account of experiences, and a place for noting reflections on the subject of enquiry, and the process of the research, Ozertugrul's creative practice offers a good reminder of the importance of self-*dialogue* as well as a practical example of how to do it. For therapists, such dialogue is—or should be—familiar, and, more broadly, is one of the reasons that the concepts and language of heuristic enquiry are similar to those from and in the theory and practice of therapy, especially, as Hiles (2001) points out, with regard to the use of the self: "In essence, [heuristic enquiry] is a research process designed for the exploration and interpretation of experience, which uses the self of the researcher." In my own research, I linked this concept and process to reflexivity, that is, *critical* self-reflection (Tudor, 2010, 2017), and hence the critical in the title of this chapter.

Heuristic research is not an excuse for self-centred, self-indulgent, individualistic reverie, with some resulting personal reflections that the researcher feels should be published. It is disciplined process of honest and courageous self-searching, which requires authentic dialogue not only with oneself (one's self) but also with others—from the "I–Researcher" to supervisors, therapists, co-participants, or co-enquirers, including imaginal ones (see Sherwood, 2019, 2021), to partners, family, and friends. As such, it is not for the faint-hearted. I have had students who chose heuristics because they thought it was easy, and then, when they experienced what was required, wished they hadn't; others who chose it quite intentionally but kept it "light"—who, in Sela-Smith's terms, were not prepared or willing to search and re-search their resistance; and others who worked thoroughly and courageously (and often didn't want to stop!) and who produced a creative synthesis of their self-enquiry that offers a contribution to others.

Tacit Knowing

According to Polanyi (1969), "While tacit knowledge can be possessed by itself, explicit knowledge must rely on being tacitly understood and applied. Hence all knowledge is *either tacit or rooted in tacit knowledge*" (p. 144). Moustakas (1990) himself and others since have considered this to be at the heart of heuristics and its epistemology: "underlying all other concepts in heuristic research, at the base of all heuristic discovery, is the power of revelation in tacit knowing" (Moustakas, 1990, p. 20). Chue (2021) describes it as an "interior terrain":

> This is the interior terrain I have been sent to venture: the rock formations, caves, stalactites and stalagmites. They are built out of each moment I have experienced, adding layer upon layer, to form the whole. This is the foundation of my "physical" inner world, the source of my being and meaning making. It is an ever-present terrain that is ineffable. (p. 14)

How you get at this unknown known varies. Chue did it through music; as far as my own doctoral study was concerned, I did it mostly through poetry (see Tudor, 2017). I have also done it through painting (see Exercise #2).

Activity 4.3 Tacit Knowing
Draw or paint a picture.

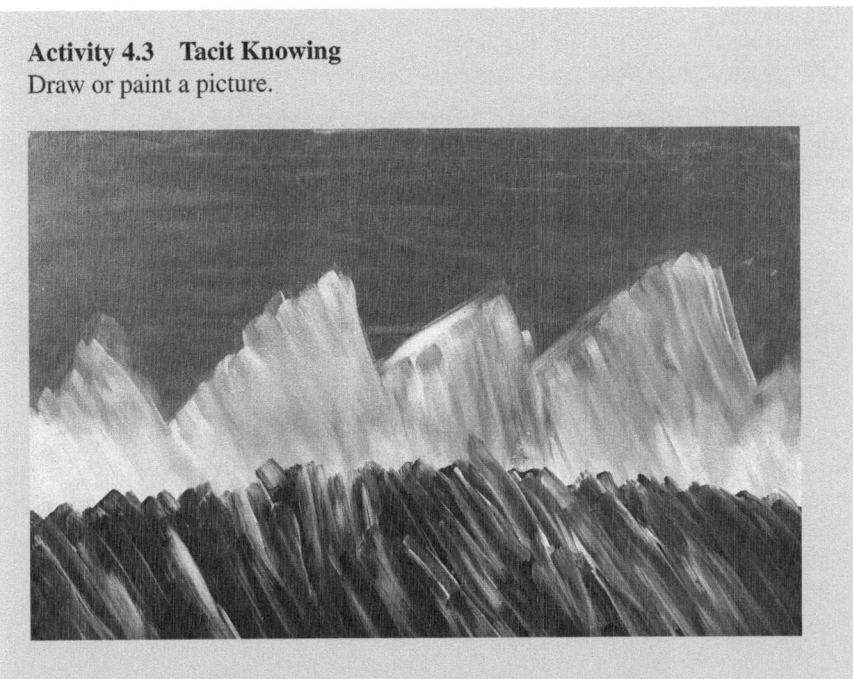

Stand back. Reflect on the experience of doing this. Give it a title.

Moustakas makes a link between tacit knowing and the immersion phase of heuristic research which he describes as "timeless" (p. 51) and guided by "intuitive clues or hunches … [and] knowledge … [that exists] within the tacit dimension" (p. 28). This, of course, raises the question of whether you can undertake heuristic in the context of a time limit such as that imposed by academic study and/or having to meet a specific deadline such as that of an examination or publication. There is no easy answer to this: some heuristic researchers consider any deadline as antithetical to having the time to explore and mine the tacit dimension, and, similarly, to allow for full immersion; others argue that, as we are all subject to time limits, this is simply another factor of which we need to take account. In this sense, this is parallel to discussions in therapy about the reality of time limits (see Strasser with Strasser, 2022; Taft, 1933/1973). Either way, I suggest that the heuristic researcher embraces the challenge of such limit(ation)s on their experience and enquiry, and addresses it in their writing.

Intuition

For Moustakas (1990), intuition is "a kind of bridge … between the implicit knowledge inherent in the tacit and the explicit knowledge which is observable and describable. [It] is the realm of the between, or the intuitive" (p. 23). My own example of this began with a poem I had written some years ago (in 2005), which I originally called "Contentment":

> Said slowly
> Contentment
> Harbours its own promise.

Whilst I quite liked this short poem, I knew that it wasn't quite right as I saved it in a file marked "Poems—In progress". Then, some five years later, towards the end of my doctoral journey, one morning while having a shower, a second verse came to me, which I added to the first, thus:

> **Contentment, and**
> Said slowly
> Contentment
> Harbours its promise.
> In turn, the harbour contains
> Its own promise of ebb, flow, and storm:
> Of rocking boats, and upsetting contents.

As I wrote later:

> To me, this speaks of necessary balance: content(ment) with discontent and, more broadly, of health and illness, of parts and wholes, of single-mindedness and group-mindedness. As Moustakas (1990) reflected: "Intuition makes possible the perceiving of things as wholes." (p. 23) (Tudor, 2017, p.165)

Hammond (2016) makes the important point that the heuristic researcher needs to value intuition and that this in itself may require something of a personal and even therapeutic journey; and, in doing so, she shares something of her own experience growing up in her family of origin of learning to override her intuition in favour of adhering to the family rules, and of relearning this as a therapist to trust her intuition.

For Sela-Smith (2002), intuition rather than formal techniques determines the steps taken in each stage or phase of heuristic research, which is another reason why these concepts, and, more generally, methodology, inform and guide the method, and, therefore, should be studied, understood, and elaborated *before* the method.

Indwelling

This concept is used by Moustakas to refer to the heuristic process of "turning inward to seek a deeper, more extended comprehension of the nature or meaning of a quality or theme of human experience" (p. 24). He continues: "It involves a willingness to gaze with unwavering attention and concentration into some facet of human experience in order to understand its constituent qualities and wholeness" (p. 24). For most of us this requires considerable discipline. In her reflections on this aspect of her heuristic process (in a diary entry), Grennell (2014) puts this well:

> I notice that I find it difficult to settle to being in a reflective mode and that the discipline required to do that is hard to grasp. It reminds me of meditating in a class years ago and how I was massively resistant as being in my body was too scary …. I still find resistance to that level of quiet and am much more comfortable in my intellect and intuition. Interesting that the method chosen for the ease it may bring is one where I am required to face in to not only my cultural identity and how that sits … but also into being quiet, allowing space and time, rather than busying myself into life. (23/01/14; original emphasis)

I love the word and concept of indwelling, with its associations of home and the sense of (the act of) residing. For some, part of the discipline of heuristics is knowing when to continue to dwell and when, as it were, to leave home. Lyons (2021) captures this well when she links this to the subject of her enquiry, that of ambivalence:

> Indwelling: I consciously lingered with the aspects of ambivalence that resonated with me, noticing what appeared in my thoughts and feelings as well as what was not there. I searched for the conditions that evoked my ambivalence and deliberately noticed its different qualities and textures—tentativeness, conflict, wobbliness and indecision. (pp. 16–17)

Focusing

In presenting this as one of the key concepts of heuristic research, Moustakas (1990) acknowledges the influence of Gendlin (1978) on the heuristic process of focusing which involves:

1. Clearing an inner space in order to tap into thoughts and feelings;
2. Getting a handle on the question;
3. Elucidating its constituents;
4. Making contact with core themes; and
5. Explicating the themes.

In the therapeutic context, it refers to the creation of inner space and the encouragement of sustained inner attention to ascertain one's thoughts and feelings. In the research context, Douglass and Moustakas (1985) write about focusing as: "a process of identifying themes and assessing connected feelings, ... [through which] a 'cognitive bodily' imaginative variation gradually unfolds and moves to refinements of meaning and perception that register as internal shifts and alterations of behavior" (p. 51). They also make the point that, together, focusing and differentiating—which they describe as "sniffing out the meanings and perceptions ... generated by focusing" (p. 52)—are ways of assessing the quality of the emergent data. In this sense, what may appear as a highly personal, self-search process that focuses on one's internal world can also contribute to how this may be of relevance to others.

In clarifying her HSSI, Sela-Smith (2002) argues that:

> Moustakas (1990) legitimized using the term *heuristics* to define the organized and systematic form for investigating human experience in which attention is focused *inward* on feeling responses of the researcher to the outward situation rather than exclusively to relations between the pieces of that outside situation. (p. 59)

And indeed, Moustakas (1990) describes the heuristic process as "autobiographic". At the same time, he notes that "with virtually every question that matters personally there is also a social—and perhaps universal—significance" (p. 15).

Reflections 4.1

Earlier (in Exercise #1), I shared a focus on friendships, love, and loss, and on a sense of ground and place, belonging and not belonging, knowing and not knowing—and uncertainty.

1. What are *your* associations with these words and themes?
2. In what ways might these words and themes be of significance to *others*?

Citing Moustakas' (1990) view that the autobiographical is also social and universal, Grennell (2014) suggests that "in focusing on my own experience I am illuminating the social and perhaps universal significance of—and for—others negotiating the hybrid cultural object" (p. 23). Finally, on this, Moustakas (1990) argues that "With new, revised, or expanded understanding, internal reorganization naturally occurs, resulting in a self-transformation that almost always has social and transpersonal implications" (p. 59).

The Internal Frame of Reference

Rogers (1951) writes about the frame of reference as "an organized pattern of perceptions of self and self-in-relationship to others and to the environment" (p. 191); another, and more literal way of describing it is as a frame or window by and through which we view, perceive, understand, and make meaning of the world. Rogers and others in person-centred psychology write about empathy in terms of understanding the client's internal frame of reference. Influenced and informed by this concept, and especially given his early emphasis on experience, Moustakas (1990) states that "Heuristic processes relate back to the internal frame of reference" (p. 26). Indeed, he emphasises this by stating that "Only the experiencing person … can validly provide portrayals of the experience" (Moustakas, 1990, p. 96). Douglass and Moustakas (1985) link this concept to the immersion phase of heuristic research (see next part), arguing that "Immersion involves self-search from the internal frame of reference" (p. 48).

Reflections 4.2

1. Think about why I refer to heuristic research method as *en*quiry rather than *in*quiry.

Having discussed heuristic methodology—or, rather a heuristic approach to methodology—in the furth and final part of the chapter, I turn to the heuristic method: as it were, the doing of the being!

Heuristic Method

From his own experience of research, Moustakas (1990) identified a number of steps or phases that form the basic research design: initial engagement, immersion, incubation, illumination, explication, and creative synthesis.

Rather than taking you, the reader/researcher, through each of these steps or phases, however, I encourage you to read Moustakas (and Douglass), as well as other heuristic researchers I cite in this chapter as each of them describes their different experiences of the various stages, many in very creative ways. Instead, in this part of the chapter, I discuss three issues regarding heuristic method that are important in thinking about how to do—and, of course, to be in and with—heuristic research, namely, the use (and abuse) of these phases and, more broadly, this aspect of the theory; a heuristic perspective on literature reviews; and the question of participants.

Stages, Phases, and Experience

One of the problems with people's approach to theory is that, in the generation after the initial theory was developed and formulated, it can become dogma (for a discussion of which, see Tudor, 2018). Phillips (1994) puts this wryly when he comments that: "Disciples are the people who haven't got the joke" (p. 162). With regard to heuristic theory, it is worth remembering that Moustakas identified the phases of research a posteriori, that is, reflecting on his experience of loneliness after the event; and, although he suggests that the phases must be completed, he also acknowledges that "the completion of the phases cannot be the focus" (p. 63). Despite this, some students believe and some supervisors insist that these phases have to be *followed* rather than *experienced*—which, for the researcher, makes the theory a priori and, thus, by definition, not heuristic. Writing about Moustakas' concepts (as described in the previous part of this chapter), Djuraskovic (in Djuraskovic & Arthur, 2010) writes that they did not occur without any order: "Instead, I had to engage in a disciplined process and follow six phases of the heuristic research" (p. 1577). In its concern with compulsion ("had to") and order ("follow"), this appears, at least to this author and researcher, to be the antithesis of the heuristic process. Compare this with Douglass and Moustakas' (1985) view that "heuristics permits and even encourages spontaneous creation of methods that will evoke or disclose experiential meanings. This license stems from the recognition that subjectivity makes to knowledge and from the dynamic nature of subjective reality" (p. 49). In other words, experience comes before—and, indeed, drives—theory and process. As Sela-Smith (2002) puts it: "what I identify as this last frontier requires setting aside the skills of controlled, objective observation and surrendering to embracing subjective experience and leaping into the unknown" (p. 54). Indeed, she heads her description of the six phases of heuristic research as *Surrender to the Six Phases of Experience* (p. 63).

Activity 4.4

1. Stay with your experience of the research enquiry.
2. Write your journal first; only later consider which phases of heuristic research you experienced.
3. Consider any resistance you have as a test of discovery. As Sela-Smith (2002) puts it: "resistance has to be confronted and overcome before full discovery can occur" (p. 58).

Reflections 4.3

1. In which order did you experience these phases?
2. Did you experience any other phases not encompassed by Moustakas' or other heuristic theory?
3. Do you consider "Illumination" to be a phase of heuristic research?

Literature View: And Re-view

There is an assumption, at least in some research circles, that a literature review has to be done in a certain way. Unfortunately (in my view), Moustakas (1990) himself contributes to this when, in Chap. 3 of his book, in a section on "Creating the research manuscript", he writes:

> Discuss the computer search, databases, descriptors, key words, and years covered. Organize the review to include an *introduction* that presents the topic reviewed and its significance; an *overview* and discussion of the methodological problems; *methods* that describe what induced you to include the published study in your review and how these studies were conducted; *themes* that cluster into patterns and which organize the presentation of findings; and *conclusions* that summarize core findings relevant to your research that differentiate your investigation from those in the literature. (p. 53–54)

Whilst there is nothing inherently wrong in this advice in the context of "present[ing] the research process and findings in a form that can be understood and utilized" (p. 53), it suggests that this kind of (literature) review is *the* way to do it, when, in fact, there are a number of different ways of reviewing literature or types of literature review. These include: the narrative (or traditional) review; the systematic review, including meta-analysis and meta-synthesis; the scoping literature review; the argumentative literature review; the integrative literature review; and the theoretical literature review (see Munn et al., 2018). Some of these methods imply a methodology (narrative, argumentative, and integrative), others may be underpinned by different methodologies. Again, the point here is for you, the reader/researcher, to have a methodology and to apply it—and herein lies the problem of Moustakas' advice as it is not based on heuristics but, rather, it appears, on the pragmatics of getting published.

If, however, we agree with Douglass and Moustakas' (1985) recognition of the significance of subjectivity (as quoted above), then we can—and should—take this license as a freedom to roam in the literature and, indeed, other media. Grennell (2014) puts this well:

> As is in keeping with heuristic research the literature discovery was not in the form of a formal literature review. The relevant literature was found by following one article or book and the references within that to the next. Intuition and interest as to which article or book I would read were the guide. (p. 26)

From a heuristic perspective, it is more consistent to refer to an initial literature *view*, which is often linked to the initial engagement with the subject of the enquiry; and a subsequent literature *re-view*, which may be experienced and elaborated as part of the explication phase. In any case, as Ferendo (2004) puts it: "the literature review must look at the traditions of the source of the researcher's experience" (p. 315). Furthermore, the heuristic approach to literature means that you have to immerse yourself in the literature and, again, this is not always easy, or, as Hammond (2016) points out, enjoyable. She writes about the experience of getting caught in the topic, in her case, shame: "In attempting to write my literature review my shame is fuelled as I struggle to find a way through the words of others, to hear my own voice" (p. 85). This is a poignant reminder of the importance of subjectivity. Chue (2021) elaborates this approach clearly:

> The heuristic research method calls for my personal experience of the literature, in which I am following my intuition as a "way of being informed, a way of knowing" (Moustakas, 1990, p. 10) to further elucidate my experience of abrupt endings. Thus, the intention is not to provide an exhaustive review, but rather *my* view of the literature that resonates most within me…. In this way, I find my voice again. *I* am calling out to the literature, feeling which of *my* echoes reverberate and resonate back to me, to firmly place where I stand against the backdrop of this historical cave. (p. 24)

Finally, in the spirit of such a review, in writing this chapter, I became curious about how heuristic researchers—or, at least, researchers who espouse an heuristic approach—did their literature reviews (views or re-views), a piece of research summarised in Table 4.2.

Table 4.2 Heuristic research studies: references to literature review

Author(s)	Research subject	Literature review (and basis)
Shantall (1999)	The experience of meaning amongst holocaust survivors	Survey (not defined), though with a focus on the growth value of suffering
Sela-Smith (2001)	Transition, transformation, and theory	Review of research which applied Moustakas' method and of Wilber's model of integral knowledge (not specified)
Atkins and Loewenthal (2004)	Lived experiences of psychotherapists working with older clients	Review (not defined)
Ferendo (2004)	Ken Wilber and personal transformation	Review of the works of Ken Wilber and their intellectual roots (not specified)
Casterline (2006)	The experience of the act of praying	Review based on a computerised search using keywords, and focusing on first-person accounts
Meents (2006)	Intuition	Review described as "interactions with literature" (p. 113); also reviews of literature on transition and transformation, HSSI, and intuition (not specified)
Djuraskovic and Arthur (2010)	Acculturation and identity construction	Search (not elaborated)
Tudor (2010, 2017)	The fight for health	Search on heuristics, paradigms, holism, and educational objectives (not specified)
Grennell (2014)	Being Māori and Pākehā (cultural hybridity)	Includes a literature whakapapa (genealogy) and review on hybrid identity, Māori experience and history, and New Zealand poetry and writing from library and databases (not specified)
Haertl (2014)	The power of the written word	Review of heuristic inquiry, and phenomenology and heuristics (not defined)
Schulz (2015)	Existential psychotherapy	Review "performed" (not elaborated)

(continued)

Table 4.2 (continued)

Author(s)	Research subject	Literature review (and basis)
Wiorkowski (2015)	The experiences of students with autism spectrum disorders	Conceptualised as part of the immersion phase (not elaborated)
Hammond (2016)	Therapists' experience of working with shame	With regard to shame (conceptualised in terms of consistency with heuristic research)
Alleyne, 2017	A psychotherapist's experience of grief	Literature on grief and working with clients who are dying searched (not specified)
Ozertugnul (2015, 2017b)	Obsessive compulsive disorder	Relevant literature on phenomenology and heuristics (not specified)
Kumar (2017)	Intimate partner violence	No reference
Harrison (2018)	Physical activity and psychotherapy	Relevant literature on exercise and psychotherapy reviewed (specified as subjective and consistent with heuristic methodology)
Yeh (2018)	Leadership practices of female faculty in higher education	Review used to expand on existing understanding of the subject, and investigated gender bias, etc. (not specified); also including reference to courage theory and leadership self-identity
Sherwood (2019, 2021)	Psychological infanticide, closed stranger adoption	Guided by an "emergent style", though including search parameters and exclusions
Shelburne et al. (2020)	Problematic eating	No reference
Williams (2020)	The experience of people of colour engaging in an asynchronous, smartphone application	Review of online health communities (not defined)
Chue (2021)	Abrupt endings	Literature view of therapists' personal experiences of abrupt endings, with exclusions (elaborated in terms of and consistent with heuristic methodology)
Ciurlionis (2021)	Humour in psychotherapy	An "idiosyncratic literature review" of humour in psychotherapeutic literature and aspects of popular culture (linked to Moustakas', 1990, concept of "internal search")
Lyons (2021)	Ambivalence in psychotherapy	Literature view of ambivalence (linked to heuristic perspectives)

Participants

When Moustakas (1990) noted that "in theory it is possible to conduct heuristic research with only one participant" (p. 47), he gave legitimacy to the value of subjectivity and laid the foundation for what Sela-Smith later developed as HSSI. However, as Sela-Smith points out, Moustakas also created a contradiction, which has led to subsequent confusion, specifically with regard to the question of having co-participants, when he stated that "a study will achieve richer, deeper, more profound, and more varied meaning when it includes depictions of the experiences of others" (Moustakas, 1990, p. 47). Critiquing this, Sela-Smith (2002) writes: "Validity of the self-experience is established by *similar* experiences of others; yet validity in subjective discovery-research is *not possible by comparing* to others' experience" (p. 76; my emphasis). She goes on to argue that, if co-participants are used in heuristic self-search enquiry, they

> are valuable as reflectors of possible areas of resistance that may be out of conscious awareness in the form of denial, projection, or incomplete search. This sends the researcher back into the self to continue the self-search into deeper or more distant tacit dimensions, thus allowing the transformation to be more expansive. (p. 78)

Ozertugrul (2017b) is extremely helpful on this point, mainly as he takes participant selection seriously and presents the logic that informs his choice in terms of familiar research concepts and language:

> As a form of phenomenological research, heuristic research uses idiographic sampling and focuses on the individual experience…. As part of heuristic research, I used purposive and criterion-based sampling. The intent was to explicate the full range of the [obsessive-compulsive disorder] experience that resides within me. The criterion is to explore an individual who has personal experience with the phenomenon …. In this heuristic self-search study, I was the researcher/participant, the single individual. (p. 219)

Ozertugrul (2017b) goes on to critique other authors for not justifying or having a rationale for including co-participants, especially if their method—and/or methodology—is HSSI, and speculates that this might be due either to a fear of the reaction from academia, including rejection; or to conforming to the established (i.e., hegemonic) view that research requires and is only valid if it has participants. Following on from the previous tables in this chapter, and in support of the validity of $n = 1$ (where n is the number of participants), Table 4.3 notes the numbers of participants in the 24 research studies reviewed, 17 of which are based on self-study or variations thereof.

One of the motivations to involve others might be to assert the greater relevance of the research to society. Indeed, a common learning outcome of research courses, dissertations, theses, and degrees is the contribution and/or relevance of the research to the discipline/profession. Again, Ozertugrul (2017a) poses a useful counterpoint to this: "How do researchers engaged in HSSI preserve self-understanding (the apparent prospect of self-search) while investing sustained attention on others' experiences?" (p. 245)

Finally, as Moustakas (1990) reminds us, if you do have co-researchers, then the (principal or primary) researcher has to experience the heuristic enquiry "not only with himself or herself, but with each and every co-researcher" (p. 32).

Activity 4.5   With Regard to Having Co-participants

1. Think about whether you need co-participants and, if so, why.
2. If so, consider Ozertugrul's (2017b) thinking on participant selection.
3. If so, also consider the time factor in facilitating your co-participants' experience of the heuristic phases.

Table 4.3 Heuristic research studies: numbers of participants/co-researchers

Author(s)	Research subject	Participants/ co-researchers
Shantall (1999)	The experience of meaning amongst holocaust survivors	5[a]
Sela-Smith (2001)	Transition, transformation, and theory	1[b]
Atkins and Loewenthal (2004)	Lived experiences of psychotherapists working with older clients	8[c]
Ferendo (2004)	Ken Wilber and personal transformation	1
Casterline (2006)	The experience of the act of praying	7
Meents (2006)	Intuition	1
Djuraskovic and Arthur (2010)	Acculturation and identity construction	7[c]
Tudor (2010, 2017)	The fight for health	1
Grennell (2014)	Being Māori and Pākehā (cultural hybridity)	1+[d]
Haertl (2014)	The power of the written word	10
Schulz (2015)	Existential psychotherapy	2
Wiorkowski (2015)	The experiences of students with autism spectrum disorders	12
Hammond (2016)	Therapists' experience of working with shame	6
Alleyne, 2017	A psychotherapist's experience of grief	1
Ozertugnul (2015, 2017b)	Obsessive compulsive disorder	1
Kumar (2017)	Intimate partner violence	1[e]
Harrison (2018)	Physical activity and psychotherapy	1
Yeh (2018)	Leadership practices of female faculty in higher education	8
Sherwood (2019)	Psychological infanticide	1
Shelburne et al. (2020)	Problematic eating	7
Williams (2020)	The experience of people of colour engaging in an asynchronous, smartphone application	6
Chue (2021)	Abrupt endings	1
Ciurlionis (2021)	Humour in psychotherapy	1
Lyons (2021)	Ambivalence in psychotherapy	1

[a]Not including the researcher/author
[b]That is, the researcher/author, unless otherwise stated
[c]Including the lead author
[d]By which I refer to the author and her social/cultural context
[e]The original work (written up in Kumar & Casey, 2017) involved ten participants but not the researcher

Summary

This chapter has offered an outline of heuristics as a research method and methodology which is especially suited to research in the psychological therapies. It has located the theory and practice of heuristic research in the wider context of research methodology and method; elaborated its key concepts; and referenced heuristic research studies. Finally, it has considered three common issues or questions with regard to heuristic research—the use of the stages or phases of heuristic research; literature reviews; and participants—in a way that is consistent with its methodology. This chapter encourages research students and supervisors to engage in heuristic research in a way of doing *and* being that is consistent with their purpose and practice and its philosophy.

References

Alleyne, B. (2017). *A psychotherapist's experience of grief: A heuristic enquiry*. Dissertation submitted in partial completion of the degree of Master of Psychotherapy, Auckland University of Technology, Auckland, Aotearoa New Zealand. https://www.openrepository.aut.ac.nz/handle/10292/10424

Atkins, D., & Loewenthal, D. (2004). The lived experience of psychotherapists working with older clients: An heuristic study. *British Journal of Guidance & Counselling, 32*(4), 493–509. https://doi.org/10.1080/03069880412331303295

Bridgman, P. (1950). *Reflections of a physicist*. Philosophical Library.

Buber, M. (1958). *I and thou*. Scribners.

Buber, M. (1961). *Tales of the Hasidim: The early masters* (O. Marx, Trans.). Schocken.

Buber, M. (1965). *The knowledge of man*. Harper & Row.

Casterline, G. (2006). *The experience of the act of praying*. A dissertation submitted in partial completion of the degree of Doctor of Philosophy, Loyola University, Chicago, IL, USA. https://www.proquest.com/docview/305319972?pq-origsite=gscholar&fromopenview=true

Chue, D. (2021). *Falling into the abyss: A heuristic self-inquiry into a psychotherapist's experience of abrupt endings*. Dissertation submitted in partial completion of the degree of Master of Psychotherapy, Auckland University of Technology, Auckland, Aotearoa New Zealand. https://www.openrepository.aut.ac.nz/handle/10292/14790

Ciurlionis, C. (2021). *In defence of a manic defence: A therapist's experience of humour*. Dissertation submitted in partial completion of the degree of Master of Psychotherapy, Auckland University of Technology, Auckland, Aotearoa New Zealand. https://www.openrepository.aut.ac.nz/handle/10292/14499

Djuraskovic, I., & Arthur, N. (2010). Heuristic inquiry: A personal journey of acculturation and identity reconstruction. *The Qualitative Report, 15*(6), 1569–1593. https://doi.org/10.46743/2160-3715/2010.1361

Douglass, B., & Moustakas, C. (1985). Heuristic inquiry: The internal search to know. *Journal of Humanistic Psychology, 25*(3), 39–55.

Ferendo, F. J. (2004). *A heuristic and hermeneutic inquiry: Ken Wilber and personal transformation*. Thesis submitted in partial fulfilment of the requirements for the degree of Doctor of Philosophy with a concentration in Psychology and a specialization in Transpersonal Psychology, Union Institute and University, Cincinnati, Ohio.

Frost, et al. (2022). Taking qualitative driven mixed methods further. In S. Bager-Charleson & A. G. McBeath (Eds.), *Supporting research in counselling and psychotherapy: Qualitative, quantitative, and mixed methods research*. Palgrave Macmillan.

Gendlin, E. (1978). *Focusing*. Everest House.

Grennell, N. (2014). *What is the experience of being both Māori and Pākehā? Negotiating the experience of the hybrid cultural object*. Dissertation submitted in partial completion of the degree of Master of Psychotherapy, Auckland University of Technology, Auckland, Aotearoa New Zealand. https://www.openrepository.aut.ac.nz/handle/10292/7710

Grennell-Hawke, N., & Tudor, K. (2018). Being Māori and Pākehā: Methodology and method in exploring cultural hybridity. *The Qualitative Report, 23*(7), 1530–1546. https://doi. org/10.46743/2160-3715/2018.2934

Haertl, K. (2014). Writing and the development of the self-heuristic inquiry: A unique way of exploring the power of the written word. *Journal of Poetry Therapy, 27*(2), 55–68. https://doi. org/10.1080/08893675.2014.895488

Hammond, M. (2016). *Therapists' experience of working with shame*. Dissertation submitted in partial completion of the requirements for the degree of Master of Health Science, Auckland University of Technology, Auckland, Aotearoa New Zealand. https://www.openrepository.aut. ac.nz/bitstream/handle/10292/10186/HammondM.pdf?sequence=3&isAllowed=y

Harrison, D. (2018). *Working (it) out: A psychotherapist's experience of exercise*. Dissertation submitted in partial completion of Master of Psychotherapy, Auckland University of Technology, Auckland, Aotearoa New Zealand.

Harrison, D., & Tudor, K. (2020). Working (it) out: An heuristic enquiry into psychotherapy and exercise. *Advances in Mind-Body Medicine, 34*(2), 14–23.

Hertwig, R., & Panchur, T. (2015). Heuristics, history of. In J. D. Wright (Ed.), *International encyclopedia of the social & behavioral sciences* (Vol. 10, 2nd ed.). Elsevier. https://doi. org/10.1016/B978-0-08-097086-8.03221-9

Hiles, D. (2001). *Heuristic inquiry and transpersonal research*. Paper presented to the Centre for Counselling and Psychotherapy Education, London, UK. http://psy.dmu.ac.uk/drhiles/ HIpaper.htm

Hill, J. (2022). *Te whakatere i ngā awa e rua (Navigating the two rivers): A heuristic investigation of Māori identity as a student psychotherapist*. Dissertation submitted in partial completion of Master of Psychotherapy, Auckland University of Technology, Auckland, Aotearoa New Zealand.

Husserl, E. (1983). *Ideas pertaining to a pure phenomenology and to a phenomenological philosophy* (F. Kersten, Trans.). Collier Books. (Original work published 1913).

Jourard, S. (1968). *Disclosing man to himself*. Van Nostrand.

Jourard, S. (1971). *Self-disclosure: An experimental analysis of the transparent self*. Wiley-Interscience.

Kumar, S. (2017). My dissertation healed me: A retrospective analysis through heuristic inquiry. *The Qualitative Report, 22*(11), 3025–3038. https://doi.org/10.46743/2160-3715/2017.3051

Kumar, S., & Casey, A. (2017). Work and intimate partner violence: Powerful role of work in empowerment process for middle-class women who experience intimate partner violence. *Community, Work & Family, 23*, 1. https://doi.org/10.1080/13668803.2017.1365693

Lyons, D. (2021). *To be or not to be (ambivalent): A heuristic enquiry into ambivalence in psychotherapy*. Dissertation submitted in partial completion of Master of Psychotherapy, Auckland University of Technology, Auckland, Aotearoa New Zealand.

Maslow, A. H. (1956). Self-actualizing people: A study of psychological health. In C. Moustakas (Ed.), *The self: Explorations in personal growth* (pp. 160–194). Harper & Brothers.

Maslow, A. H. (1966). *The psychology of science*. Harper & Row.

Maslow, A. H. (1971). *The farther reaches of human nature*. Viking.

McCann, M. (2022). *Invisible wounds: A heuristic exploration of unintentional racial microaggressions and their relationship to unconscious racialisation*. Dissertation submitted in partial completion of Master of Psychotherapy, Auckland University of Technology, Auckland, Aotearoa New Zealand.

McCann, M., & Tudor, K. (2022). Unintentional racial microaggressions and the social unconscious. *International Journal of Applied Psychoanalytic Studies, 19*(2), 202–216.

Meents, J. (2006). *Acres of diamonds: A heuristic self-search inquiry into intuition*. A thesis submitted to the Faculty of Graduate Studies in partial fulfilment of the requirements for the degree of Doctor of Philosophy, University of Calgary, Alberta, Canada.

Merry, T. (2004). Supervision as heuristic research inquiry. In K. Tudor & M. Worrall (Eds.), *Freedom to practise: Person-centred approaches to supervision* (pp. 189–199). PCCS Books.

Moustakas, C. (Ed.). (1956). *The self: Explorations in personal growth*. Harper & Row.

Moustakas, C. (1961). *Loneliness*. Prentice-Hall.

Moustakas, C. (1967). Heuristic research. In J. Bugental (Ed.), *Challenges in humanistic psychology* (pp. 100–107). McGraw-Hill.

Moustakas, C. (1990). *Heuristic research: Design, methodology and applications*. Sage.

Moustakas, C. (1994). *Phenomenological research methods*. Sage.

Moustakas, C. (2000). Heuristic research revisited. In K. J. Schneider, J. F. T. Bugental, & J. F. Pierson (Eds.), *The handbook of humanistic psychology: Leading edges in theory, research, and practice* (pp. 263–274). Sage.

Munn, Z., Peters, M. D. J., Stern, C., Tufanaru, C., McArthur, A., & Aromataris, E. (2018). Systematic review or scoping review? Guidance for authors when choosing between a systematic or scoping review approach. *BMC Medical Research Methodology, 18*(143), 143. https://doi.org/10.1186/s12874-018-0611-x

Ozertugrul, E. (2015). *Heuristic self-search inquiry into one experience of obsessive-compulsive disorder*. Unpublished doctoral dissertation, Walden University, Minneapolis, MN, USA.

Ozertugrul, E. (2017a). A comparative analysis: Heuristic self-search inquiry as self-knowledge and knowledge of society. *Journal of Humanistic Psychology, 57*(3), 237–251. https://doi.org/10.1177/0022167815594966

Ozertugrul, E. (2017b). Heuristic self-search inquiry into one experience of obsessive–compulsive disorder. *Journal of Humanistic Psychology, 57*(3), 215–236. https://doi.org/10.1177/0022167815592503

Patton, M. Q. (2002). *Qualitative research and evaluation methods*. Sage.

Phillips, A. (1994). On flirtation. Faber & Faber.

Polanyi, M. (1962). *Personal knowledge: Towards a post-critical philosophy*. Routledge.

Polanyi, M. (1964). *Science, faith and society*. University of Chicago Press.

Polanyi, M. (1966). *The tacit dimension*. Doubleday.

Polanyi, M. (1969). In M. Grene (Ed.), *Knowing and being*. University of Chicago Press.

Rogers, C. R. (1951). *Client-centered therapy*. Constable.

Rogers, C. R. (1969). Toward a science of the person. In A. J. Sutich & M. A. Vick (Eds.), *Readings in humanistic psychology*. Macmillan.

Rogers, C. R. (1985). Toward a more human science of the person. *Journal of Humanistic Psychology, 25*(4), 7–24.

Schulz, C. (2015). Existential psychotherapy with a person who lives with a left ventricular assist device and awaits heart transplantation: A case report. *Journal of Humanistic Psychology, 55*(4), 429–473. https://doi.org/10.1177/0022167814539192

Sela-Smith, S. (1998). *Regaining wholeness: A heuristic inquiry into childhood sexual abuse*. Unpublished master's thesis, Saybrook Graduate School, San Francisco, CA, USA.

Sela-Smith, S. (2001). *A demonstration of heuristic self-search inquiry: Clarification of the Moustakas method*. Unpublished doctoral dissertation, Saybrook Graduate School, San Francisco, CA, USA.

Sela-Smith, S. (2002). Heuristic research: A review and critique of Moustakas's method. *Journal of Humanistic Psychology, 42*(3), 53–88. https://doi.org/10.1177/0022167802423004

Shantall, T. (1999). The experience of meaning in suffering among Holocaust survivors. *Journal of Humanistic Psychology, 39*(3), 96–124. https://doi.org/10.1177/0022167899393009

Shelburne, S., Curtis, D., & Rockwell, D. (2020). Spontaneous transformation and recovery from problematic eating: A heuristic inquiry. *Journal of Humanistic Psychology, 39*(3), 96–124. https://doi.org/10.1177/0022167820945803

Sherwood, V. (2019). *Understanding psychological infanticidal experiences of adopted children as illuminated by a study of nineteenth century baby-farming: An heuristic inquiry*. Thesis submitted in completion of a Doctor of Philosophy, Auckland University of Technology, Auckland, Aotearoa New Zealand.

Sherwood, V. (2021). *Haunted: The death mother archetype*. Chiron.

Strasser, A., & Strasser, F. (2022). *Time-limited existential therapy: The wheel of existence*. Wiley.

Taft, J. (1973). *The dynamics of therapy in a controlled relationship*. Macmillan. (Original work published 1933).

Tudor, K. (2010). *The fight for health: A heuristic enquiry into psychological well-being*. Unpublished context statement for a PhD in Mental Health Promotion by Public (Published) Works, School of Health and Social Sciences, Middlesex University, London, UK.

Tudor, K. (2017). The fight for health: An heuristic enquiry. In K. Tudor (Ed.), *Conscience and critic: The selected works of Keith Tudor* (pp. 143–168). Routledge.

Tudor, K. (2018). *Psychotherapy: A critical examination*. PCCS Books.

Valéry, P. (1957). In J. Hyties (Ed.), *Ouevres [Works]* (Vol. 1). Gallimard.

Williams, N. F. (2020). Going "beyond the surface" in an app-based group: A heuristic inquiry. *Journal of Humanistic Psychology*, 1–24. https://doi.org/10.1177/0022167820974503

Wiorkowski, F. (2015). The experiences of students with autism spectrum disorders in college: A heuristic exploration. *The Qualitative Report, 20*(6), 847–863. https://doi.org/10.46743/2160-3715/2015.2163

Yeh, T.-J. (2018). A heuristic study on the leadership practices of female faculty in higher education. *The International Journal of Organizational Innovation, 11*(2), 245–259. http://www.ijoi-online.org/

Chapter 5
Autoethnographic Psychotherapy Research: A Methodology that Keeps Our 'Heart in Mind'

Saira Gracie Razzaq

Learning Goals

- To understand the criteria for producing an autoethnographic account.
- To become familiar with Autoethnographic Psychotherapeutic Research and how to put it in practice.
- To reflect on how we can write an Evocative Autoethnographic account and consider the relational ethics within the research process.
- To feel encouraged to engage in Autoethnographic Psychotherapeutic Research journey.

Autoethnographic Psychotherapy Research: A Methodology That Keeps Our 'Heart in Mind'

Words are free, paper and pencils are plentiful, but the right words are hard to find. Engaging texts don't pretend to be perfect. Instead, engaging texts are honest. Rather than burying passion, these texts speak 'from the heart', centralising the subjective and constructing a space in which 'others might see themselves' (Pelias, 2005, p. 419).

S. G. Razzaq (✉)
British Psychological Society, London, UK

© The Author(s), under exclusive license to Springer Nature
Switzerland AG 2022
S. Bager-Charleson, A. McBeath (eds.), *Supporting Research in Counselling and Psychotherapy*, https://doi.org/10.1007/978-3-031-13942-0_5

First-Person Research

Autoethnography originally arose from the field of anthropology, ethnography (people and cultures with their customs, habits, and differences), and sociology. It is a first-person, insider account that can differ from a personal narrative and auto-biography, as it locates literature to self-experience that intends to illuminate an epiphany or powerful experience to make meaning. This often reveals a conflict of culture and/or self within dominant and discursive narratives. Autoethnography is a novel approach that straddles a range of disciplines and uses varied theoretical and methodological approaches, with a range of emphasis on 'auto', the representations of self, 'ethno', the personal experience that examines cultural beliefs, practices, and identities (Ellis & Bochner, 2002), and finally 'graphy' which both represents research and the research audience.

I felt inspired when I discovered autoethnography, as I had been wrestling with the daunting array of methodological approaches and only a few of which really spoke to me. I was somewhat baffled by dominant discourses, distancing academic texts and conceptually rigid frameworks that kept me out rather than the reflexive relationality of the psychotherapeutic training. I also felt constrained by the types of stories that were made available to me in the therapeutic world. I wanted to use other interdisciplinary forms to produce research that invited the reader close and offer a relational home for storied contexts which can be regained by amplifying silent narratives that enhance clinical practice through sensitive research. Whilst holding in mind as Pennycook (1994) suggests that 'voice is not just a non-silence, a [writing] of words. . it is a place of struggle in the space between language, dis-course, and subjectivity' (p. 311). This also speaks to how we grapple and engage in our writings as we seek for what 'exists in struggle, searching for what it may come to realize. It becomes a small, nervous solution, offered with humility. Its ideas slide into cautious claims, noting its limitations' (Barone & Eisner, 2012, p. 666). I wanted to integrate what *we do as therapists with what we do as researchers*, and certainly this does not mean research is therapy, but good research can be *therapeutic*, when it seeks to transform wounds and deepen psychological understanding.

Evocative Research

Evocative Autoethnographic Psychotherapy Research (APR) most closely resem-bles therapy, in its accessibility, its call for connection and is restorative in its capac-ity to heal. Isn't this what good therapists do? Many therapists are 'seekers', we seek out the metaphors and stories of our clients that hold together a presence and comprehension that otherwise might be missed. This is because cultural, and sub-jective knowledge is often tacit, deeply embedded and not explicitly defined and it requires an internal connection to clarify the conditions in which understanding can take place (Gadamer, 1975, p 295). There is an attempt to bring together a multiplicity of discourses into a more unified framework (Denzin et al., 2008) with the rigour and scholarship of Psychotherapy and Counselling Psychology theory and research interlinked with the subjectivity of resonant emotional narratives.

The *interaction* between Evocative Autoethnography and Psychotherapy as Autoethnographic Psychotherapy Research (APR) is the integration of the intrapsychic and psychological realm that is centrally configured as both theoretical and deconstructive of existing concepts within a social, political, and societal context as illustrated in Fig. 5.1. This nuanced relational possibility invites *the wounded voice* of the researcher and collaborator, moving across subjectivities and self-states that are often not present in theoretical descriptions to create another dimension of voicing. In the spirit of Saldaña's (2016) ideas of being on the lookout for 'buried treasure' (p. 289) to discover important epistemological insights to serve us in understanding our emotional human geography and map its breaches. This experiential process becomes an embodiment of awareness and psychological meaning of the subjective and relational self as APR complements existing knowledge by capturing the liminal and transitional journey of the researcher. Rather like the experience of crossing untraversed spaces and places, that move from a transitional state to one in which there is a felt sense of an organising experience coming from dynamic transformation which is experienced within the therapeutic dyad. Vulnerability is not a passing indisposition in research, it's often not a choice, but a present and abiding undercurrent and without it we can become closed off to the

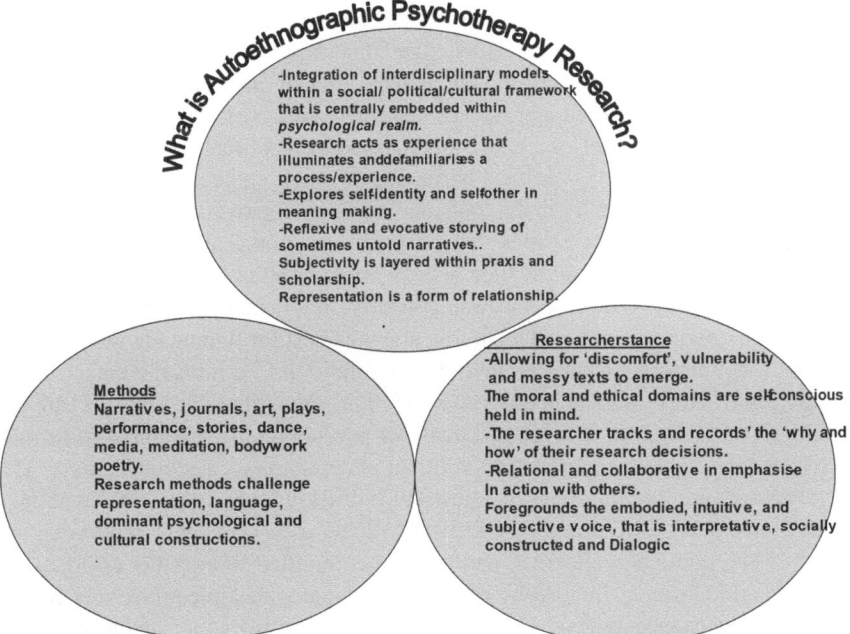

Fig. 5.1 What is APR?

very complexities that we are trying to excavate in ourselves and in our subject of interest. This coupled with the intensive experience of examining what seems unspeakable or difficult to name can bring about transformational change for the researcher and researched.

> If you feel a pull to write an autoethnography, you will engage in an experiential interpretative methodology embedded in scholarship and praxis which nurture the creative imagination and give primacy to the researcher's subjectivity. Despite its emphasis on experiential processes within Psychotherapy and Counselling Psychology practice, autoethnographic methodologies have been a surprisingly neglected area of research.

> How do you define research? What are the commonly held requirements, and how may, or may not, autoethnography fit in here. For reflection points, read about the four processes to engage (4 Ps) with the approach further down.

Honouring Differences and Sometimes Opposing Views

There is an attempt to capture the marginal discourses that Foucault (1977) describes as the insurrection of subjugated knowledge. This is often outside dominant psychological theory, representation, and knowledge to reclaim, through self-reflective responses, the representational spaces have marginalised those at the borders (Tierney & Lincoln, 1997). This involves honouring difference, and sometimes opposing views, whereby dominant narratives of psychotherapy theory and knowledge can be challenged to help the 'outsider' better understand the rupturing experience upon the self. Here stories can be transformational and become a site of empowerment and resistance as they become more accessible and less deniable. In the current landscape of co-occurring, collective traumas, the pandemic, multiple oppressions, serious ecological anxieties, and the quest for finding identity, we need research methodologies that can help define conditions for human connectedness, healing, and safety, as Denzin and Lincoln (2003) say within the ethics of care and kindness. APR suggests that we can consider psychotherapy research as a form of activism that is a humanitarian and political undertaking as a moral witness. This involves not just 'calling out' of injustices but a kind of 'calling in', evoking a bridge to contact. APR draws from Denzin's (2018, p. 97) concepts of research that speak to the political, collective, and that are committed to unsettle, critique, and challenge the assumed, inviting moral and ethical dialogue while reflexively clarifying one's own stance, engendering resistance, demonstrating care, interpretive representations, and authentic capacities.

Understanding Autoethnography

Autoethnography is a constructivist post-modernist methodology that overlaps with narrative and autobiographic methods. Bouchner (2017) states: The truths of auto-ethnography exist between storyteller and story listener; they dwell in the listeners' or readers' engagement with the writer's struggle with adversity, the heartbreaking feelings of stigma and marginalisation, the resistance to the authority of canonical discourses, the therapeutic desire to face up to the challenges of life and to emerge with greater self-knowledge, the opposition to the repression of the body, the difficulty of finding the words to make bodily dysfunction meaningful, the desire for self-expression, and the urge to speak to and assist a community of fellow sufferers. Autoethnographic stories call for engagement, identification, and resonance. They do what other work in the human sciences can't do, or chooses not to do—to provide 'a means for the readers own moral experience' and 'show us how to feel the sufferings of others' by privileging emotions and emotionality (Denzin, 1997, pp. 201–202).

Autoethnography employs creative analytic practices (CAP) that are a type of critique and resistance in diverse forms such as novels, fiction, poems, prose, script, song, performance, art, photography, documentaries, images, or performance narratives and attempts at generating *feeling* with a story rather than being told about it (Denzin & Lincoln, 2003). Writing is a form of inquiry to search for thick descriptions (Geertz, 2000) while crafting a story that can contribute to deeper understandings and mean-making using messy texts (Lather, 2001). This method views data as social facts that are situated representations as the broad intention is not to arrive at universal claims or assemble a site of generalised definitive hypotheses. Instead, it explores contextual and localised knowledge that is inclusive of diversity, respectful of historical contexts and value systems.

Arthur Bouchner (2017) suggests that; 'the truths of autoethnography exist between storyteller and story listener; they dwell in the listeners or readers engagement with the writer struggle with adversity. The heart-breaking feelings of stigma and marginalization, the resistance to authority of canonical discourses, the therapeutic desire to face up to the challenges of life and to emerge with greater self-knowledge...Autoethnography calls for engagement, identification and resonance' (p. 75). He suggests that it requires a willingness to remain open and engage in active dialogue with these stories, whilst being available to 'otherness' and the ethics of a moral imagination.

Autoethnography has many forms and overlaps various styles; Bochner and Ellis (2016) have identified sixty forms and terms with similar meanings to autoethnography such as literary autoethnography, poetic autoethnography, meta-autoethnography (Ellis, 2004), performance autoethnography (Denzin, 2018). To cite a few brief examples of various autoethnographies, Kiesinger's (2002) work on the multi-interpretative positions experienced in anorexia allows for an engagement with the text that helps the audience to experience her world, filling the gaps with one's own experience and understanding. Garratt's (2014) Psychoanalytic

Autoethnography explored the embodied masculinity of competitive natural body-building that revealed the ambivalence of the ideal body reflected in the loss and fragmentation associated with socially conditioned roles. Toyosaki's et al. (2009) work on the resituating whiteness as a social paradox to epistemologically engage with a complex analysis of whiteness by using 'community autoethnography' to call for social justice and advocate for change. Crossley's (2000) work on trauma narratives with HIV positive individuals suggests there is a quest for a moral imperative and ethical practice of the self in relation to trauma. As reliable witnesses, this can validate suffering and pain, and make change more possible. Fox's (1996) innovative work on sexual abuse presents a triad of three voices in three separate columns, her own as researcher, the 'victim's voice', and the convicted sex offender. The material was drawn from therapy sessions that she accessed as a participant observer. This created a varied and ambiguous representation of a complex subject that was dialogic, relational, and emotive.

Collaborative forms of Autoethnography

Whilst duoethnography is a form of collaborative autoethnography that is a multi-collective and multi-dialogic process that deconstructs preconceived views and cultural contexts and one's narrative relationship to a research theme (Norris et al., 2012). Such as Dunne and Ly-Donpvan (2021) work, which offers an intersectional layered account of identities to untangle the lived multifaceted experience of (step)m(Other)ing that deconstructs the sometimes pejorative and essentialising cultural constructions of stepmothers. Ellis and Bochner's (2002) duo-autoethnography presented their termination story written in script form in their co-mingled voices. These co-constructed narratives highlight a relationality and mutual experience, that explore one's humanness, conflicts, and ambiguities of being in relationship with other, as jointly authored, and contextual in emphasis, where researcher and researched can share control over voice and representation.

Principles of APR

Bager-Charleson and McBeath (2020) argue that quantitative research seeks to *confirm* meaning whilst qualitative research seeks to *explore* experience and meaning, both offering a useful vantage point. APR is firmly a qualitative methodology that attempts to 'use' emotional involvement within research rather than trying to escape or contain it.

> **Box 5.1 Activity: Using Emotional Involvement**
> Can you think of an example where your emotional involvement has been part of your research?
>   Thinking in terms of 'being alongside the questions' may help. I am sharing some of my thoughts from my own research below:
>   *Be alongside the questions themselves as if they were written in ancient language. Don't search for the answers, live the questions, trusting that someday you will live your way into the answers. In speaking and sharing these vulnerable storied worlds, we risk bruising and face being misunderstood but when the spring arrives, what is formed is an embodied capacity for empowerment and tenderness as a surprising, creative bridge to consciousness and spirit, and for research that has space for healing and heart.* (Razzaq, 2007, 2017, from a conference presentation)
>
> • **What might 'being alongside the questions' mean to you?**

APR asks us to acquire the characteristics of psychological narrator and storyteller to explore with artfulness, emotionality, politic, ecology, and embodiment as we access hidden and often unknown subjectivity.

I developed APR as an approach from the research I undertook explored the imprint of racist trauma within my family group and how psychotherapy professionals known to me considered racist trauma in their clinical work and its impact on their own life stories. There seemed to be leakages and confusion in my understandings about racism(s) experienced by my family that I consciously knew little about that I could no longer avoid. This internal tug to respond (Pizer, 2016) was in part, what I retrospectively realised, drove me to become a therapist. The project was a recreation and reclaiming of a less than conscious experience, made available by accessing incoherent parts through self-conscious inquiry. This described how racist trauma *felt and what it means to try to be present and available to it as a therapist.* The research project then became a place to find these lost accounts that became a narrative dynamic or *narrative quintessence* in an 'an effort to avert the critical gaze from the racial object to the racial subject from the described to the imagined, to the describers to the imaginers, the serving to the served' (Morrison, 1992, p. 22). It involved testifying and externalising oppressive experiences as well as demonstrating the need to embrace the intersubjective space in-between the divisions as a therapeutically available surface (White, 1995).

Within the research, the professional and family group read each other's and my account and dialogued with these texts and their own text, rendering their voices against others whilst in dialogue with mine. I did this in the hope that evocative narratives could generate conversations and dialogues about racialised subjectivities. The conversational interviews were transcribed and thematised, and I translated some of the interviews into stories with the collaborators, some of the collaborators wrote their own storied accounts arising from the dialogues. I did not want to produce a theorising abstract clinical text, but the possibility of filtering the experiences of racism that used my vulnerability to induce the vulnerability of the reader, to make a resonating connection. This is an attempt at enabling rather than constraining the researcher whereby 'vulnerability becomes the new capacity' that is modelled and internalised through the research process. We can firmly place the authority of survivorship, human suffering and hold the deep subjectivity of the narrator and witness account to identifying cultural and psychotherapeutic insights. As research knowledge, APR is not just a methodology but as a *set of attitudes towards the self and Other* through the development of an autoethnographic stance and attitude as a way of being in the world. This means being autoethnographic with self when thinking about clients and research, provide a temporal framework into the subjective that otherwise would have been difficult to know. The analytic interpretations that might emerge from this process become a therapeutically available terrain enhancing both the research endeavour and our capacities in the consulting room.

I am convinced there is a need for further research methodologies and epistemologies to access and describe what takes place when we are doing work with Otherness, difference, identity, intersectionality, psychological suffering, and trauma. Denzin and Lincoln (2003) ask, who is the Other? Can we ever truly authentically name the Other's experience and how do we include the voice of the Other within our texts? In my experience, psychotherapy sometimes struggles to explain Otherness and its injurious effects from the inside, APR feels like as a suitable and respectful method of exploration to create understandings into what is perceived as the effects of the internalisation of dominant oppressions, stereotypes, and Othering. To challenge and highlight prevailing psychological theories and practice, by developing a greater capacity to find a way to live with ambiguity and mess. Where research taps into powerful material that is sometimes enacted, denied, and entangled and that resists simple understandings. This process reflects the conflictual concepts in dialectic tension as a place for our uncertainties and the relationship between author and reader to create the 'experience of being there', provoking curiosity and possible unsettlement. We are helped by LaCapra's (1994) ideas of empathetic unsettlement; '… affect the mode of representation in different, nonlegislated ways, but still in a fashion that inhibits or prevents extreme objectification and harmonizing narratives… One's own unsettled response to another's unsettlement can never be entirely under control, but it may be affected by one's active awareness of, and need to come to terms with, certain problems related to one's implication in, or transferential relation to, charged, value-related events and those involved in them' (p. 40–41). Empathetic forms of understanding are facets that emerge from narrative accounts that can be indirectly experienced, even if stories are dissimilar to our own. The researcher is given a different way to receive and understand insights that can engage implicit right brain to right brain processes and empathetic awareness.

Herman (1997) argues that only 'when truth is finally recognised, survivors can begin their recovery' (p. 1). This means exploring the lived experience of survivorship where we might contest and erase some of the breaches of Othering as often 'trauma cannot be grasped because there are neither words nor categories of thought adequate to its representation' (Laub & Auerhahn, 1993, p. 301). APR as a framework honours the intersectional stance of the multiplicities of oppressions and how they interrelate, intersect, and interweave by seeking out the inclusion of the theorising voice of the Other. This becomes a construct of psychological knowledge and Self/Other experience that evoke the 'moral third'. This is a remembrance of the human community and the dignity we accorded to our fellow human beings (Benjamin, 2007). This suggests that the interaction between autoethnography and psychotherapy research is a journey of personal discovery and a self-reflective process that requires a 'thirdness' which is a psychological space facilitated by mutual recognition of being able to relate to the other's mind while allowing for the separateness and difference. As Benjamin (2007) says; 'we might say that the third is that to which we surrender, and thirdness is the intersubjective mental space that facilitates or results from surrender. In my thinking, the term surrender refers to a certain letting go of the self, and thus also implies the ability to take in the other's point of view or reality. Thus, surrender refers us to recognition—being able to sustain connectedness to the other's mind while accepting his separateness and difference. Surrender implies freedom from any intent to control or coerce' (p. 2).

Residing in and Around Ambiguities

The task hence is not to resolve ambiguities but reside in and around them to bring about heightened engagement and awareness of Self/Other contact to extend forms of empathy and an internal connection to the Other and a way for 'naming the unnameable, marking the unmarked, seeking the invisible' (Twine & Warren, 2000, p. 20). This method might support the process of repair within one's own story and critically evaluates the complexity and uncertainties we face in talking about ourselves and others. We face the fundamental contradictions of what it is to be human and act as a reliable witness to the testimonials that helps create a relational home for life narratives to cohere. Research as experience can provide, as Schwandt (1996) suggests, an embodied coherence and expansiveness that is impactful, authentic, and beautiful when undertaken with fidelity and relevance. Writing as a mode of inquiry, testimony, and survivorship becomes an embodiment of awareness and wisdom that attempts to validate and humanise experiences.

APR in Action

> Your pain is the breaking of the shell that encloses your understanding—*Gibran*

APR is highly intentional but is not explicitly structured. There are however some principles which I hope to capture in this section. Below are some ways in which APR can be implemented and used, starting with the questions in the reflection Box 5.2.

Box 5.2   Activity: You and APR
Doing APR often involves exploring some of these questions:

- Why are you writing this story?
- How are you willing to examine it and what might be the impact of this work?
- How has this experience shaped you or your life as a therapist?
- What are your assumptions about this narrative and how willing are you to be surprised?
- What are some of the 'unvoiced' research questions connected to this project?

Think about a story you want to tell, and question; can you *feel and press at the boundaries of the* story?

As an APR research practitioner, you might seek out areas of practice that are unformulated in some way that might feel ambiguous or unresolved to. Your search might challenge traditional forms of representation and the praxis of stuck places (Lather, 2001). You can, for instance, draw from what Hochschild (1994) describes as magnified moments or emotionally charged episodes in your practice or personal journey, questioning how this work might offer insights and contribute to the field of therapy? APR can be done by the lone researcher exploring self-other experience and in writing their own narrative account however, this process comes alive in collaboration and in action with others, where representation appears as relationship (Gergen & Gergen, 2002).

Engaging with the 4 'P's

The APR researcher might begin by using a reflexive journal (Etherington, 2004) to record the researcher journey and any transferential responses to the research or if viewing the research from an imaginal perspective, reflecting on which ancestral figures come to mind that might be championing or guiding the work from the sidelines? I would encourage research dialogues with supervisors and peers to elicit and identify what I describe as the 4 'P's, Pitfalls, Passions, Possibilities, and the Production of the project.

For example, the implications of insider research might for example challenge the notion of 'special insider status'. We cannot represent or speak for any group, but we can bring our unique representation to light, and recognise its impact and potential value. These are limitations which need to be addressed as part of our transparency. Autoethnographies are often also accused of being rooted in sentimental self-indulgence and narcissism. I am unapologetic about this as it is the same critique that is sometimes levelled at therapy. Indeed, evidence suggests that when self-narratives cohere, it seems to be associated with improved psychological capacities and mental health outcomes, as storytelling is fundamental to the human need to organise experience, and this can bring about possible psycho-social change.

In the early stages of your research, it is helpful to review the existing psychological literature in the field to identify both the body of work already undertaken and any potential gaps in our understanding. I would also recommend identifying how you want to analyse your data as part of your research design, as I am not convinced that we can analyse our own subjectivity through conventional methods. You will be required to enter the ongoing tensions between contrasting ontological and epistemological positions and think carefully about the prism you employ to capture your findings. You can use more traditional methods for analysing your data like thematic analysis, grounded theory, narrative analysis, and phenemological methods or stay closer to the spirit of the autoethnographic endeavour and explore more novel approaches.

Seek Out and Gather Evocative Stories

Stories are living things and their real life begins when they start to live in you. They never stop growing stories are subversive because they come from the other side and we can never inhabit all sides at once. If we are here, story speaks for there. They are the freest invention of our deepest selves. (Okri, 1997, p. 44)

Your Writing

How do you *write* an APR? In clarifying and identifying what kind of autoethnography style that you would like to bring to life, this is best done by reading as many autoethnographies as you can, as well as seeking out art and literature that communicate a story that has impact. It is often challenging to write evocatively and engagingly, and you might begin by experimenting with the quality and expression of your voice and write in a way that is in 'relationship' and in dialogue with the reader. You can use dramatic dialogue, showing rather than telling (Ellis, 2004) as you *live and feel with the story*. This can give space for the experience of 'Other' as ambivalent, specific, and complex that is open to multiple interpretations and a multiplicity of voices that are textual. This form of narrative writing as inquiry cannot be neatly chronologically ordered when temporality is itself may be disjointed and scattered. As Denzin and Lincoln (2002) suggest we might aspire to writing that is embodied, visceral, nonlinear, making new textual epiphanies.

This may involve the practice of overwriting, which is to layer narrative storying to redefine meaning, each layer is superimposed on other layers that alters and expands on the multiplicity of identities, rather like the therapeutic encounter in which layers of meaning, symbols, and language unfold. Another option is the interweaving of stories from a sequential model allowing each co-researcher to write their experience, the next co-researcher adds to and develops the story from their unique perspective, adding depth in a relational and collaborative emphasis between the researcher and researched.

Interviewing

The interviews within APR are active, intentional, and contextual; where stories can evolve and where meaningful dialogue allows for the research encounter to become a mutual learning ground. The engagement with research participants is an ongoing negotiation and process of meaning-making so they are described as 'co-researchers or collaborators' or make up an autoethnographic team. Collaboration can also be done partially, where different co-researchers collaborate on different aspects of the research process, for example some of the collaborators in my research wrote their own interpretive and artistic autoethnography that emerged from research dialogues rather than constricting academic prose. The need to attend to issues of power within the research project is hence important and this includes exploring your authorial intentions, reflexivity, voice and the emotional salience, and valence of stories (Ivanic, 1998). For example, who becomes a character in our account and who appears less perceptibly? Denzin and Lincoln (2003) describe collaborators as stakeholders within the research.

> **Box 5.3   Reflections Around Collaborators**
> Questions linked to my authorial intentions may involve wanting to know if I got close to my collaborator's subjectivity. How, if at all, did I miss them? Was this process overwhelming or limiting for them? What if anything surprised or changed something for them from the research experience?

An 'Intertextual' and Authentic Representation

APR produces an intertextual and authentic representation of a multivocal and polyvocal self in which the intersubjective narratives emerge but they are incomplete as important things are left unsaid within research process that continued to be unnarratable or withheld. By intertextual I mean to how self-experience, learning, and literature have influenced the researcher and how this conveys meaning within the project.

Within my own experience, I found that I struggled with the obligations and charged relationships that come from witnessing the testimonies and grappled with how traumatic and painful events interrupt experience and present difficulties in representational forms of writing (Lacapra, 1994). It is difficult to capture and be with the *incomprehensibility of the experience* that can remain in a raw uncon-structed state when researching sensitive subjects. The consequences of this are that some narratives cannot be coherently symbolised and many research conversations remain partial. As Bolkowsky (1987) suggests, the questions always seemed imper-tinent, gratuitous, insensitive. The answers always seemed incomplete, like shad-ows that are simultaneously real and unreal. Nothing is certain, no words adequate; there lurk an infinite and unfathomable number of meanings that are inexplicable and ungraspable (p. 218). This certainly echoed the intertextual experience as researcher that I grappled with as illustrated below:

> I have felt like a pioneer journeying to distant territories of the familiar with a compass that kept on moving me off course, pushing me further towards what seemed just out of reach, when I tried to capture the unvoiced narratives from my family's experience of racist trauma as we began to describe and record the fragmented and sometimes unspoken effects of deeply felt trauma. There were circles of repetitions. These repetitions embodied the voice of trauma and by removing this density and confusion for the benefit of the reader to orga-nise and clarify, I was struck there was much being was lost which was sometimes incom-prehensive, authentic, and fragmentary nature of the racist experience. The ontological multiplicity of subjectivities I inhabited within the narrative were as witness, testifier and narrator, inducing conflicting feelings of both failing and privilege at being invited into lost worlds/memories that were recovered and lost again as I tried to describe them for the story to make sense. This bewildering process of feeling lost and getting lost as a methodological stance meant that I was forced to seek out disjunctions in trying to inhabit new spaces and pathways. The broken remains of these understandings meant using archaeological imagin-ings by exposition and compassionate understanding. It requires that we feel lost at times, unsettled, and even derailed by what we find and feel. (Razzaq, 2007, p. 8)

In trying to deconstruct dominant knowledge about racism using autoethnography, I sometimes felt like I was being pushed onto the margins by dominant discourses that seemed to limit and discount. One reviewer stated, 'I do not think that readers on racism and psychotherapy will be at all interested in the details of debates over autoethnography and where it fits in with other research methodologies. Nor am I convinced that the concept of trauma is a useful way of making sense of the kind of constant everyday painful experiences that are associated with being on the receiv-ing end of racist attitudes. Trauma is a concept that has generally been associated with single powerful events (e.g. definitions of PTSD). The author may be in danger of losing the distinctive value of an autoethnographic approach (i.e. the creation of a richly textured account) by wrapping it up in a single concept in this way'. Another reviewer suggested that the autoethnographic parts should be erased, 'I would sug-gest a stronger focus on racism and trauma literature and theory with only a very brief sprinkling of your own story, I would be happy to have it reviewed'. I was anxious that this work would not find a suitable home, yet I was resolute, as the most painful experiences generated for the collaborators were their experiences being invalidated and silenced. The grief experienced in racist trauma is often voice-less and its unspoken nature can leave one feeling powerfully isolated. I bring this example by way of saying that when we use innovative and more radical practices and constructs there are sometimes challenges along the way. This means grappling with adversity and critical evaluation when trying to deconstruct the privileging of existing assumptions and paradigms. I also recognise that APR like other methodologies can potentially reproduce the very power structures it seeks to challenge by privileging academic structures over other forms of dialogue.

Creative Analytic Practices

Remember everyone who touches you affects your healing. (Franks, 2002, p. 369)

Creative Analytic Practices capture research conversations and allow for stories themselves to act as both product and text (Ellis, 1997, 1999, 2004, 2007. This can form the 'data analysis' or what I prefer to call 'human storying'. These methods can involve using clay, artwork, writing, poetry, performance, song, meditation, drama, somatic resonance, and photographs that can activate right brain interactions that are beyond and beneath words, and nonverbal bodily based affective material within the implicit can capture and tap into the novel and unexpected, contained within a research framework. These potential deep research experiences and creative forms such as drama, poetry, multi-voiced or co-narratives involve relationality and resonance that sometimes relate to Gendlin's idea of 'felt sense' (1996, p. 32). I used photos to elicit memories within some research dialogues and one of my collaborators made artwork to express his emotional responses to our research conversations which he described as 'dramatic and fierce' embodied representations of racism. Within the research conversations themselves, I noted any poetic expressions, styles of speech, words, and syntax that allowed multiple selves and voices to emerge. The collaborators within the research wrote a collective poem that was an interweaving of communal multi-voicing. I take from Buechler's (2004) idea that poetry asks us to 'bear the ambiguity of the unfinished thought. We have to wade into a poem, letting it wash over us, feeling it out. If we demand that it immediately surrender its meaning to our forces of reason, we are likely to get nowhere' (p. 234). One of the collaborators within the family group found the research process became a vehicle that helped him acknowledge his pain and this was reparative. He felt less alone when he imagined his story maybe useful to others who might be struggling to heal and beyond, as it is taken into the wider field. As Brison (1999) says, 'Individualized stories become collective one and are essential to avoid the dehumanizing abstractions that allow people to forget or trivialize the suffering of others' (p. 34).

In fact, the Viva process could not be concluded without taking the collaborators with me, through the representation of food, music, tapestry, and poetry on the examination day, the memories of this are savoured with gladness and gratitude. I recall a journey that *could not have been done alone and that ultimately made me feel less alone*. Research that engages with representation, therapeutic possibilities, and the transformative or subversive aspects of stories and re-authoring the self often feels overwhelming and complex. Research is also sometimes isolating and difficult to endure; therefore having collaborators provided both accountability and an assembly of relationships that can be sustaining. Some of them made up an 'internal chorus' that cheered me on which Buechler (2004) has developed to support the challenges of being a therapist that I believe is also applicable to the researcher's journey. The internal chorus is the 'internalized voices help us bear the strains of our work... My own internal chorus includes many of my teachers, analysts, and supervisors, as well as theoreticians who have influenced me through their writing and includes the poets, painters and pets, as kind of assembly of wise elders ...all of whom taught me something about living life as a human being... those who have been kind or at the very least it can make us feel less lonely. Our internal chorus light the path, it's a compass, driving away some fears of the dark but not always telling us which way to go...so we can respond to the other, even when you feel besieged, exhausted, in danger of retaliating' (p. 111).

Resonance and Impact

APR and other qualitative methodologies have no claim of mainstream generalisability and validity has been reconceptualised. Denzin and Lincoln (2003) emphasise textual reflexivity, textual self-exposure, multiplicity of voices, and a diverse range of literary representation. In conjoining forms of representation, the researcher mediates against their own interpretations and authority by the participants writing their own accounts, as in the research I undertook, the therapist's written autoethnographies mediated against the all-powerful and all-knowing researcher voice and by generating stories from varied sources. The researcher takes the research findings/narrations back to the collaborators to assess truth claims and attention is paid to the ethical dilemmas and contingencies faced in this process. The methods of representation are varied and interpretative in nature, where narratives can be co-joined and co-written collaborations or distributed representations between collaborators should include an analysis of the consequences of these alternative forms of relational research. The researcher's inquiry should strive to include the collaborators being encouraged to challenge interpretations and question how the data might be heard.

The audience becomes a witness to the testimony of the researcher and collaborators and through this, they themselves become implicated in what they are witnessing as part of the experience as a vehicle to be named and heard. This reciprocal relationship with the audience is one marked by mutual responsibility and participation that become part of an ongoing conversation of the work, hoping for readers to bring the same careful attention to your words in the context of their own lives (Denzin & Lincoln, 2003). As Ellis & Bochner (2000) suggest validity strives for verisimilitude, credibility, and is an interpretative activity as the focus shifts to readers and the extent to which they think the writing is meaningful to them. Does the work resonate, or does it speak to the reader of lives known and unknown? How is the work relational and collaborative? How is it useful and impactful in the wider context? Reliability in the research is local and based on specific interactions with others in the research field (Kiesinger, 2002).

Relational Ethics

We intentionally try and generate research that is galvanising and impactful as we question how can one be a non-exploitative researcher (Pillow, 2003) and examine how researcher's privilege might influence and impact upon those you intend to research. APR acts on a continuum allowing the researcher to select their level of comfort with the use of self-disclosure and interpretation of socio-cultural-political-intrapsychic self in context. In the early stages it is worthwhile reflecting on the implications of expressing vulnerability and pain in our writing and in taking authorship of such stories means examining the effects of exposure, disclosure of others and ourselves. Indeed, it can feel taboo to name one's experiences openly, initially for me it felt like contravening boundaries and risking exposure for myself and others. What are the ethics of taking this into the public world? What would the research do to our relationship? Would I be derided and discounted by the 'therapeutic community' for revealing not just myself but my family? However, there is a desire to start conversations that are not easily spoken, embedded within an optimistic spirit of wanting to ask, 'how can we make a connection' and 'how can I make the implicit explicit'. This means holding the relational ethics of honesty, mourning and the tensions of considered self-disclosure feel less prohibitive for me now, as this method uses the perspective and action of the subjects as a point of departure and ongoing co-collaboration is necessary. Also, the complexities inherent in struggling with fragmentation and reparation have helped establish coherent connections amongst life events and closely align with my therapeutic contact. APR invites intentional self-disclosure that can accelerate meaning and generativity that is humanising if used discriminatingly and ethically.

Within this there may be a need to place the ethical consequences of self-disclosure and self-representation first, as a powerful emotional instrument of insight and healing. Tolich (2010) suggests we investigate if those within the text have rights and hold in mind that the researcher should not publish anything they would not show those within the writing. He lists ethical guidelines for writing an evocative autoethnography to support the researcher through these complex waters. I also found Clandinin and Connelly's (2004) question: do we own the story because we tell it, helpful to hold in mind. This means recognising that stories can be equally misappropriated and used to oppress. Those who appear in such stories can be aggrandised, valorised, and made into a reluctant or unwanted hero. This means exploring the problematic nature of self-representation and being interested and transparent about ethically important moments in research (Guillemin, 2004). Being ethical in psychotherapy is the obvious adherence to the code of conduct promulgated by BPS, UKCP, and so on and the ethics of our contexts—but this is not only what makes a psychotherapist ethical. What it does not provide us with is what it means to be with another human being, as ethical codes cannot do our questioning, and responding for us. Our ethics are an active dynamic process as we acknowledge our relationships and interpersonal bonds to others with reflection and negotiation, and the possible changing nature of relationships both interpersonal and professional (Ellis, 2004).

Summary

Meaningful research requires that we both acknowledge both our privilege and make space for our courage. APR requires courage and the use of one's vulnerability which is why this method is not suitable for everyone, as it demands we seek and embrace our ache and pain and we burn it as fuel for our journey, as a painstaking form of excavation that brings a visceral experience into a place of existence and availability. As a result, I began to believe that the obstacles that we sometimes find along the way could contribute to the richness of one's existence. I have realised I have been writing my research for much of my life. Now that it is committed to paper, I can see how it has helped me to be more compassionate therapist and find a place to give my story a home. By expanding on the concept of Autoethnographic Psychotherapeutic Research and how to implement it in practice, this chapter aims to support you along a similar journey.

References

Bager-Charleson, S., & McBeath. (2020). *Enjoying research in counselling and psychotherapy qualitative.* Quantitative and Mixed Methods Research.
Barone, T., & Eisner, E. (2012). *Arts based research.* Sage.
Benjamin, J, (2007) *Intersubjectivity, Thirdness, and mutual recognition from a talk given at the institute for contemporary psychoanalysis.* Los Angeles, CA. https://icpla.edu/wp-content/uploads/2013/03/Benjamin-J.-2007-ICP-Presentation-Thirdness-present-send.pdf.
Bolkowsky, S. (1987). In J. In Kauffman (Ed.), *Loss of the assumptive world, a theory of traumatic loss* (p. 218). Brunner Routledge Taylor Francis Group.
Bouchner, A. (2017). Heart of the matter, a mini manifesto for autoethnography. *International Review of Qualitative Research, 10*(1), 67–80. https://doi.org/10.1525/irqr.2017.10.1.67
Brison, S. J. (1999). *Aftermath: Violence and the remaking of a self.* Princeton University Press.
Buechler, S. (2004). *Clinical values emotions that guide psychoanalytic treatment.* Routledge.
Clandinin, J. D., & Connelly, M. F. (2004). *Narrative inquiry: Experience and story in qualitative research.* Wiley Jossey Bass.
Crossley, M. (2000). *Introducing narrative psychology: Self, trauma, and the construction of meaning.* Open University Press.
Denzin, N. K. (1997). *Interpretive Ethnography: Ethnographic Practices for the 21st Century.* Thousand Oaks, CA: Sage. https://doi.org/10.4135/9781452243672
Denzin, N. K. (2018). *Performance (auto) ethnography: Critical pedagogy and the politics of culture.* Taylor & Francis.
Denzin, N. K., & Lincoln, Y. S. (Eds.). (2002). *The qualitative inquiry reader.* Sage Publications.
Denzin, N. K., & Lincoln, Y. S. (2003). *Collecting and interpreting qualitative research materials.* Sage.

Denzin, N. K., Lincoln, Y. S., & Smith, L. T. (Eds.). (2008). *Handbook of critical and indigenous methodologies*. Sage.

Dunne, T., & Ly-Donpvan, C. (2020). Wicked stepmother, best friend, and the unaccounted space between: A critical duoethnography of (step)m(other)ing in blended families. *Journal of Autoethnography, 2*(1), 55–74. https://doi.org/10.1525/joae.2021.2.1.55

Ellis, C. (1995). *Final negotiations; a story of love, loss and chronic illness*. Temple Press.

Ellis, C. (1997). *Evocative autoethnography: Writing emotionally about our lives in representation and the text: Re-framing the narrative voice*. SUNY Press.

Ellis, C. (1999). He(art)ful autoethnography. *Qualitative Health Research, 9*, 653–657.

Ellis, C. (2004). *The ethnographic I, A methodological novel about autoethnography*. Altamira.

Ellis, C. (2007). Telling secrets, revealing lives: Relational ethics in research with intimate others. *Qualitative Inquiry, 13*(1), 3–29.

Ellis, C., & Bochner, A. (2000). Autoethnography, personal narrative, reflexivity: Researcher as subject. In N. K. Denzin & Y. S. Lincoln (Eds.), *Sage handbook of qualitative research* (pp. 733–768). Sage.

Ellis, C., & Bochner, A. (Eds.). (2002). *Ethnographically speaking: Autoethnography, literature and aesthetics*. Altamira Press.

Ellis, C., Boucher, A., & Berry, K. (2006). Implicated audience members seeks understanding; re-examining the gift of autoethnography. *International Journal of Qualitative Methods, 5*(7), 119.

Etherington, K. (2004). *Becoming a reflexive researcher - using our selves in research*. Jessica Kingsley Publishers.

Foucault, M. (1977). *Discipline and punish: The birth of the prison* (A. Sheridan, Trans.). New York: Vintage.

Fox, K. (1996). Silent voices: A subversive Reading of child sexual abuse. In C. Ellis & A. Bochner (Eds.), *Composing ethnography*. AltaMira.

Franks, A. (2002). Between the ride and the story: Illness and Remoralisation. In C. Ellis & A. Bochner (Eds.), *Ethnographically speaking: Autoethnography, literature and aesthetics* (pp. 357–371). Altamira Press.

Gadamer, H. (1975). *Truth and method*. Continuum.

Garratt, D. (2014). Psychoanalytic-autoethnography: Troubling natural bodybuilding. *Qualitative Inquiry, 21*, 343–353.

Gendlin, E. (1996). *Experiencing and the creation of meaning: A philosophical and psychological approach to the subjective*. North-western University Press.

Gergen, K. J., & Gergen, M. M. (2002). Qualitative inquiry: Tensions and transformations. In N. K. Denzin & Y. S. Lincoln (Eds.), *The landscape of qualitative research: Theories and Issues* (pp. 575–610). Sage.

Guillemin, M. (2004). Ethics, reflexivity, and "ethically important moments" in Research. *Qualitative Inquiry, 10*, 261.

Herman, J. L. (1997). *Trauma and recovery: From domestic abuse to political terror*. Basic Books.

Hochschild, A. 1994. The commercial spirit of intimate life and the abduction of feminism: Signs from women's advice books. Theory, Culture and Society, 11(2): 1–24.

Ivanic, R. (1998). *Writing and identity: Discourses construction of identity in academic writing*. John Benjamin.

Kiesinger, C. (2002). My Father's shoes: The value of narrative reframing. In C. Ellis & A. Bochner (Eds.), *Ethnographically speaking: Autoethnography literature and aesthetics* (pp. 94–114). Alta Mira Press.

Lacapra, D. (1994). *Representing the holocaust, history, theory trauma*. Cornell University Press.

Lather, P. (2001). Postbook: Working the ruins of feminist ethnography. *Journal of Women in Culture and Society, 27*, 199–227.

Laub, D., & Auerhahn, N. (1993). Knowing and not knowing massive psychic trauma: forms of traumatic memory. *International Journal of Psychoanalysis, 74*, 287–302.

Morrison, T. (1992). *Playing in the dark, whiteness and the literary imagination*. Harvard University Press.

Norris, J., Sawyer, R. D., & Lund, D. E. (Eds.). (2012). *Duoethnography. Dialogic methods for social, health, and educational research.* Left Coast Books.

Okri, B. (1997). *A way of being free.* Weindenfield and Nicholson.

Pelias, R. J. (2005). Performative writing as scholarship: An apology, an argument, an anecdote. *Cultural Studies, Critical Methodologies, 5,* 415–424.

Pennycook, A. (1994). Towards a critical pedagogy for teaching English as a worldly language. In A. Pennycook (Ed.), *The cultural politics of English as an international language* (pp. 295–327). Longman.

Pillow, W. S. (2003). Confession, catharsis or cure? Rethinking the uses of reflexivity as methodological power in qualitative research. *The International Journal of Qualitative Research in Education, 16*(2), 175–196.

Pizer, S. (2016). Put down the duckie. In A. R. Ben-Shahar (Ed.), *When hurt remains: Relational perspectives on therapeutic failure.* Routledge.

Razzaq, S. (2007), *An autoethnographic exploration into transforming the wounds of racism: Implications for psychotherapy.* Doctor in psychotherapy by professional studies. (A joint programme between the National Centre for Work based Learning Partnerships Middlesex University and Metanoia Institute.

Razzaq, S. (2017) Autoethography workshop presentation at The Metanioa Research Academy Conference

Saldaña, J. (2016). *The coding manual for qualitative researchers* (3rd ed.). Sage.

Schwandt, T. A. (1996). Farewell to criteriology. *Qualitative Inquiry, 2*(1), 58–72. https://doi.org/10.1177/107780049600200109

Tierney, W., & Lincoln, Y. (Eds.). (1997). *Representations and the text: Re-framing the narrative voice.* State University of New York Press.

Tolich. (2010). A critique of current practice: Ten foundational guidelines for autoethnographers. *Qualitative Health Research, 20*(12), 1599–1610. https://doi.org/10.1177/1049732310376076

Toyosaki, S., Pensoneau-Conway, S. L., Wendt, N. A. & Leathers, K. (2009). Community autoethnography: Compiling the personal and resituating whiteness. *Cultural Studies Critical Methodologies, 9*(1), 56–83.

Twine, F., & Warren, J. (Eds.). (2000). *Racing research, researching race: Methodological dilemmas in critical race studies.* University Press.

White, M. (1995). *Re-authoring lives: Interviews and essays.* Dulwich Centre.

Part II
Quantitative Research

Chapter 6
Quantitative Practice-Based Research

Emily Banwell, Terry Hanley, and Aaron Sefi

Learning Goals

After reading this chapter you should be able to:

- Know which types of research questions, within real-world counselling and psychotherapy practice, can be answered with quantitative methods
- Understand how studies within the field are designed, by looking at two example studies
- Understand how quantitative findings are used to inform practice
- Critically evaluate the extent to which quantitative research methods can 'humanise numbers'

Introduction: Key Concepts in Quantitative Research

What Is Quantitative Research?

Quantitative research refers to the collection and interpretation of numerical data. The data used in quantitative research usually comes from:

- Statistics
- Routinely collected **demographic** data

E. Banwell • T. Hanley (✉)
University of Manchester, Manchester, UK
e-mail: Terry.Hanley@manchester.ac.uk; emily.banwell@manchester.ac.uk

A. Sefi
Kooth, London, UK
e-mail: aaron@kooth.com

S. Bager-Charleson, A. McBeath (eds.), *Supporting Research in Counselling and Psychotherapy*, https://doi.org/10.1007/978-3-031-13942-0_6

- Survey responses
- Assessment measures, completed either by the client or a practitioner

Descriptive and Inferential Statistics

How do we use this data to draw meaningful conclusions for our research? What can we identify from the data that we have for each **variable**? A variable is a characteristic or quantity that has been measured to obtain the data. These can include demographics like age, gender, or ethnicity, as well as responses to items within a questionnaire. For example, how many clients within the **sample** rated their therapeutic session as 'excellent'? An **independent variable (IV)** is a variable that might have an influence on the outcome. For example age, gender, or whether (or not) a client received a certain type of therapy. A **dependent variable (DV)**, on the other hand, can be seen as more of an output: essentially *depending* on the values of the IV. This could be therapeutic outcomes, or responses to a measure. **Descriptive statistics** allow us to summarise data based upon its properties, and begin to identify patterns within. The three main types of descriptive statistics are as follows:

1. Measures of **frequency**—used to establish how often a response or characteristic features in the data. This is usually established with counts, percentages, or frequencies.
2. Measures of **central tendency**—used to find out how typical a certain response or characteristic is. This can be done by calculating the **arithmetic mean** (summing the responses under the variable of interest, and dividing it by the number of responses), the **mode** (the most common response), or the **median** (the response that lies at the middle of the distribution so that there is an equal likelihood of a value falling either higher or lower than this).
3. Measures of **dispersion**—used to show how data is spread. Data that is very spread out can influence how the mean average is interpreted—we might ask 'how representative of the data set is this mean?' **Outliers**, data points that are considered extreme scores, might distort the mean somewhat. Dispersion can be examined by looking at the **range** (the difference between the highest and lowest values), and the **standard deviation** (the average of the squared differences from the mean). The standard deviation provides an indication of how far most values deviate from the mean. This is best explained alongside the concept of a **normal distribution** curve (Fig. 6.1). This represents a situation where data is clustered around a middle point. An example of data that tends to be normally distributed is Intelligence Quotient (IQ) score. Most people's scores are clustered around the 100 value, with fewer scoring either very low or very high.

Inferential statistics allow relationships between variables to be investigated. This allows *inferences* to be made from the sample that can be applied to the general **population**.

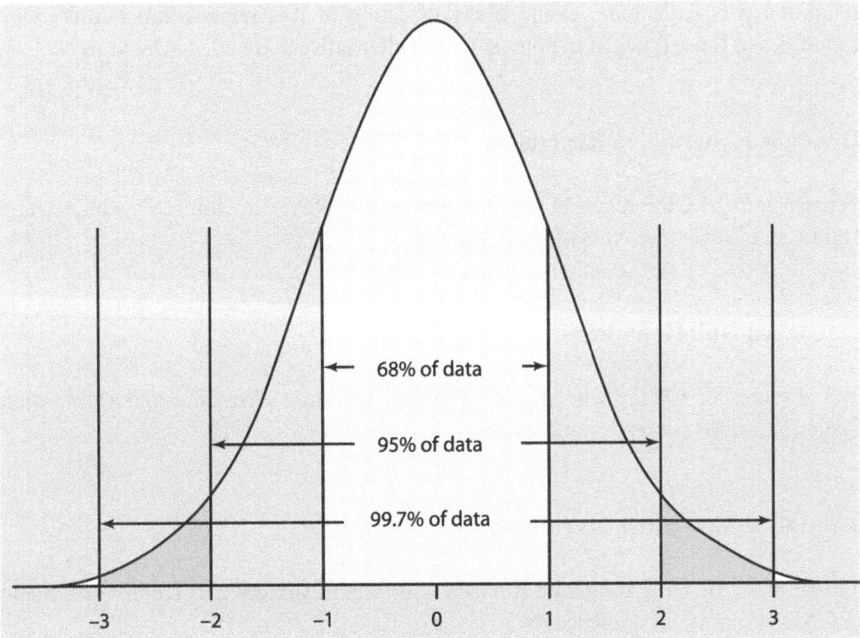

Fig. 6.1 Example of a normal distribution, adapted from McBeath (2020)

Table 6.1 Examples of parametric and non-parametric tests

	Hypothesis tests	Regression analyses
Parametric tests	t-Tests	Linear regression
	Analysis of variance (ANOVA) tests	Logistic regression
Non-parametric tests	Wilcoxon signed rank test	Non-parametric regression analyses
	Mann-Whitney U test	

Hypothesis Tests

There are two main types of inferential statistical tests, which can be conducted to investigate, commonly with the use of **statistical packages**, the **research questions** that we have. Table 6.1. shows just some examples of these tests.

The first key type of inferential test is a **hypothesis test**. A hypothesis is a prediction, made on the basis of previous evidence, that we wish to test with our research. When planning research, it is important to clearly lay out what the two possible overarching **conclusions** that we can draw from our research are: essentially, whether or not we find support for our hypothesis. The **null hypothesis** states that no relationship between variables exists. When this is not the case, the **alternative hypothesis** is accepted, stating that this predicted relationship was evidenced. Each hypothesis can be **one-tailed** or **two-tailed**. A one-tailed hypothesis predicts that a relationship in only one direction is expected. With a two-tailed hypothesis, a relationship is expected, yet the likely direction of this relationship is unknown. Examples of these types of hypotheses, both alternative and null, can be found below.

One-tailed Alternative Hypothesis

Ten sessions of CBT result in lower scores on the Revised Children's Anxiety and Depression Scale (RCADS) for adolescents.

One-tailed Null Hypothesis

Ten sessions of CBT do not reduce Revised Children's Anxiety and Depression Scale (RCADS) scores for adolescents.

Two-tailed Alternative Hypothesis

Ten sessions of CBT influence Revised Children's Anxiety and Depression Scale (RCADS) scores for adolescents.

Two-tailed Null Hypothesis

Ten sessions of CBT have no effect on adolescents' Revised Children's Anxiety and Depression Scale (RCADS) scores.

How do we know that a true relationship exists between variables? Sticking to the simple example outlined in the above hypotheses, how would we identify whether a true difference in RCADS score exists when comparing them before and after a course of CBT? Inferential hypothesis tests are used to investigate the assumptions and predictions that we have. **Parametric** hypothesis tests work with the premise that variables from the population sample follow a normal distribution. These typically involve comparing mean scores of participant groups or timepoints. When there are two means to compare, a **t-test** is conducted, and an **analysis of variance (ANOVA)** is conducted when more than two means need to be compared. These tests exist in several forms, depending on if the two means come from the same or different participants. Whilst more intricate forms of each exist, the key distinction is as follows. If an individual's scores, taken at several timepoints, are compared, a *paired samples t-test* or a *within-subjects ANOVA* is chosen. If we are comparing two types of individuals, for example if we wanted to test if scores on a measure, completed once, differed between those with a diagnosis of depression and those without, an *independent samples t-test* or a *between-subjects ANOVA* is the appropriate test.

It is worth reminding you here that parametric tests are used under the main assumption that data points are normally distributed within the sample. In the instance that this assumption is not met, a **non-parametric** equivalent may be employed to help investigate our hypotheses. The **Mann-Whitney U test** (for independent samples) and the **Wilcoxon signed rank test** (for a within-subjects study design) compare *medians* rather than *means*, and aim to identify, based on these, differences between variables. Whilst parametric tests have a stronger ability to detect differences, and are therefore preferable, non-parametric alternatives are also valuable when the data is not suitable for these.

Regression Analyses

The other key type of inferential tests, as you can see from Table 6.1, are tests of **regression**. These tests are used to investigate the effects that variables have on each other. In essence, does a change in one variable lead to a change in the other, and to what extent? An example investigation might be whether the number of therapeutic sessions has an influence on scores of a mental health symptom measure. The most frequently used of these regression methods is **linear regression**. This method is used to quantify how many units of change in the IV result in a change in the DV.

Statistical Significance

How do we interpret the results of these statistical tests? The key piece of information that tells us whether a difference, a relationship, or an effect is found is the **significance value.** This value, known as a **p-value,** is a probability statement, that when interpreted tells us whether the null hypothesis should be rejected or accepted. The p-value, which appears in the output of statistical tests conducted in most software packages, is given as a figure from 0–1, signifies the probability that the results we see are down to chance, or if there is indeed a true observation to be made as a result of the comparisons made in the test. Within psychology, a significant value of $p = <0.05$ is deemed to be statistically significant. This value signifies a 1 in 20 chance of the null hypothesis being true. Anything above 0.05 suggests that our results are due to chance, and that the null hypothesis should be accepted. Anything below suggests that a systematic relationship between variables is present, which is unlikely to be down to chance alone. In this case, the null hypothesis is usually rejected.

What Types of Questions can be Answered with Quantitative Research Methods?

With qualitative research, which uses data collection methods like interviews, focus groups, or observations, we usually wish to explore our participants' lived experiences and personal stories: what a phenomenon, situation, or identity means to

Table 6.2 The three main types of quantitative research questions

Type of research question	Questions relating to…	Example question
1. Descriptive research questions	• How many…? • How often…? • What percentage of…?	How many 18–25 year olds received CBT in your practice in 2019?
2. Comparative research questions	• What is the difference between…?	What is the difference in therapeutic outcome between depressed and non-depressed clients?
3. Relationship-based research questions	• How are X and Y associated? • What is the relationship between…?	What is the relationship between annual income and depression?

them. Quantitative studies, on the other hand, typically answer three main types of questions outlined in Table 6.2.

Sometimes, qualitative and quantitative questions are present within the same study. Known as **mixed methods** studies, the two lines of enquiry can be included either as separate elements, where qualitative and quantitative investigations are conducted side-by-side to approach a topic from different angles, or they can be sequentially linked. This can be where themes or discussion points raised in qualitative data are further explored quantitatively, or alternatively where a more detailed qualitative insight is required to delve deeper into responses that were provided quantitatively. It is common, especially in people-focussed fields like counselling, for quantitative studies to follow or prelude qualitative research in this way. An example of this can be found later on in this chapter under 'Developing a Theory of Change', and more information on mixed-methods study designs can be found in Hanson et al.'s (2005) paper (see 'further reading').

Humanising Numbers

You might be asking, as a researcher of counselling practice, 'how is my client represented in a quantitative study of their data?' It is easy to see, especially when compared to qualitative research, how all the terms you have learned above, like 'variable', 'statistical test', 'p-value', seem a little depersonalised. How, then, is the 'person' represented in quantitative work? If the richness of your clients' unique experiences is something that you wish to capture, we must admit, a qualitative approach is probably the one you are looking for. However, the key way in which a client, or participant, can be represented within a dataset is with the type of analytical **design** used. In a **between-subjects** design, participants are assigned, either deliberately or as a natural consequence, to one condition only. The participants in each condition are then compared. An example of this would be comparing age groups, or genders, on how they respond to a question. Alternatively, in **within-subjects** designs, often used for **longitudinal** studies, the same group of subjects is examined more than once, and their responses are compared each time. An example of this would be issuing an outcome measure at several times across the therapeutic process, to examine how their responses change. A **mixed-factors** design combines elements of both. Here, a researcher might compare responses to a measure over time (the **within-subjects** element), however they might also be interested in how any changes might differ depending on gender (the **between-subjects**) element. Our earlier section on *hypothesis tests* gives a brief explanation of how these types of research design impacts which statistical tests are purposefully chosen to answer the questions that we have. Our two examples of practice-based counselling research studies, later on in the chapter, will shed more light on how personalised measures can be measured statistically.

What Is Practice-based Quantitative Research, and What Can It Tell Us?

So how does this all link to the counselling field? What can the numerical or statistical data that is collected by our services tell us? What insights can be gained, and how can it help improve things going forwards? As you are probably aware, therapeutic practice has the potential to generate large amounts of numerical data. Lots of information is recorded, and outcome and experience measures are completed frequently. This data has the potential to tell us:

- What is working, and what is not working, including for whom, and why…
- which can, in turn, show us where time, effort, money, or further research attention should be dedicated

The latter point is worth expanding on here. As well as having utility within our own practice, our research can generate new knowledge that can contribute to the wider research field. The insights that we gained can potentially, if we have enough **statistical power,** be **generalised** or **transferred** to the wider population. If we find out, for example, that a certain type of person responds to a treatment in a particular way, other practitioners might be able to extend this knowledge to their own work. At a wider level, this type of applicability can lead to wider scale funding and policy changes as well as stimulating further research. Indeed, most researchers know that research tends to produce more questions and 'unknowns' than it answers! This can be within the field of counselling and psychotherapy research, or findings may be more widely transferable, into the fields of mental health, psychology, or digital health, to name just a few examples.

Activity 6.1   What Kinds of Numerical Data Do You Collect in Your Practice or Workplace?

Spend 5 minutes thinking about the numerical data that is collected within your practice or workplace. Note down the answers to the following questions:

- What type of data is this?
- How is it collected? By whom?
- Who does the data come from? What ethical issues should be considered before using it in research?

Once you have your list information, now move to consider what you might be able to do with it. Consider:

- What types of questions could you answer with this data?
- How could these answers guide practice going forward? Who might they help?
- What steps could you take to ensure that the person is represented in the research?

As a final part of this activity, consider if there are types of information that you are not collecting. Consider:

- What type of data could be collected? Would it be easy to collect?
- Do you think that doing so would be beneficial? Why?
- What types of questions could you answer with this potential data?
- How could these answers guide practice going forward? Who might they help?

Quantitative Research in Practice

The following sections of this chapter reflect upon a series of collaborative projects between academics based at the University of Manchester in the UK and professionals working for the online counselling and support service, Kooth. Kooth's main service offers text-based counselling and support for young people aged between 11 and 25. It is free and anonymous at the point of access to young people, with individuals only having to give very limited information to access support. It received approximately 1700 log-ins per day in 2019 and this increased to over 3000 log-ins on the day schools were shut due to COVID-19 restrictions in March 2020. Kooth also offer services for adults. Both the services for young people and adults have a humanistic underpinning, prizing the uniqueness of those accessing the services and believing that positive growth can occur if the right environment is provided (Bugental, 1964), and offer pluralistic support that is responsive to the people who access them (Cooper & McLeod, 2011).

The roots of the projects reported here are underpinned by the hope to gain a greater understanding of the growing practice of offering web-based support to young people and young adults. In particular, we were interested in pooling together our different perspectives of this work to more fully understand how young people make use of the resources on offer and what might be viewed as successful service engagement. This endeavour comes, in part, because of the observed limitations of existing frames of understanding successful therapeutic work in this context. For example, attempting to make use of commonplace outcome measures for therapy in this context proved problematic due to the varied ways that individuals made use of the resources on offer to them (Sefi & Hanley, 2012).

Developing a Theory of Change

Given the above, a series of work was undertaken to develop a **Theory of Change** (ToC) for Kooth. A ToC can be defined as 'a sequence of events that is expected to lead to a particular desired outcome' (Davies, 2012, p. 1). It involves investigating ways of working in great detail with a view to identifying which activities offered by a service lead to which outcomes (Kail & Lumley, 2012). For us, this meant developing a core working group of academics, service managers, and professionals to discuss the work being entered into. From this, four service pathways were identified based upon the ways that young people were using the website. These were (i) Therapeutic content and peer support, (ii) Reactive/responsive therapeutic support, (iii) Structured therapy, and (iv) Ongoing therapeutic support. See Fig. 6.2 for brief descriptions of these pathways.

Once the service pathways had been identified and described, the group then moved to the task of identifying what successful engagement may look like in each of these. This led to the articulation of a ToC for each pathway. Once these were created these were shared and discussed for coherence with a wider group of professionals and a panel of young people. Due to space, it is not possible to describe the full ToC here (this can be found in this publication: Hanley et al. (2019)), but the process highlighted the complexity of each pathway and the way that they require different ways of monitoring the work that individuals are engaged in. It also highlighted the way that the Kooth resource might be viewed as a multifaceted ecosystem. Indeed, ultimately, we described Kooth as a Positive Virtual Ecosystem (+VE) to reflect the caring and supportive multifaceted resource that it is. This initial statement has subsequently evolved and been developed into a statement related to Kooth's work with adult populations too (Noble et al., 2021).

As with all exploratory research, the development of the ToC raises more questions than it provides answers. Whilst they offer rich understanding of what clients want from the different resources and helped to articulate what successful support might look like, they raise numerous questions about how this success might be monitored. It is at this point that the projects described in this chapter start to develop and a second chapter of the ToC work begins. Within this new phase, the project has moved to proactively develop tools and resources that appropriately capture the changes occurring in peoples' lives whilst they are in contact with the service. As

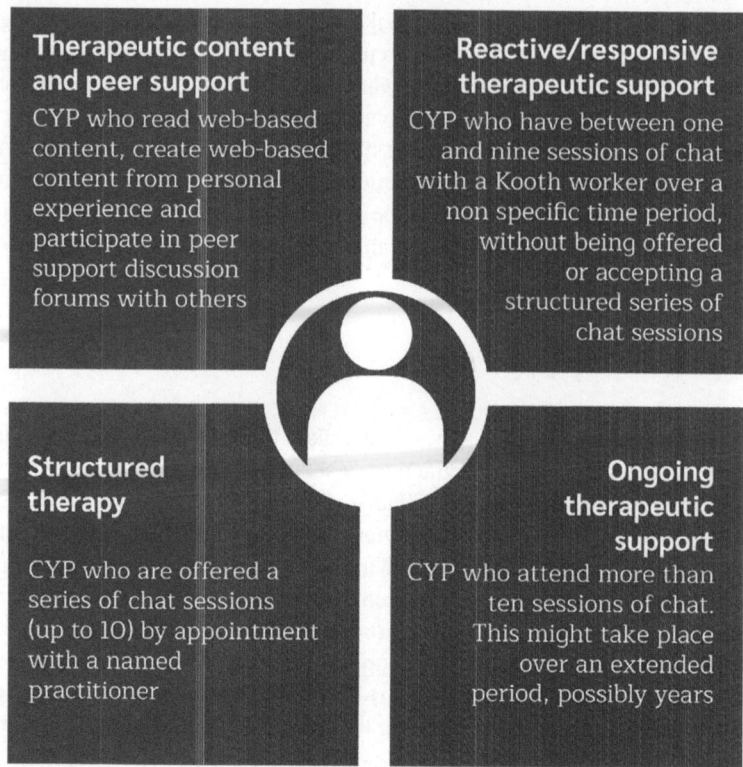

Fig. 6.2 The four service pathways of Kooth

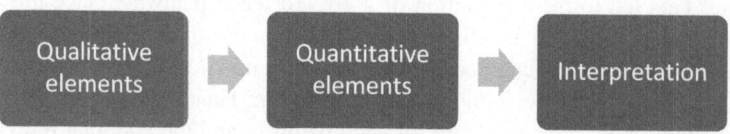

Fig. 6.3 The exploratory sequential mixed methods design

such, whilst separated for practical reasons, the work here may be viewed as an exploratory sequential mixed methods research project (Hanson et al., 2005), with the qualitative ToC work being complemented with a series of quantitative projects aiming at testing the evaluative tools that are being embedded into the online resource (see Fig. 6.3). Ultimately, the combination of the qualitative and quantitive elements will be viewed and interpreted together with a view to considering the utility of the ToC that are being proposed.

Before moving on to describe and discuss two of the projects that have emerged within the second phase of the ToC work, it is important to revisit the ethos of the service. As noted above, it is underpinned by humanistic principles and offers pluralistic support—it does not believe that one size of therapy can fit all. This stance to therapeutic work and support means that, unlike many psychological services, it does not have a primary focus upon pre-existing diagnostic categories. In contrast, the service prizes the idea that individuals have agency and are able to articulate their own wants from the services that they access. This position means that many of the **nomothetic psychometric measures**, that have predetermined questions and are often used to capture change in specific symptoms in therapy, do not have the same currency. Instead, **idiographic measures**, that rely on the client articulating what they want from the resources they are accessing, provide a more flexible and responsive way of monitoring change. These latter tools therefore support researchers in capturing more personalised numerical data that can reflect change in therapeutic work. The studies that follow make use of one idiographic measure, a Goal-Based Outcome (GBO) measure, and a purpose-built nomothetic/idiographic hybrid measure, the Session Wants and Needs Outcome Measure (SWAN-OM). Both place the individual's goals at the centre of (i) the therapeutic work and (ii) its evaluation.

We will now outline two examples of practice-based research, one that involved adult clients, and one focussed on young people. As you read through, try to think about the different research designs that are used, and how well the person is represented in each piece of research—how well are the numbers 'humanised'?

Study 1: The Use of Goal-based Outcome Measures in Digital Therapy with Adults: What Goals Are Set, and Are They Achieved?

Background and study rationale: Service-users who are clear on why they are attending therapeutic sessions tend to have more favourable outcomes than those who are not (Geurtzen et al., 2020). Goal-focussed therapy, especially when goals are set alongside a practitioner (Tryon et al., 2018), has shown a number of positive outcomes in research conducted to date, however much of this research was in children and young people's (CYP) counselling settings (Jacob et al., 2017, 2020). There is a clear lack of knowledge about how adults engage with therapeutic goal setting, including the types of goals they set, and their engagement with and attainment of these goals. Findings from CYP research can only be tentatively transferred to adult populations. More specific investigation is needed to identify whether goal-focussed therapy is a useful means of progress for adults who receive psychotherapy. This includes research into their engagement with idiographic goal-based outcome measures (GBOs; (Law & Jacob, 2015), as a means of recording progress made towards goal actualisation. With web-based therapy becoming an increasingly popular alternative to face-to-face sessions, exploring these topics within this context will provide a timely and relevant addition to this emerging body of literature.

Research objectives: This study looked at how GBOs were used to monitor progress made within a pluralistic web-based therapy platform for adults. We presented the following research questions for investigation:

- What broad patterns of usage, by adults, of a web-based GBO can be found?
- In adults who have set goals in the service, is there movement towards achieving their goals when monitored using a GBO?

- Does this goal progress vary depending upon the types of goals that are articulated?
- Does the service-user's level of engagement with the service increase the potential for successfully achieving their therapeutic goals?
- Does goal movement vary between self-set and collaboratively set goals?
- Do key presenting issues in service-users influence goal movement?

What data did we have available? In this study, we analysed routine GBO data variables from 557 adults who engaged with a web-based therapy service. The service-user's age and gender were collected when they signed up to the service, and once they began setting goals with the GBO, each goal was categorised into a topic. When they revisited the system to record goal progress, this was measured on a scale of 1–10. We also looked at whether their goals were self-set with no input from a practitioner, or if they were made in collaboration with a practitioner. If a service-user displays a presenting issue such as anxiety, depression, or suicidal ideation, during an interaction with a practitioner, this is also recorded.

How can we use this data to answer the research questions? Based on these different types of data, quantitative statistical tests were used to answer the research questions we had. Questions on demographics and frequencies can often be answered with simple percentages, and the presentation of central tendencies such as mean averages with accompanying standard deviations. These simple methods told us how many goals were set and achieved. Patterns of service engagement and their relationships with goal progress were explored with a correlation analysis, and one-way ANOVA tests allowed us to compare the mean goal movement of service-users with the presenting issues of depression, anxiety, self-harm, and suicidal thoughts.

What did we find? The 557 users collectively set 1242 goals. This meant that a mean average of 2.23 goals were set per person. Only 442 of these users engaged with goal setting for more than one day, however, so the remainder of the analyses were carried out with these users only. 31.6% of the goals set by the 442 returning users were recorded as fully achieved, and the mean average movement was 4.35 out of a possible 10. Goals relating to signposting were frequently set, and good progress was made towards achieving these. Goals set in collaboration with a practitioner were also attained to a higher level than those set alone. Those who set more goals and had more interactions with a practitioner made more progress, and those with anxiety seemed to make better progress than those with other presenting issues.

Conclusions: Although nuances associated with the online environment need to be considered if the findings of this study are to be generalisable to other therapeutic settings, we suggested that GBOs appear to be a useful way of monitoring therapeutic progress with adults within the digital context.

How well was the person represented in this study? When compared to other therapeutic outcome measures, that often focus on symptoms, behaviour change, or functioning change (Wolpert et al., 2012), the GBO is a more idiographic measure (Jacob et al., 2020). Users can record their own goal progress interactively, and the measure is suitable for use with any topic of goal. In our data set, 34 unique goal topics were recorded, ranging from emotional exploration, to career changes, to dealing with suicidal thoughts. However, we did note that goals were categorised by the practitioner rather than the service-user, and because of this, important factors such as immediate distress were lost when this categorisation occurred. Presenting issues were also recorded in a similar way. This raises the important question of whether the person and their goals were truly captured by this measure, and subsequently in the data. Could collaborative goal categorisation, as well as goal setting, ameliorate this?

What were the strengths and limitations of this study? This piece of research was a broad exploration, meaning that a number of important variables were assessed within one single study. This produced a number of interesting and useful insights. However, deeper, focussed investigations into each element might be warranted to further harness the mechanisms of GBO use with adults. The idiographic nature of measures like the GBO can make progress measurement difficult, particularly when the flexibility offered results in sporadic completion. The drop-in nature of digital therapy, aligned with an idiographic ethos, also impacts this, meaning that therapy is unstructured, with little follow-up. We will explore these ideas in greater depth towards the end of this chapter.

Study 2: The Session Wants and Needs Outcome Measure for Single-session Web-based Therapeutic Support: A Mixed-methods Investigation into the Use of Free-text Responses

Background and study rationale: Brief psychotherapeutic interventions, such as single-session therapeutic support (SST; Talmon, 1990), can go some way towards ameliorating some of the widespread issues associated with the provision of comprehensive and appropriate mental health care to children and young people (CYP; NHS Digital, 2021). The unsuitability of commonly used therapeutic outcome measures for SST (Hymmen et al., 2013) led to the development of the Session Wants and Needs Outcome Measure (SWAN-OM) by de Ossorno Garcia et al. (2021). This measure, designed for use by CYP, aims to harness the user's reasons for approaching the SST session, and allows them to rate the extent to which they feel their therapeutic wants or needs have been met. These aims can be articulated through a number of pre-set responses, or an alternative free-text option can be chosen, which was added to enhance the idiographic value of the measure. This paper investigates how this free-text option is engaged with in web-based CYP SST, thus providing a vital contribution towards the ongoing development of the SWAN-OM.

Research objectives:

1. Did pre-set and free-text wants and needs differ, in terms of the extent to which they were recorded as met during SST…

   • Within sessions where a free-text want or need was chosen alongside a pre-set want or need
   • Between sessions where only pre-set wants or needs were selected, compared with those where at least one want or need was articulated through free-text

2. Do any demographic characteristics differentiate service-users who chose to articulate their want or need through free-text?
3. Does the articulation of multiple wants and needs influence how likely they are to be met in SST?

- Did the number of articulated wants and needs per SWAN-OM influence how likely they were to be met in SST?
- Did wants and needs articulated by users who completed multiple SWAN-OMs differ from those articulated by users who only completed one SWAN-OM in terms of how likely they were to be met in SST?

4. How were wants and needs articulated through SWAN-OM's free-text option? An exploratory, data-driven approach was taken by:

- Qualitatively analysing the wants and needs articulated through free-text, in an inductive manner
- From this exploration, quantitatively analysing any differences in SST outcomes between qualitatively identified types or categories of free-text answer

What data did we have available? The data extraction spanned an eight-month period and comprised 1255 SWAN-OM completions by 1009 users. The start of this time-period represented the first availability of the free-text function, and by the end of August, the completion rate was deemed sufficient for analyses to commence. The data set covered the age, gender, and ethnicity of the user completing each SWAN-OM, plus how many, and which, wants and needs were selected. If the free-text option was chosen, their answer was available for qualitative analysis. The corresponding SWAN-OM score for each want or need was included for comparison. From these scores, we were able to calculate average scores for each user, both overall, and for pre-set answers only.

How can we use this data to answer the research questions? We took a mixed-methods approach to analyse our data. The quantitative data did not fit the assumptions required to carry out parametric statistical tests. For this reason, a series of non-parametric tests were carried out. The free-text responses yielded brief responses for qualitative analysis. Despite their brevity, research suggests that useful insights can still be gained from this type of short response (Rich et al., 2013). In our research, this data was examined to find points of interest that could then be compared with the use of further non-parametric quantitative tests.

What did we find?

1. SWAN-OM scores corresponding to each articulated want or need did not differ based upon whether they were expressed through pre-set or free-text options.
2. Investigating demographic differences with the aim of identifying a 'typical' free-text user found that whilst articulation method did not differ by gender or ethnicity, SWAN-OMs completed by those aged 14 and under were more likely to contain wants and needs articulated through free-text, than those completed by other age groups.
3. The number of wants or needs expressed also bore no relation to SWAN-OM score, nor did the completion of multiple SWAN-OMs.
4. Free-text answers were most commonly used to express wants and needs relating to mental health and coping. Responses were divided based upon expressed immediate risk, and clarity of goal focus. Neither showed a significant relationship with SWAN-OM score, or with multiple completion.

Conclusions: Analysis of SWAN-OM data, including that which pertains to the free-text articulation option, provided useful insight into how the function was engaged with by CYP in web-based SST. The results show how multiple uses of SWAN-OM, and multiple goal selection, had no effect on score variability. Whilst we found no indication that free-text articulations were any more likely to be met than pre-set goals, it can be concluded that they are equally as useful, especially for younger users who tend to choose this option more readily. This highlights the value of personalisation items in digital instruments and web-based therapies, and the importance of idiographic approaches to SST.

How well was the person represented in this study? The data used in the study was analysed as completions of the SWAN-OM measure, rather than as person-level data. It was common that one individual had completed the measure several times. This meant that the same individual appeared several times within the demographic data, and that perhaps the essence of *who* completed the measure was inaccurate. However, it is possible that the qualitative element of the study mitigated this short-coming somewhat. Qualitative analysis is widely regarded as deeper, and more focussed on individuals and their experiences, than quantitative. Analysing this data in a non-numerical way may means that the individuals' unique reasons for completing the SWAN-OM were harnessed in a deeper, more personalised way than the pre-set responses. But, as only a small proportion of SWAN-OMs (n=70) contained at least one free-text want or need, the study's ability to fully represent 'the person' is still questionable.

What were the strengths and limitations of this study? The use of non-parametric tests, whilst unavoidable, limited the complexity of the analyses that we were able to run. This is because the use of parametric tests allows more complex and power-ful statistical models to be built. In terms of the free-text responses which were analysed qualitatively, responses varied greatly in terms of richness—some were extremely vague and short. This may have limited our ability to categorise the responses meaningfully. When more free-text data is obtained as time goes on, con-ducting another qualitative analysis might result in more robust categorisation.

Activity 6.2

In another study we wanted to find out who used GBO in a web-based univer-sity therapy service. We also wanted to find out about what types of goals the students were setting. Take a look at the two different visual presentations of data below (labelled A & B) and think about these questions:

1. What are the researchers trying to show with each visualisation?
2. What are the main advantages and disadvantages of presenting data in each way?

(continued)

Activity 6.2   (continued)
   Data visualisation A)

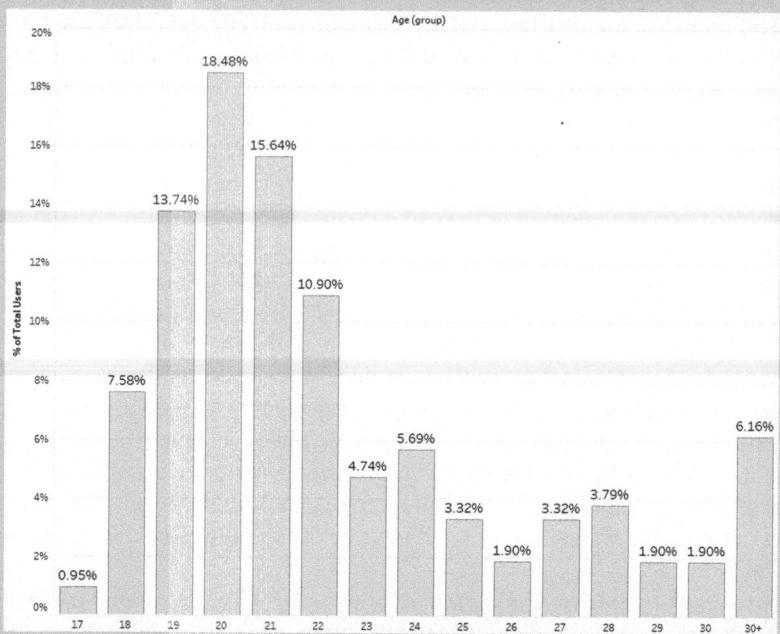

Data visualisation B)

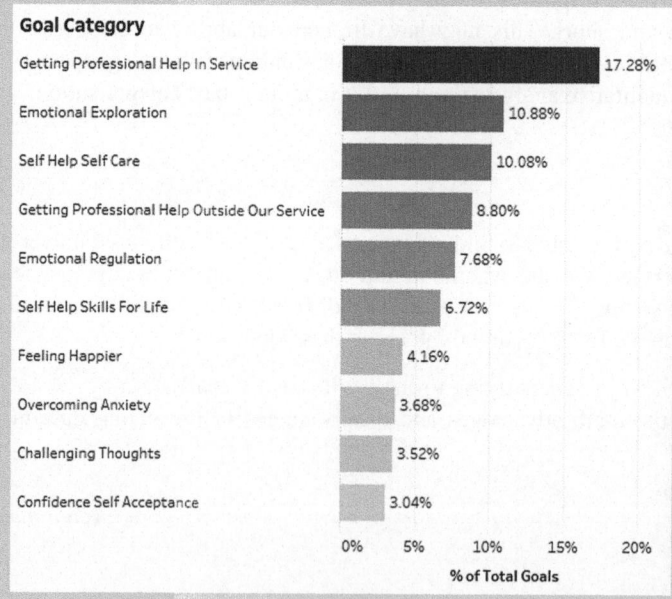

- Qualitative methods can add personalisation, and mixed-methods research is undeniably useful within this field. However, when a person can express exactly what they wish, data is often inconsistent in quality, and therefore difficult to analyse. The resulting 'chaotic' data set might therefore lack robustness, and weaken the inferences we can make.
- Practice-based research can sometimes be burdensome for the therapist and client due to the number of measures being used. These therefore need to be designed to be user-friendly and skilfully integrated into therapeutic work.

Fact Box 6.1   Glossary

Alternative hypothesis: accepted when a predicted relationship or pattern was supported by the data. The opposite of the **null hypothesis**

Analysis of variance (ANOVA): a statistical test where two or more means are compared, to establish whether they significantly differ from one another

Arithmetic mean: the average of a set of values. It is calculated by summing all values, and dividing them by the number of values

Between-subjects design: a study design where participants are assigned to one condition only

Central tendency: how 'typical' a certain response or characteristic is compared to the rest of the sample

Conclusion: the overarching 'message' of your research after your data has been analysed

Dependent variable (DV): a variable where values are impacted by another (independent) variable

Demographic: a core characteristic of a sample or population

Descriptive statistics: a statistic that summarises the data based on its properties

Design: the overall strategy adopted to answer a study's research questions

Dispersion: how data is 'spread out'

Frequency: how often a response or characteristic features in the data

Generalisability: the extent to which a study's findings or conclusions can be applied to other populations or situations

Idiographic measures: measures where outcomes are recorded in ways that are personalised and relevant to the individual

Independent variable (IV): a variable where values are not impacted by another variable

Inferential statistics: used to make predictions from, or test relationships within, the data

Hypothesis test: testing a prediction to establish whether or not it is supported

Longitudinal: where data is collected at several time points to assess whether a relationship or pattern can be found

---

(continued)

(continued)

Mann-Whitney U test: a non-parametric test used to establish differences between two independent groups. It compares medians rather than means

Median: when values of a variable are laid out in order, the median is the value that lies exactly at the mid-point. This means that there is an equal likelihood of a value falling either higher or lower than this

Mixed-factors design: a study design where at least one IV is a within-subjects factor, and at least one is a between-subjects factor

Mixed methods research: studies that require a mixture of quantitative and qualitative research to answer their research questions

Mode: the most common value or score within a variable

Nomothetic measures: measures where predetermined, standardised questions are used to assess symptoms, progress, or other outcomes

Non-parametric test: statistical tests that do not make assumptions about the distribution or parameters that the data falls within

Normal distribution: a distribution whereby values fall symmetrically around the mean value. That data follows this approximate pattern is a key assumption of parametric statistical tests.

Null hypothesis: the opposite of an **alternative hypothesis**, whereby no significant difference, pattern, or relationship is found within the sample

One-tailed hypothesis: a prediction where a change in one direction is expected

Outliers: an observation that lies far away from other values within the data set

P-value: the probability of obtaining results at least as extreme as those that were actually observed. Used to indicate **statistical significance**

Parametric test: statistical tests that make assumptions about the parameters or distribution of the data

Population: the entire group that the research aims to draw conclusions about by examining a **sample**

Range: a measure of dispersion that examines the difference between the highest and lowest values

Regression: statistical tests that are used to investigate the effects that variables have on each other

Research question: the key line(s) of enquiry of your research

Sample: a subset of a **population** that data is available from for analysis

Standard deviation: an indication of how far most values deviate from the mean

Statistical package: a software programme designed to conduct statistical tests. SPSS, R, and Microsoft Excel are some examples of these

Statistical power: the extent to which a true deviation from the null hypothesis can be found given the current size of the sample

(*continued*)

(continued)
　　Statistical significance: a relationship that is statistically significant is unlikely to have occurred by chance, and therefore is likely to represent a true difference.
　　T-test: a statistical test where two means are compared, to establish whether they significantly differ from one another
　　Theory of change: a theory of how, why, and under which circumstances, a particular change may happen
　　Transferability: the extent to which findings of a study conducted under experimental settings can be applied to real-world settings
　　Two-tailed hypothesis: a prediction where a change in either direction is expected
　　Variable: a phenomenon that is measured within research
　　Wilcoxon signed rank test: a non-parametric test used to establish differences in a within-subjects design. It compares medians rather than means
　　Within-subjects design: a study design where the same group of subjects is examined more than once, and their responses are compared each time

Further Reading
There are lots of areas that people might want to follow up after reading this chapter. Here we recommend a few sources that we hope will help individuals to deepen their understanding of some of the key topics discussed.

1. Hanley, T., Sefi, A., Grauberg, J., Prescott, J., & Etchebarne, A. (2021). A Theory of Change for online therapy and support services for children and young people: A collaborative qualitative exploration. JMIR Pediatrics and Parenting, 4(1), e23193. https://doi.org/10/gjg5hw

To start with, readers may want to take a look at the paper that provides a summary of the theory of change that has been articulated for Kooth. This is a freely available journal article.

2. Barkham, M., & Mellor-Clark, J. (2003). Bridging evidence-based practice and practice-based evidence: Developing a rigorous and relevant knowledge for the psychological therapies. Clinical Psychology & Psychotherapy, 10(6), 319–327. https://doi.org/10.1002/cpp.379

Our second recommendation is to delve deeper into the world of practice-based research. Barkham and Mellor-Clark provide a brief, but very useful overview of the way in which evidence-based practice and practice-based evidence interact.

3. Hanson, W. E., Creswell, J. W., Clark, V. L. P., Petska, K. S., & Creswell, J. D. (2005). Mixed methods research designs in counseling psychology. Journal of Counseling Psychology, 52(2), 224–235. https://doi.org/ 10.1037/0022-0167.52.2.224

Our final recommendation directs people to a paper to learn more about mixed-methods research design in the counselling and psychotherapy professions. This is a useful introductory paper, but there are now some excellent textbooks on this topic.

Summary

This chapter introduces the way that counsellors and psychotherapists might make use of practice-based evidence in their work. It begins by providing an overview of some core principles of quantitative research before considering how these might be used to answer descriptive, comparative, or relationship-based research questions. Following on from this, we discuss an adventurous project attempting to articulate a theory of change for online therapeutic services. The overarching mixed-methods design is described before going on to discuss the way that quantitative methods have been used to complement earlier qualitative research. Here two examples of projects have been provided. Throughout this work, the research team have attempted to keep the individuals seeking support at the fore of what is being measured. As such, the studies report the use of an idiographic measure (the GBO) and a hybrid nomothetic/idiographic measure (the SWAN-OM) in real-world therapeutic work. Both these studies highlight the utility of using these measures in web-based therapeutic work. To end, we reflect upon the strengths and limitations of this work, concluding that while quantitative research is always reductive, there are ways of collecting numerical information that can place the individuals seeking support in the driving seat of what is being assessed. Whilst this adds an element of complexity to the understanding gained from such measures, we believe that this can help to humanise the numbers being collected and has the potential to enhance the therapeutic work engaged in.

References

Bugental, J. F. T. (1964). The third force in psychology. *Journal of Humanistic Psychology, 4*(1), 19–26. https://doi.org/10.1177/002216786400400102

Cooper, M., & McLeod, J. (2011). *Pluralistic counselling and psychotherapy*. Sage.

Davies, R. (2012). *Criteria for assessing the evaluability of a theory of change* (pp. 1–6). file:/// Users/mewxsth3/Downloads/Davies_Evaluability20of20ToCs.pdf

de Ossorno Garcia, S., Salhi, L., Sefi, A., & Hanley, T. (2021). The session wants and need outcome measure: The development of a brief outcome measure for single-sessions of web-based support. *Frontiers in Psychology, 12*, 4900. https://doi.org/10.3389/fpsyg.2021.748145

Geurtzen, N., Keijsers, G. P. J., Karremans, J. C., Tiemens, B. G., & Hutschemaekers, G. J. M. (2020). Patients' perceived lack of goal clarity in psychological treatments: Scale development and negative correlates. *Clinical Psychology & Psychotherapy, 27*(6), 915–924.

Hanley, T., Sefi, A., Grauberg, J., & Prescott, J. (2019). *A positive virtual Ecosystem: The theory of change for Kooth*. Xenzone.

Hanson, W. E., Creswell, J. W., Clark, V. L. P., Petska, K. S., & Creswell, J. D. (2005). Mixed methods research designs in counseling psychology. *Journal of Counseling Psychology, 52*(2), 224–235. https://doi.org/10.1037/0022-0167.52.2.224

Hymmen, P., Stalker, C. A., & Cait, C.-A. (2013). The case for single-session therapy: Does the empirical evidence support the increased prevalence of this service delivery model? *Journal of Mental Health, 22*(1), 60–71. https://doi.org/10.3109/09638237.2012.670880

Jacob, J., Costa da Silva, L., Sefi, A., & Edbrooke-Childs, J. (2020). Online counselling and goal achievement: Exploring meaningful change and the types of goals progressed by young people. *Counselling and Psychotherapy Research, 21*(3), 502–513.

Jacob, J., De Francesco, D., Deighton, J., Law, D., Wolpert, M., & Edbrooke-Childs, J. (2017). Goal formulation and tracking in child mental health settings: When is it more likely and is it associated with satisfaction with care? *European Child & Adolescent Psychiatry, 26*(7), 759–770.

Kail, A., & Lumley, T. (2012). *Theory of change: The beginning of making a difference*. New Philanthropy Capital.

Law, D., & Jacob, J. (2015). *Goals and goals based outcomes (GBOs): Some useful*. information Third Edition CAMHS Press.

McBeath, A. G. (2020). Doing quantitative research with a survey. In S. Bager-Charleson & A. G. McBeath (Eds.), *Enjoying research in counselling and psychotherapy*. Palgrave Macmillan.

NHS Digital. (2021). *Mental health of children and young people in England 2021—Wave 2 follow up to the 2017 survey*. NHS Digital. https://digital.nhs.uk/data-and-information/publications/statistical/mental-health-of-children-and-young-people-in-england/2021-follow-up-to-the-2017-survey

Noble, J., de Ossorno Garcia, S., Gadd, L., & Gillman, A. (2021). *Theory of change Kooth for adults*. NPC. https://doi.org/10.13140/RG.2.2.23036.05764

Norcross, J. C., & Wampold, B. E. (2018). A new therapy for each patient: Evidence-based relationships and responsiveness. *Journal of Clinical Psychology, 74*(11), 1889–1906.

Rich, J. L., Chojenta, C., & Loxton, D. (2013). Quality, rigour and usefulness of free-text comments collected by a large population based longitudinal study—ALSWH. *PLoS One, 8*(7), e68832. https://doi.org/10.1371/journal.pone.0068832

Sefi, A., & Hanley, T. (2012). Examining the complexities of measuring effectiveness of online counselling for young people using routine evaluation data. *Pastoral Care in Education, 30*(1), 49–64.

Talmon, M. (1990). *Single-session therapy: Maximizing the effect of the first (and often only) therapeutic encounter* (p. xxi, 146). Jossey-Bass.

Tryon, G. S., et al. (2018). Meta-analyses of the relation of goal consensus and collaboration to psychotherapy outcome. *Psychotherapy, 55*(4), 372–383.

Wolpert, M., Ford, T., Trustam, E., Law, D., Deighton, J., Flannery, H., & Fugard, R. J. B. (2012). Patient-reported outcomes in child and adolescent mental health services (CAMHS): Use of idiographic and standardized measures. *Journal of Mental Health, 21*(2), 165–173.

Chapter 7
Dilemmas and Decisions in Quantitative-Driven Online Survey Research into Researchers' Mental Health and Support

Cassie Hazell and Clio Berry

Learning Goals

After reading this chapter, you should be able to:

- Understand the process of identifying the constructs of interest and planning their measurement
- Understand how surveys can be used to collect quantitative, qualitative and mixed-methods data
- Have an awareness of the major ethical issues related to online survey research and potential mitigations
- Have an awareness of the different strategies that can be used to improve participant recruitment and retention
- Make your online survey ready for distribution
- Produce and enact an appropriate analysis plan that addresses your research questions
- Reflect on the different stories that you can tell with your data
- Understand important considerations in creating a publication plan

C. Hazell (✉)
University of Surrey, Guildford, UK

Brighton and Sussex Medical School, Brighton, UK
e-mail: cassie.hazell@surrey.ac.uk

C. Berry
Brighton and Sussex Medical School, Brighton, UK
e-mail: C.Berry@bsms.ac.uk

© The Author(s), under exclusive license to Springer Nature
Switzerland AG 2022
S. Bager-Charleson, A. McBeath (eds.), *Supporting Research in Counselling and Psychotherapy*, https://doi.org/10.1007/978-3-031-13942-0_7

Introduction

Surveys are a powerful way of turning 'fuzzy' phenomena into something tangible and measurable, and allowing the collection of lots of data from lots of people within a short period of time. Surveys are predominantly used as a quantitative method, but can also be used for qualitative and mixed-methods research. Surveys can be administered in various forms: in-person, telephone or video-calling, on paper, and using digital technologies, for example, computers and mobile devices. The increased availability of digital technologies has made online research more attractive (Callegaro et al., 2014), and increasingly utilised by academic researchers (Evans & Mathur, 2018). This chapter focuses on our online survey into understanding doctoral researcher mental health needs among doctoral researchers, which included 4608 participants; 3352 PhD students and 1256 working professionals.

Compared to other methods, online survey research tends to be cheaper (Dillman et al., 2014); for less time and fewer resources are needed to collect data (Greenlaw & Brown-Welty, 2009). Sample sizes can therefore be greater. Greater sample sizes are further facilitated by the fact that online surveys allow people to participate in their preferred location, at their preferred pace (O'Brien et al., 2014), and because the possibility of anonymity facilitates collecting data on more sensitive or potentially controversial topics (Hood et al., 2012). Moreover, research suggests that online surveys can be useful in rapidly recruiting particularly narrow or unique populations (Miller et al., 2020; Wright, 2005). Nonetheless, the impersonal nature of online surveys can undermine participants' motivation to complete the survey (Hood et al., 2012). Research suggests that online samples are not necessarily any less representative than those otherwise recruited (Miller et al., 2020), yet selection bias is an important consideration (Ball, 2019; Hlatshwako et al., 2021). Digital exclusion does still exist (Watts, 2020), and a proportion of the population, especially older people and those living rurally, may not be able or willing to access an online survey. Moreover, researchers lack control over online survey completion; they are unable to provide a quiet, distraction-free environment, or prevent potential 'sham' responses (Pozzar et al., 2020). Despite these potential drawbacks, online survey research remains a powerfully pragmatic, efficient, and cost-effective means of conducting research.

This Chapter

In this chapter we will, as mentioned, use the U-DOC (Understanding DOCtoral researcher mental health needs) project to illustrate and reflect on the stages of making, launching, and analysing an online survey. The U-DOC project was funded from 2017 to 2020 by the Office for Students and Research England, forming one of 17 'catalyst' projects designed to focus on the mental health and wellbeing of doctoral researchers. The rationale for our project was borne from local evaluation and reviewing the literature. We found that the evidence on the mental health of doctoral researchers was disparate and comparatively neglected, with specific evidentiary gaps around mental health problem prevalence, and potential causes and protective factors. We believed that these gaps would be best initially addressed using a primarily quantitative mixed-methods online survey. In this chapter, we provide illustrative examples from U-DOC of the dilemmas we faced pertaining to online survey research, and our associated decision-making processes. We hope that readers will emerge from reading this chapter more confident in their ability to identify and resolve some of their own dilemmas in online survey research.

Stage One: Making the Survey

Dilemma One: What Did We Want to Know and How Could We Know It?

What can be known, and how to know it, is an incredibly complex question spanning epistemological, ontological and discipline- and construct-specific considerations. Such considerations are fundamentally important to ensure that we conduct high-quality, internally consistent, and worthwhile research. We take a broadly critical realist approach to our research. We understand this to reflect a realist ontology with a robust relativist epistemology (McEvoy & Richards, 2003); that is, that an objective reality exists independent of humans perceiving it, yet is experienced through the veil of human perception and interpretation (Danermark et al., 2002; Fletcher, 2017). Critical realism focuses on the identification of causal mechanisms, observable through their effects (McEvoy & Richards, 2003). These causal mechanisms are considered contextually dependent (McEvoy & Richards, 2003), reflecting an important interplay between social structures and human agency and action (Danermark et al., 2002; Fletcher, 2017). We, therefore, chose to design a primarily quantitative survey in U-DOC to enable us to test whether our data would support proposed causal mechanisms. Additionally, we wanted to use both quantitative and qualitative data to generate a nuanced understanding of the contextual-dependence of such mechanisms, for example, as affected by doctoral researcher demography and PhD study characteristics (e.g. Berry et al., 2021a, 2021b). The decision to take a primarily quantitative mixed-methods approach was further shaped by the traditional prominence of quantitative research in policy and practice.

The selection of constructs and measurement approaches must be theoretically informed. Research which is not clearly theoretically driven can inadvertently lead to poor findings and poor practice; including spurious and non-replicable results, poor integration with existing evidence and failing to advance theory (Burghardt & Bodansky, 2021). For the U-DOC survey, we were informed by multiple theories. The mental health symptoms we first selected to measure were informed by understandings of the most common mental health problems affecting the general population and students, that is, anxiety and depression (Jenkins et al., 2021; MHFA England, 2020). We next selected to measure suicidality due to theory suggesting key risk factors that aligned with known aspects of the doctoral experience (e.g. isolation; Cornette et al., 2009), and its associations with mental health problems (World Health Organisation (WHO), 2021). The selection of correlates was informed by our broad social, positive and clinical psychology approach—with the 'clinical' bit adopting a broad cognitive behavioural model of mental health symptoms (Beck & Bredemeier, 2016). The selection of social correlates was informed by our interests in social recovery theory and the interplay between mental health symptoms and behavioural functioning (Fowler et al., 2019), theoretical understandings of loneliness (Hawkley & Cacioppo, 2010) and the social cure approach to health (Jetten et al., 2012).

Under a critical realist approach, we believe that measuring things is basically possible (albeit always with inherent errors and inaccuracies) and that (well) measured things, including psychological and social phenomena, have some basis in an objective reality (Danermark & Ekström, 2002). We understand complex constructs to be 'latent' variables—themselves not directly observable, but which can be approximated through considered measurement (Kline, 2011). Multiple similar or related questionnaire items can be used to try and collectively capture this complexity (Allen et al., 2022). In the U-DOC survey, we assessed the merit of questionnaires based on their face and content validity (e.g. whether the items appear to measure what they intend to measure Connelly, 2022), reliability (e.g. good internal consistency Tavakol & Dennick, 2011) and participant burden. We additionally thought it pertinent to use measures prioritised by key stakeholders. For example, we selected measures of depression and anxiety that have been nationally adopted by NHS clinical policy and services, that is, the Patient Health Questionnaire-9 (PHQ9; Kroenke et al., 2010) and the Generalised Anxiety Disorder-7 (GAD7; Spitzer et al., 2006). We felt that the ability to explicitly map doctoral researcher mental health problem prevalence against standard accepted thresholds for specialist psychiatric or psychological therapies referral would make our findings difficult to ignore.

We selected our measurement tools to facilitate our broad theory-testing approach, that is, we sought to test whether our data seemed to 'fit' with identified theoretical models and the specific hypothesised associations between different variables there within (Oberauer & Lewandowsky, 2019). We collected qualitative data primarily for the purposes of triangulating such findings, that is, seeing whether the qualitative data 'agreed' with the patterns observed in the quantitative data (Duffy, 1987). However, triangulation can additionally offer opportunities to further our understanding and develop new theories (Olsen et al., 2004). We collected the two types of data concurrently, that is, in the same survey, but we collected qualitative data after the quantitative data within this survey to avoid any priming effects. We achieved this through dividing the survey into 'conceptual chunks' (e.g. 'mood', 'supervisory relationship'), presenting participants with quantitative measures and then qualitative questions on the same 'topic' before moving on to another. We used focused qualitative questions that were clearly tied to the preceding quantitative items, that is, reminding participants that they had just answered a series of questions about a particular topic and then asking them to describe how that topic impacted on their PhD studies and vice versa.

We noted early on that there appeared to be a lack of epidemiological research focused on doctoral researchers (Hazell et al., 2020). This population is poorly delineated in existing epidemiological surveys, for example, national birth cohort studies and similar. The lack of such evidence impedes the ability to infer causal associations between exposures and outcomes. We could not rectify the issues with population cohort research, but we did institute the design feature of a comparison group. A non-doctoral comparison group felt particularly important in the context of apparent growing mental health problems for young people and students more generally (UCAS, 2021). We were interested in whether PhD study itself appears causative of mental health problems (Hazell et al., 2021). The best test of this claim would be to randomly allocate people to do or not do a PhD and compare their outcomes. As this is impractical, a naturally occurring non-exposed (i.e. non-doctoral) comparison offers some protection against confounding. Confounding (Fig. 7.1) occurs when a third variable that is associated with (or causes) both the independent (IV; proposed cause) and dependent variable (DV; proposed outcome) leads to a spurious association between IV and DV (Type I error), or masks a true association (Type II error) (Grimes & Schulz, 2002). It is important to choose appropriate selection criteria for the comparison sample, so that the two groups are matched in terms of potential confounds. Typically, few selection parameters are actually used in practice, because lots of inclusion and exclusion criteria can limit and lengthen sample recruitment. We set selection criteria for the control group in relation to participant age, UK residence, being educated to at least undergraduate degree level, and being employed on a contract of at least 0.6 whole time equivalent, which is the minimum requirement for a part-time PhD in the UK.

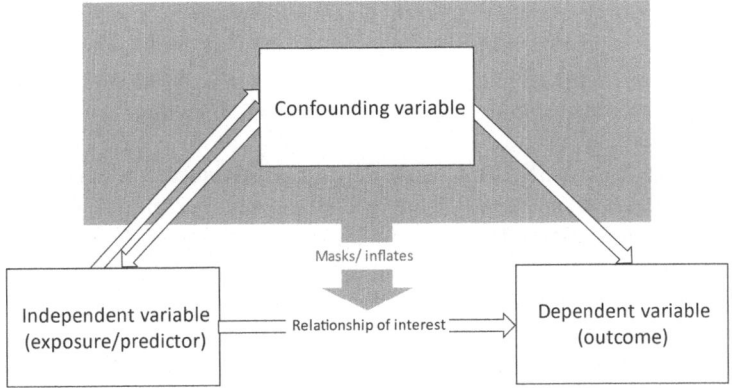

Fig. 7.1 Confounding

Activity 7.1

An assumption of online surveys is (typically) that we are using questionnaires to measure latent constructs, for example, we used the PHQ-9 to measure depression. Creating an online survey, therefore, requires you as a
researcher to engage in a matching process of identifying the constructs you
want to measure and then finding questionnaires that capture these appropriately, comprehensively and reliably. There may be multiple questionnaires
that posit to measure your construct of interest but will conceptualise it in
slightly different ways. The final decision of which questionnaire(s) to choose
may be influenced by many factors; including each questionnaire's theoretical
stance, psychometric properties, utility, cost or adherence to norms within
your field. Please consider the following:

What construct are you trying to measure?	What are the potential questionnaires you could use?	Which questionnaire(s) are you going to use and why?
–	–	–
–	–	–
–	–	–
–	–	–
–	–	–

Dilemma Two: What Could and Should We Ask Participants to Do?

Our second dilemma was how to meet our survey aims whilst preserving the comfort and wellbeing of participants. This dilemma involved considerations of ethical issues around what it is permissible to ask of research participants, how to
ensure participants understand their involvement and related rights, how to minimise any risks associated with participation, and how to safely and securely manage research data. Like all other types of research study, online surveys should be
conducted in accordance with relevant locally applicable ethical and data protection regulations.

The potential for participant anonymity in online survey research offers an
ethical (and practical) advantage. That is, if no personally identifying information
is collected from participants, then there are no risks associated with its retrieval,
storage or usage. Consent is an important consideration, irrespective of whether
participation is or is not anonymous. Consent in online surveys is typically not
taken as a signature (which would be non-anonymous), as many people do not
have the hardware or software needed to provide this, but instead using a tick box

consent form built in to the survey itself. It is possible on most survey platforms to add an option that prevents participants from progressing with survey participation until consent is provided.

The right for persons to withdraw their participation and data is a fundamental consideration (The British Psychological Society, 2021). In one sense, withdrawing from an online survey is easier than for other studies, as participants need to simply close their internet browser window. However, where data are collected anonymously, as in U-DOC, they cannot therefore be later identified in order to withdraw them. There are methods available to try and resolve this issue, for example, timestamping participation, or inviting participants to create (and remember) a unique identifier. We elected not to use such methods in U-DOC due to their margin for error in the accurate identification and selection of data to be withdrawn, especially in a large-scale survey. Participant information documents should be used to make participants clearly and explicitly aware at outset of their rights and any restrictions in relation to data identification and withdrawal. Moreover, some survey platforms automatically save responses as they are provided on a page-by-page or question-by-question basis, meaning responses are recorded even if the participant has not reached the end of the survey and pressed the final 'submit' button. Without information to the contrary, participants may assume that if they close the browser window before completing the survey their responses may not be recorded or used. In the U-DOC project, we chose to use all data collected, saving responses on a page-by-page basis, for this uses all data that the participant has taken the time to provide. Participants must be transparently informed of this at the outset where this is the case.

When conducting face-to-face research, it is possible to observe participants' behaviour and reactions and respond accordingly to any signs of distress (Draucker et al., 2009)—this is obviously not possible with online surveys. Your research ethics committee will want to see that you have considered this by trying to minimise the risk of causing distress, whilst planning strategies for managing any distress which does occur. It is important to consider whether the potential benefits from your research are balanced against the potential risks. The questionnaire should always only ask for the minimum personal and sensitive information needed to achieve its aims. The selection of participants and questionnaire items should be carefully considered to minimise the risk of distress. The information sheet should forewarn participants, using clear language, about the topics covered so that they can make an informed choice about whether the survey is likely to negatively affect them (Knapp et al., 2011). Participants should be provided with information on relevant support organisations within study documents (i.e. participant information sheet and debrief) as a minimum (The British Psychological Society, 2021). We additionally recommend linking to support information on every page of the survey, for example as a footer, negating participants needing to memorise the information given at the start of the study or having to complete a study so as to view the information in the debrief.

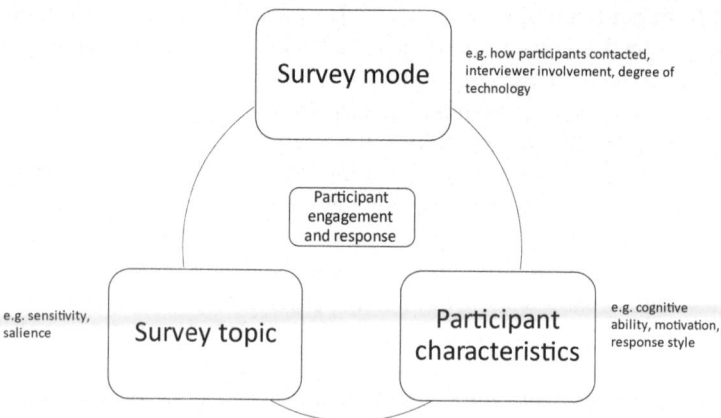

Fig. 7.2 Influences on survey participant engagement and response

Dilemma Three: How Could We Facilitate Participant Engagement?

Our third dilemma was how to optimise participant survey engagement, that is, promote retention and response quality. Engagement is influenced by characteristics of the survey and its participants (see Fig. 7.2), and by interactions between the two (Hood et al., 2012). For example, most people will be more likely to answer sensitive questions honestly when data are collected remotely without the presence of a researcher (Hood et al., 2012), yet people with neurocognitive difficulties may be more likely to complete a survey, including sensitive questions, in a face-to-face research encounter. Considerations regarding survey mode characteristics (also see dilemma two), and survey design and content, are all vital in promoting retention and enhancing response quality (Hood et al., 2012).

Retention in the context of an online survey differs to most other studies. With the majority of online surveys, the researcher and participant will never have direct contact, so the usual approaches, such as establishing rapport (Leonard et al., 2003), mean something different in this context. Most online surveys have a single data collection time point so while the means of retaining participants are more limited, the period over which it is ideal to retain them is shorter, that is, preventing drop-out before participants reach the end of the survey.

Response quality can be understood as the mitigation of error. Any survey item response comprises the true score, plus measurement error. Measurement error can be random or systematic. Random error reflects unknown and unpredictable deviations from true responses that are inherent to the measurement process, for example, relating to natural fluctuations and environmental changes. Conversely, systematic error reflects persistent and consistent biases in measurement caused by design, sampling, or other research conduct problems; for example, issues with a survey measurement tool that particularly affect one sub-group of participants. Random error decreases as the sample size increases, yet systematic error does not—and can actually increase. Response error can occur at any stage of responding; survey item comprehension, information retrieval, decision-making and response formulation (Tourangeau et al., 2000). Thus, strategies for enhancing response quality should consider both types of error and their mitigation across the stages of responding.

Participant burden is inversely associated with retention and response quality (Deutskens et al., 2004; Roberts et al., 2019). If the burden of a survey is high enough, especially where participants are less motivated and/or the survey appears to have less credibility, then participants may drop out. Alternatively, participants may continue the survey but resort to 'satisficing', that is, only superficial engagement with the survey items (Roberts et al., 2019). Satisficing, in turn, increases the impact of respondent's own characteristics on their survey responses, and thus, the influence of their own response style becomes greater. Response style refers to individuals' habitual patterns of responding that occur irrespective of content (Roberts, 2016). For example, some individuals are 'acquiescent', tending to score high agreement with all items, some are 'dis-acquiescent', tending to disagree, and some are 'mild' scores, who tend to avoid the extremes of any response scale (see Fig. 7.3). Response style not only influences the actual absolute scores of survey instruments, but can also influence the associations between different variables, and thus its effects should be minimised (Roberts, 2016). For reducing participant burden, convenience is key. Brief, easy to navigate, and simple to understand surveys improve recruitment, retention and response quality (Deutskens et al., 2004). It can help to reflect on your research questions and consider what items are essential to answer these, or, if you have more than one research question, considering whether these be addressed using multiple short surveys. There are situations, however, where you do need to ask participants for a lot of data in a single survey in order to answer your research questions—this was our situation in the U-DOC project. We had received funding for a time-limited project that could cover the delivery of one survey. We also were interested in the interactions between all of the variables of interest,

This chapter is very informative

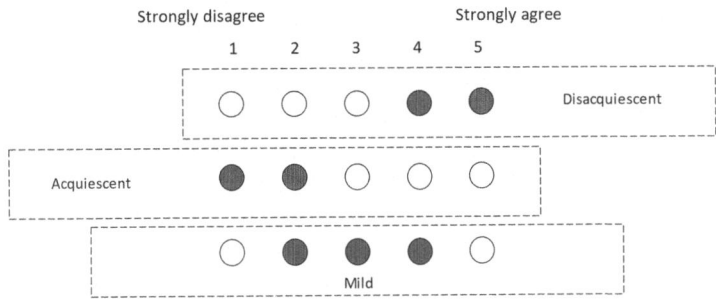

Fig. 7.3 Survey response style

therefore, splitting the questionnaires into multiple smaller surveys was not possible. We instead had to find other ways to make the survey as low burden as possible so as to minimise drop-outs and enhance response quality.

A common strategy to aid recruitment and retention of participants is the use of incentives, such as a prize draw offered to participants directly or to gatekeepers (Draper et al., 2009). Incentives should reflect reimbursement (i.e. giving people an appropriate award in exchange for the time and effort they are expending) rather than payment (i.e. giving people a fee that is unrelated to the participant burden) (Draper et al., 2009). Incentives can become ethically problematic where: (a) the participant is dependent on the researcher in some way; (b) the project is very high risk; or (c) the participant does not want to participate but could be convinced if the incentive is big enough (Grant & Sugarman, 2004). Incentives should be commensurate and not coercive. Overly generous incentivisation will likely attract people who are financially vulnerable and who might take less heed of any inherent risks (Tishler & Bartholomae, 2002). In the U-DOC project, our recruitment targets were high, so we did not have the funds to reimburse each participant. We initially opened recruitment via social media and university mail-outs, offering participants the opportunity to enter a prize draw to win one of two smart tablets.

The choice of the online survey hosting platform involves consideration of functionality, resourcing, and research ethics. Academic institutions often have preferred platforms that comply with their data protection and security requirements. For U-DOC, we selected our university's preferred platform, Qualtrics, for these reasons. Moreover, this platform offers credibility, technical support, and good functionality—including a range of different question types and multiple personalisation tools to facilitate the creation of a survey that is professional in its appearance. Formal language, logos, naming the research team and institution, and providing contact details, are important aspects of the information provided at the start of the survey to enhance credibility. Taking time to consider simple aspects of the survey presentation, such as a clear font and complimentary colour schemes, can reduce the time and effort needed to complete the survey (Hood et al., 2012). Participants can move more quickly through the survey if questions are formatted to avoid the need to scroll up and down or go back and forth between pages in order to answer them. The formatting should be suitable for completion on a range of devices. Displaying questions in a table or grid can be problematic and can increase the probability that participants select responses according to their habitual response style. Ideally, survey items should be presented one by one, with each item then forming a single page of the survey. Extensive piloting can help identify any aspects of the survey that are creating burden, or otherwise increasing the likelihood of response error. Piloting typically involves the research team completing the survey several times, selecting different answers, on different devices. If possible, piloting the survey with the intended end-user is additionally recommended, that is, one or more people from your target population (van Teijlingen & Hundley, 2001). This facilitates the identification of potential issues relating to the likely characteristics of your intended respondents, and could be used to explore how such characteristics may impact on and interact with the survey mode and topic (Hood et al., 2012).

Stage Two: Launching the Survey

Dilemma Four: Who Did We Want to Find and How Could We Find Them?

Research suggests that online recruitment methods, including email, social media and survey services, are more effective and cheaper than offline methods (Christensen et al., 2017). Online recruitment methods can broadly be divided into two categories (Antoun et al., 2016); those that 'pull in', where potential participants are already looking for research opportunities, and those that 'push out', where adverts are placed in the hope of attracting potential participants. Examples of 'pull in' platforms are survey sites like Amazon Mechanical Turk, Prolific and Qualtrics XM; and examples of 'push out' platforms include social media adverts (e.g. Facebook, Twitter, Instagram) and Google Ads. 'Pull in' methods tend to be more efficient and cost-effective, for you are reaching a sample of people who are seeking out opportunities to take part in research surveys. However, these methods perform worse with respect to sample representativeness. In our study, we were fortunate to have the funding to use both of these approaches to recruitment, that is, advertising the study via general social media platforms as well as specific survey participation platforms. Where using both approaches is not possible, then the method should be selected according to scientific and pragmatic considerations, for example whether efficiency or sample representativeness matters more.

Recruitment using 'push out' methods does nonetheless still confer risks to sample representativeness. Email can be a quick means of reaching people where you have access to a mailing list, yet using email alone can attract a generally older sample (Nolte et al., 2015). Social media platform advertising can be effective at reaching high numbers of people (Blumenberg et al., 2019), yet may result in a younger age bias (Nolte et al., 2015). The effectiveness of individual social media platforms in aiding recruitment will fluctuate as their popularity and usership change. Being aware of such trends will enable you to make decisions on what platforms are most appropriate to meet your recruitment needs. Hlatshwako and colleagues have provided a helpful framework for the mitigation of selection bias and otherwise increasing the rigour of online surveys (Hlatshwako et al., 2021). Additional threats more specific to online survey research include the risk of bogus responding and bots, that is, fraudulent accounts that complete the survey using automation; a particularly pertinent risk for surveys involving reimbursement. Bogus or non-human responses are obviously not valid and inclusion in your analysis would lead you to draw incorrect conclusions. One research group found that within seven hours of posting their paid survey on social media, almost 95% of responses were considered either fraudulent or suspicious (Pozzar et al., 2020). These responses were identified via inconsistencies in answering, duplicate answers or irrelevant content. This study provides helpful recommendations for preserving sample legitimacy (Pozzar et al., 2020).

An aspect of recruitment from specialist groups that is often overlooked is gate-keeping (Lindsay, 2005). Gatekeepers are those organisations or persons giving access to potential participants; for example, teachers who can help recruit students, or doctors who can help recruit their patients. Within the U-DOC project, relevant gatekeepers included doctoral schools across the UK. We curated a list of all UK universities and the email addresses of their doctoral schools via web searches. Using this database, we emailed asking for their support with recruitment. When approaching gatekeepers, it helps to keep requests simple, doing as much of the 'heavy lifting' for them as possible, and highlighting benefits for the gatekeeper themselves. For example, we kept our email brief but did include a draft email that doctoral schools could copy and paste to their mailing lists and attached a study flyer that they could print out or send on. In terms of benefits, we offered doctoral schools the opportunity to register for project updates and, upon request, receive data on the prevalence of mental health problems for their region. We were fortunate to have the support of many doctoral schools who disseminated our study information to their PhD cohorts.

The key to recruiting participants is spreading the word far and wide, ensuring that as many people see/find out about your study as possible. This does not mean, however, that everyone who sees the study advert can or should take part. The target sample for the survey can be described in terms of their eligibility criteria, broken down into either the characteristics participants should (inclusion criteria) and should not (exclusion criteria) have. To avoid wasting people's time, a summary of these criteria should be included in study advertisements and checked within the survey using an eligibility assessment. For example, multiple choice questions that participants are required to answer to proceed with the survey can ensure those who take part are eligible. In U-DOC, ineligible participants were then shown a message thanking them for their time and informing them that the study was not the right fit for them.

Activity 7.2

One of the reasons that researchers opt for online survey studies is that it has the potential for a lot of data to be collected in a short period of time. However, realising this benefit requires an effective recruitment strategy. What will your recruitment strategy for your research look like? For example:

- What strategies have you used in the past? Were these effective?
- Are there any new strategies that you can try?
- Where are the people you are trying to recruit? How can you make sure they see your study advert? How does your intended target population think you can best recruit them (if you can discuss with someone who fits this profile)?
- Who are the gatekeepers that you could engage with to promote your survey? Is there anything that could make your research more visible?
- What can you include on your study advert to make it easy and attractive for people to take part?
- Are you making the most of the full range of ways that you can connect with people online?
- Could your recruitment strategy bias your sample? How can you address this?

Stage Three: Analysing the Survey

Dilemma Five: Did We Actually Find the Participants that We Wanted to Find?

We achieved our recruitment targets but it took longer than we first anticipated. Meeting our target meant that all of our planned analyses would have sufficient statistical power. However, an inherent risk with all survey research in which any form of convenience (including snowball) sampling methodology is used is that your sample population does not necessarily represent your target population well (Jager et al., 2017). The potential impact of such selection bias is that it undermines the generalisability of your findings to other populations and settings (Blair & Zinkhan, 2006).

As expected, we do consider selection bias an issue for the data we collected in the U-DOC project. Females are generally more likely to take part in research surveys than males (Smith, 2008), and we found the same gender bias in our sample. A bias in the sample may lead you to re-open recruitment, targeting the subsample that you are lacking. Alternatively, you may wish to enter any biased characteristics into the analysis as covariates. At minimum, you should acknowledge such sample issues as a limitation in your study report. We did not have capacity to re-open the survey and instead included all key demographics as covariates in the analysis and identified issues of selection bias in publications arising. Reporting of online survey research must include detailed descriptions of the sampling and recruitment methods used (ideally with an indication of response rate if possible) and the resulting population of participants (including details of non-completion and missing data) to enable readers to understand the potential for bias.

The high potential for incompleteness, or otherwise missing data, is one of the most frustrating aspects of online survey research (Galesic, 2006). It is easier to withdraw from an online survey than most other study designs, increasing the chance of people exercising that right and withdrawing before they have completed any of the questionnaires (Hoerger, 2010). In addition, as participants are not supervised while completing the survey, there is a greater potential for questions being missed or skipped (Mirzaei et al., 2022). Reducing the amount of missing data in the survey dataset can be addressed using the same strategies employed to reduce dropouts. If appropriate, you can also use the survey settings to ensure that participants must answer all questions before progressing to the next page.

The first consideration when managing missing data is identifying whether it is missing at random or if there is a pattern to it (Papageorgiou et al., 2018). If there is a pattern to the missing data, then this suggests there may be a systematic explanation that may reflect a bias in the data (Tremblay et al., 2010). To assess this within our survey, we modelled whether participant demographics (e.g. gender, age, ethnicity, participant group), or other study variables, predicted whether data were missing or present for each study variable. We found that none of the characteristics entered predicted whether data were missing or not. We therefore concluded that data were likely to be missing at random and did not present a serious threat to the integrity of our analysis. If we had identified any significant relationships, then steps would need to be taken to try to offer some mitigation, for example, entering significant characteristics as covariates or using additional statistical corrections.

The management of missingness in statistical analysis typically either takes the form of using only present data in analysis (e.g. listwise or pairwise deletion; Peugh & Enders, 2004), replacing the missing values (imputation; Brick & Kalton, 1996) or using the present values to maximise the inferences made about missing data should it have been present (Full Information Maximum Likelihood or FIML; Field, 2013). An account of approaches to handling missing data can be found in a book chapter by Graham et al. (Graham et al., 2013). In the U-DOC project, we had only a small amount of item-level missing data. We wanted to make the most of the data we had and retain as much of it as possible. Therefore, we either used pairwise deletion or, when conducting analysis using packages that offered this option, Full Information Maximum Likelihood (FIML) approaches.

Both data coding and missing data protocols are integral to the data cleaning process. Data cleaning is a necessary first step in the analysis. It is the process of preparing the data set for analysis. In addition to handling missing data and scoring the variables, other steps in the data cleaning process may include deleting non-responses, removing participants who are ineligible, and deleting participants who did not complete the consent statement. As is good practice when working with large datasets, we recommend using version control and saving a clearly labelled new version of the data file every time an edit is made. Doing so will mean that, in the event of any errors, you will not have to start from scratch and can simply return to the previous version of the dataset.

Dilemma Six: We Have the Data: Now What Do We Do With It?

The analysis approach chosen will depend on the type of data collected and the research question(s). We conducted a mixed-methods online survey, so we had the option of using quantitative or qualitative methods alone, or combining them. We have utilised all of these analysis approaches within the U-DOC project, choosing the one that allowed us to best answer each specific research question. For one of our papers, we wanted to find out if there was a difference in the severity of mental health difficulties between PhD students and our control group of working professionals (Hazell et al., 2021). Looking at differences between groups in relation to continuous dependent variables is a question that lends itself to quantitative approaches such as t-tests or ANOVAs (Field, 2013). Providing a full account of these statistical tests is beyond the scope of this chapter and questions related to this are better answered by statistics textbooks. But before you can look into how to do these tests though you need to identify what test you need to do.

There are some key decisions that we made a priori related to analysis that then determined the type of test we needed to conduct. For example, are there any potential confounding variables that you want to control for in your analysis? Ideally you want to try to identify and control for potential confounding variables in your design or analysis (or both!). This facilitates a truer test of the association between your independent and dependent variable. We first attempted to match our two participant groups on some basic potential confounds, for example, education and occupational activity. We then measured and included in our analyses all key demographic variables as covariates as we know that the risk of mental health difficulties can vary in relation to demographic characteristics, such as age, gender and ethnicity. Also, do you want to explore more than one dependent variable in your analysis and, if so, would a composite of these dependent variables be informative? In our between-groups comparison paper, we had four dependent variables and wanted to also create a composite of these scales reflecting general poor mental health. We therefore entered all of the dependent variables into a single model, that is, a MANCOVA. It should be noted that, before embarking on any quantitative analysis, it is important to check that your data are suitable for the test you wish to conduct. To conduct analyses like t-test or ANOVAs, the data must meet parametric test assumptions (Field, 2013). Where assumptions are violated, then the data can be transformed or alternative analysis approaches can be utilised (Field, 2013). Such assumptions do not need to be met when conducting non-parametric tests such as chi-square or Mann-Whitney U tests (Field, 2013).

In another of our papers, we adopted a mixed-methods analysis approach. In this analysis, we wanted to learn about PhD student experiences of stigma within their university, and also its relationship to attendance behaviours, specifically absenteeism and presenteeism (Berry et al. 2021a). Mixed-methods research can broadly take two forms: (1) convergent: also thought of as triangulation, whereby you are using quantitative and qualitative approaches to answer the same question with the goal of drawing a singular harmonious conclusion; or (2) divergent: whereby you study the same phenomenon but use quantitative and qualitative approaches separately, making use of the relative strengths of each methodology and acknowledging that contradictory or differing findings may occur (Fetters et al., 2013). For a more detailed account of mixed-methods research please see Doyle et al. (2009) and part three of this book. Our analysis aligned more to the convergent triangulation approach, for we collected quantitative and qualitative data in one questionnaire designed to answer the same core research questions around whether, and if so, how, perceived and experienced stigma were experienced by PhD students and whether, and if so, how, stigma was associated with attendance behaviours (see Fig. 7.4). We analysed the quantitative data and qualitative data separately, but contemporaneously, moving between the two to facilitate co-evolving understandings. The quantitative analysis comprised a structural equation model, which specified the measurement of perceptions and experiences of mental health stigma in the university setting (measurement model) and associations between stigma and attendance behaviours (structural model). The qualitative analysis comprised framework analysis, a derivative of thematic analysis (Braun & Clarke, 2013), and sought to understand perceptions and experiences of mental health stigma in the university setting and their associations with attendance behaviours; that is, analogous to the

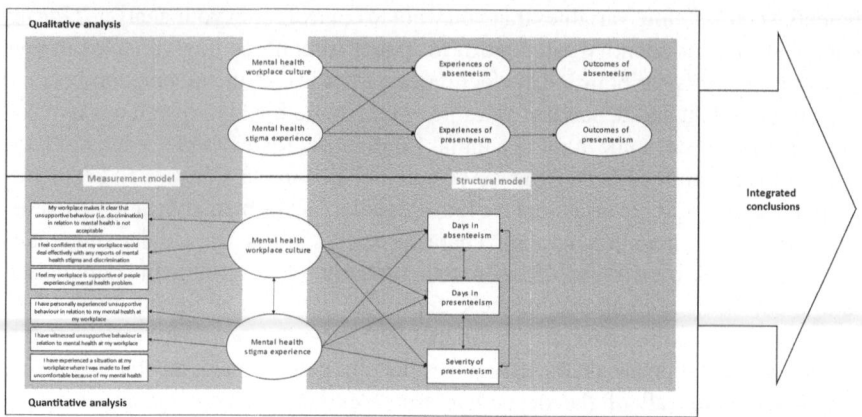

Fig. 7.4 Mixed-methods analysis of doctoral student perceptions and experiences of mental health related-stigma and its associations with attendance behaviours

measurement and structural model respectively (see Fig. 7.4). We additionally aimed to understand the potential influences of gender, ethnicity and pre-existing mental health problems (quantitative and qualitative analysis) and to identify novel qualitative themes. We then sought to identify convergence and divergence in conclusions that could be drawn following from the quantitative and qualitative analyses (O'Cathain et al., 2010). We have also used the U-DOC data to conduct a purely qualitative study. We wanted to explore PhD students' lived experience of suicidality and therefore approached this using qualitative methods alone, analysing the free-text responses using thematic analysis (Braun & Clarke, 2013). For more information on qualitative methods see parts one and three of this book.

Dilemma Seven: How Do We Let People Know What We Found?

The most common method of communicating online survey research results is via academic publications. With any project, it is important to devise a publication plan. A publication plan details what papers you plan to publish, who will lead them and otherwise be involved, and where (and perhaps when) you would like to submit them. Where you have multiple planned papers, it is important to divide them up appropriately and then find them each a home where they are likely to be seen by the intended audience. This division should be scientifically driven, that is, 'chunking' analyses into meaningful and coherent stories, as opposed to needless 'salami-slicing'. For example, we could have decided to divide our main survey paper comparing mental health symptoms severity between PhD students and working professionals according to the type of mental health problem being investigated, that is, a paper on depression symptoms and a separate paper on anxiety symptoms. We decided not to do this as we are able to tell a richer and more impactful narrative about the mental health of PhD students when looking at these symptoms all together in a single paper.

Sharing your findings outside of academia is equally, if not more, essential. Public engagement is an important aspect of the research cycle (Grand et al., 2015). Effective public engagement involves communicating your research using non-technical and accessible language—also sometimes referred to as 'lay' language. Examples of public engagement activities and outputs include public seminars, blog posts, media interviews and public reports. In the U-DOC project, we have shared our findings via the traditional academic platforms (i.e. papers and conference presentations), but we have also welcomed and sought out public engagement opportunities. We have presented at public engagement events and festivals, written several blog posts, and been interviewed about our work by media outlets. Each of these opportunities has helped us learn more about our own research—for example, the comments on our blog posts give us insight into what others think of our findings and how they make sense of them; and the interviews give us the opportunity to see our research through another's eyes. Public engagement also helps to raise the profile of your work which can open the door to future collaborations, further funding and career development opportunities.

Dilemma Eight: When Does It End?!

The U-DOC project produced a large dataset that could be used to test many hypotheses and answer many research questions. We are fortunate to have such a rich dataset, but it can be difficult to know when the project has come to an end. The papers thus far have been driven by the interests of our research team but there are a number of other questions that could be explored. Ethically, there is an imperative to explore all of these questions and learn everything we can from the data given so generously by the participants. Yet some of the potential research questions fall outside of our expertise and we continue to welcome opportunities to share our data with collaborators for further exploration. We are able to do this because our data were collected anonymously, and we gathered consent from participants to share these anonymous data for research purposes.

Further exploration can be facilitated by making a dataset accessible to others via a data sharing repository, such as Open Science Framework. We have not yet shared our database as we have projects currently ongoing. However, we plan to make our dataset available to others as soon as we can. A further key consideration in our ongoing work and future collaborations is at what point may data become obsolete? There is no single answer to this question and should instead be considered in light of the related context and culture. Where the data are taken from a rapidly changing setting, their shelf-life may be short, whereas for contexts that are slow-moving, the data may be valid for a long time.

Activity 7.3

Research is akin to story-telling—you pose a question, seek to answer this, and reflect and comment on the process and your learning. Online surveys like the one we conducted within the U-DOC project allow you to tell multiple stories. The potential stories that can be told are dictated by the nature and number of questions asked and the range of analytic approaches available. What are the different stories that you could tell from your online survey research? Are these stories complimentary or contradictory? Which stories are the most compelling and why? You might find it helpful to reflect on this final question in light of how different stories could:

- Best advance our understanding(s);
- Address gaps in available evidence;
- Lead to significant real-world impact;
- Align best with your research interests and expertise;
- Give you data that can direct future research studies and grant applications.

Summary

Online surveys are an increasingly popular research method that can support the collection of quantitative, qualitative, and mixed-methods data. They offer researchers the potential to create large datasets over short periods of time. Nonetheless, using online surveys to their full potential requires a number of thoughtful and considerate design decisions that strike a balance between the needs of researchers and those of participants. That is, it can be tempting to overload online surveys so as to answer a wide range of research questions—but this has negative implications for the participant experience. We have used our experience of the U-DOC survey to illustrate this decision-making journey, from the point of online survey conception through launching and analysis. We have emphasised the importance of carefully specifying your research question, thoughtfully identifying constructs and related measurement tools, accurately identifying your target population and appropriate recruitment strategies, ethically minimising participant burden and maximising motivation, mindfully planning your analyses and considering missing data. We hope that this chapter will have helped you to reflect on your own research ideas, make informed choices when designing your own online surveys, and ultimately produce high-quality and ethical research that will advance psychological science.

References

Allen, M. S., Iliescu, D., & Greiff, S. (2022). Single item measures in psychological science. *European Journal of Psychological Assessment, 38*(1), 1–5. https://doi.org/10.1027/1015-5759/A000699

Antoun, C., Zhang, C., Conrad, F. G., & Schober, M. F. (2016). Comparisons of online recruitment strategies for convenience samples: Craigslist, Google AdWords, Facebook, and Amazon Mechanical Turk. *Field Methods, 28*(3), 231–246. https://doi.org/10.1177/1525822X15603149

Ball, H. L. (2019). Conducting online surveys. *Journal of Human Lactation, 35*(3), 413–417. https://doi.org/10.1177/0890334419848734

Beck, A. T., & Bredemeier, K. (2016). A unified model of depression: Integrating clinical. *Cognitive, Biological, and Evolutionary Perspectives, 4*(4), 596–619. https://doi.org/10.1177/2167702616628523

Berry, C., Niven, J. E., Chapman, L., Valeix, S., Roberts, P., & Hazell, C. M. (2021a). A mixed mixed-methods investigation of mental health stigma, absenteeism and presenteeism among UK postgraduate researchers. *Studies in Graduate and Postdoctoral Education, 12*(1), 145–170.

Berry, C., Niven, J. E., & Hazell, C. M. (2021b). Personal, social and relational predictors of UK postgraduate researcher mental health problems. *BJPsych Open, 7*(6), e205. https://doi.org/10.1192/BJO.2021.1041

Blair, E., & Zinkhan, G. M. (2006). Nonresponse and generalizability in academic research. *Journal of the Academy of Marketing Science, 34*(1), 4–7. https://doi.org/10.1177/0092070305283778

Blumenberg, C., Menezes, A. M. B., Gonçalves, H., Assunção, M. C. F., Wehrmeister, F. C., & Barros, A. J. D. (2019). How different online recruitment methods impact on recruitment rates for the web-based coortesnaweb project: A randomised trial. *BMC Medical Research Methodology, 19*(1), 1–9. https://doi.org/10.1186/s12874-019-0767-z

Braun, V., & Clarke, V. (2013). *Successful qualitative research: A practical guide for beginners.* Sage. http://eprints.uwe.ac.uk/21156/3/SQR

Brick, J. M., & Kalton, G. (1996). Handling missing data in survey research. *Statistical Methods in Medical Research, 5*(3), 215–238. https://doi.org/10.1177/096228029600500302

Burghardt, J., & Bodansky, A. N. (2021). Why psychology needs to stop striving for novelty and how to move towards theory-driven research. *Frontiers in Psychology, 12*, 67. https://doi.org/10.3389/FPSYG.2021.609802/BIBTEX

Callegaro, M., Jon Cohen, G., Elizabeth Dean, S., Harwood, P., & Josh Pasek, T. (2014). *Mobile technologies for conducting, augmenting and potentially replacing surveys: Report of the AAPOR task force on emerging technologies in public opinion research.* www.aapor.org

Christensen, T., Riis, A. H., Hatch, E. E., Wise, L. A., Nielsen, M. G., Rothman, K. J., Sørensen, H. T., & Mikkelsen, E. M. (2017). Costs and efficiency of online and offline recruitment methods: A web-based cohort study. *Journal of Medical Internet Research, 19*(3), e58. https://doi.org/10.2196/jmir.6716

Connelly, L. M. (2022). Understanding research. Measurement instrument validity. *MEDSURG Nursing, 31*(1), 64–65. https://web.p.ebscohost.com/abstract?direct=true&profile=ehost&scope=site&authtype=crawler&jrnl=10920811&AN=155300022&h=evWO%2FnjPmz%2Bv8Exx5QpuPWg8W3nx6fdF%2BL%2FVS0%2FxZDpvUXrqNb8PYBANvyp5G1W5HjjEuCEdy4CnpH7LFm%2Fx5A%3D%3D&crl=c&resultNs=AdminWebAuth&resultLocal=ErrCrlNotAuth&crlhashurl=login.aspx%3Fdirect%3Dtrue%26profile%3Dehost%26scope%3Dsite%26authtype%3Dcrawler%26jrnl%3D10920811%26AN%3D155300022

Cornette, M. M., Deroon-Cassini, T. A., Fosco, G. M., Holloway, R. L., Clark, D. C., & Joiner, T. E. (2009). Application of an interpersonal-psychological model of suicidal behavior to physicians and medical trainees. *Archives of Suicide Research, 13*(1), 1–14. https://doi.org/10.1080/13811110802571801

Danermark, B., & Ekström, M. (2002). *Explaining society: Critical realism in the social sciences.* Routledge.

Danermark, B., Ekström, M., & Karlsson, J. C. (2002). *Explaining society: Critical realism in the social sciences.* Routledge.

Deutskens, E., de Ruyter, K., Wetzels, M., & Oosterveld, P. (2004). Response rate and response quality of internet-based surveys: An experimental study. *Marketing Letters, 15*(1), 21–36.

Dillman, D. A., Smyth, J. D., & Christian, L. M. (2014). *Internet, phone, mail, and mixed-mode surveys: The tailored design method.* Wiley.

Doyle, L., Brady, A. M., & Byrne, G. (2009). An overview of mixed methods research. *Journal of Research in Nursing, 14*(2), 175–185. https://doi.org/10.1177/1744987108093962

Draper, H., Wilson, S., Flanagan, S., & Ives, J. (2009). Offering payments, reimbursement and incentives to patients and family doctors to encourage participation in research. *Family Practice, 26*(3), 231–238. https://doi.org/10.1093/fampra/cmp011

Draucker, C. B., Martsolf, D. S., & Poole, C. (2009). Developing distress protocols for research on sensitive topics. *Archives of Psychiatric Nursing, 23*(5), 343–350. https://doi.org/10.1016/j.apnu.2008.10.008

Duffy, M. E. (1987). Methodological triangulation: A vehicle for merging quantitative and qualitative research methods. *Image: The Journal of Nursing Scholarship, 19*(3), 130–133. https://doi.org/10.1111/J.1547-5069.1987.TB00609.X

Evans, J. R., & Mathur, A. (2018). The value of online surveys: A look back and a look ahead. *Internet Research, 28*(4), 854–887. https://doi.org/10.1108/IntR-03-2018-0089

Fetters, M. D., Curry, L. A., & Creswell, J. W. (2013). Achieving integration in mixed methods designs - principles and practices. *Health Services Research, 48*(6 PART2), 2134–2156. https://doi.org/10.1111/1475-6773.12117

Field, A. (2013). *Discovering statistics using IBM SPSS.* SAGE.

Fletcher, A. J. (2017). Applying critical realism in qualitative research: Methodology meets method. *International Journal of Social Research Methodology, 20*(2), 181–194. https://doi.org/10.1080/13645579.2016.1144401

Fowler, D., Hodgekins, J., Berry, C., Clarke, T., Palmier-Claus, J., Sacadura, C., Graham, A., Lowen, C., Steele, A., Pugh, K., Fraser, S., & French, P. (2019). Social recovery therapy: A treatment manual. *Psychosis, 11*, 261–272.

Galesic, M. (2006). Dropouts on the web: Influence of changes in respondents' interest and perceived burden during the web survey. *Journal of Official Statistics, 22*(2), 313–328.

Graham, J. W., Cumsille, P. E., & Shevock, A. E. (2013). Methods for handling missing data. In J. A. Schinka, W. F. Velicer, & I. B. Weiner (Eds.), *Handbook of psychology: Research methods in psychology.* Wiley.

Grand, A., Davies, G., Holliman, R., & Adams, A. (2015). Mapping public engagement with research in a UK university. *PLoS One, 10*(4), 1–19. https://doi.org/10.1371/journal.pone.0121874

Grant, R. W., & Sugarman, J. (2004). Ethics in human subjects research: Do incentives matter? *The Journal of Medicine and Philosophy: A Forum for Bioethics and Philosophy of Medicine, 29*(6), 717–738. https://doi.org/10.1080/03605310490883046

Greenlaw, C., & Brown-Welty, S. (2009). A comparison of web-based and paper-based survey methods: Testing assumptions of survey mode and response cost. *Evaluation Review, 33*(5), 464–480. https://doi.org/10.1177/0193841X09340214

Grimes, D. A., & Schulz, K. F. (2002). Bias and causal associations in observational research. *The Lancet, 359*(9302), 248–252. https://doi.org/10.1016/S0140-6736(02)07451-2

Hawkley, L. C., & Cacioppo, J. T. (2010). Loneliness matters: A theoretical and empirical review of consequences and mechanisms. *Annals of Behavioral Medicine: A Publication of the Society of Behavioral Medicine, 40*(2), 218–227. https://doi.org/10.1007/S12160-010-9210-8

Hazell, C. M., Chapman, L., Valeix, S. F., Roberts, P., Niven, J. E., & Berry, C. (2020). Understanding the mental health of doctoral researchers: A mixed methods systematic review with meta-analysis and meta-synthesis. *Systematic Reviews, 9*(1), 197. https://doi.org/10.1186/s13643-020-01443-1

Hazell, C. M., Niven, J. E., Chapman, L., Roberts, P. E., Cartwright-Hatton, S., Valeix, S., & Berry, C. (2021). Nationwide assessment of the mental health of UK doctoral researchers. *Humanities and Social Sciences Communications, 8*(1), 8–16. https://doi.org/10.1057/s41599-021-00983-8

Hlatshwako, T. G., Shah, S. J., Kosana, P., Adebayo, E., Hendriks, J., Larsson, E. C., Hensel, D. J., Erausquin, J. T., Marks, M., Michielsen, K., Saltis, H., Francis, J. M., Wouters, E., & Tucker, J. D. (2021). Online health survey research during COVID-19. *The Lancet Digital Health, 3*(2), e76–e77. https://doi.org/10.1016/S2589-7500(21)00002-9/ATTACHMENT/DACDFE51-523B-4EFB-AC39-E798FA533B66/MMC1.PDF

Hoerger, M. (2010). Participant dropout as a function of survey length in internet-mediated university studies: Implications for study design and voluntary participation in psychological research. *Cyberpsychology, Behavior and Social Networking, 13*(6), 697–701.

Hood, K., Robling, M., Ingledew, D., Gillespie, D., Greene, G., Ivins, R., Russell, I., Sayers, A., Shaw, C., & Williams, J. (2012). Mode of data elicitation, acquisition and response to surveys: A systematic review. *Health Technology Assessment, 16*(27), 1–161. https://doi.org/10.3310/hta16270

Jager, J., Putnick, D. L., & Bornstein, M. H. (2017). More than just convenient: The scientific merits of homogeneous convenience samples. *Monographs of the Society for Research in Child Development, 82*(2), 13–30. https://doi.org/10.1111/mono.12296

Jenkins, P. E., Ducker, I., Gooding, R., James, M., & Rutter-Eley, E. (2021). Anxiety and depression in a sample of UK college students: A study of prevalence, comorbidity, and quality of life. *Journal of American College Health, 69*(8), 813–819. https://doi.org/10.1080/07448481.2019.1709474

Jetten, J., Haslam, C., & Haslam, A. S. (Eds.). (2012). *The social cure: Identity, health and well-being.* Psychology Press. https://books.google.co.uk/books?hl=en&lr=&id=EeB4AgAAQBAJ&oi=fnd&pg=PR3&dq=The+social+cure:+Identity,+health+and+well-being.&ots=OZ8Ny-jXCU&sig=w8YpkrvAj79W3nW_Yfgomh2onc0#v=onepage&q=The

Kline, R. B. (2011). *Principles and practice of structural equation modeling* (3rd ed.). The Guildford Press. https://doi.org/10.1080/10705511.2012.687667

Knapp, P., Mitchell, N., Raynor, D. K., Silcock, J., Parkinson, B., Holt, J., Birks, Y., & Gilbody, S. (2011). Can we improve recruitment to trials and informed consent by improving participant information sheets? - a nested RCT. *Trials, 12*(S1), 1–2. https://doi.org/10.1186/1745-6215-12-s1-a123

Kroenke, K., Spitzer, R. L., Williams, J. B. W., & Löwe, B. (2010). The patient health questionnaire somatic, anxiety, and depressive symptom scales: A systematic review. *General Hospital Psychiatry, 32*(4), 345–359. https://doi.org/10.1016/j.genhosppsych.2010.03.006

Leonard, N. R., Lester, P., Rotheram-Borus, M. J., Mattes, K., Gwadz, M., & Ferns, B. (2003). Successful recruitment and retention of participants in longitudinal behavioral research. *AIDS Education and Prevention, 15*(3), 269–281. https://doi.org/10.1521/aeap.15.4.269.23827

Lindsay, J. (2005). Getting the numbers: The unacknowledged work in recruiting for survey research. *Field Methods, 17*(1), 119–128. https://doi.org/10.1177/1525822X04271028

McEvoy, P., & Richards, D. (2003). Critical realism: A way forward for evaluation research in nursing? *Journal of Advanced Nursing, 43*(4), 411–420. https://doi.org/10.1046/j.1365-2648.2003.02730.x

MHFA England. (2020). *Mental health statistics.* MHFA England.

Miller, C. A., Guidry, J. P. D., Dahman, B., & Thomson, M. D. (2020). A tale of two diverse qualtrics samples: Information for online survey researchers. *Cancer Epidemiology Biomarkers and Prevention, 29*(4), 731–735. https://doi.org/10.1158/1055-9965.EPI-19-0846/70558/AM/A-TALE-OF-TWO-DIVERSE-QUALTRICS-SAMPLES

Mirzaei, A., Carter, S. R., Patanwala, A. E., & Schneider, C. R. (2022). Missing data in surveys: Key concepts, approaches, and applications. *Research in Social and Administrative Pharmacy, 18*(2), 2308–2316. https://doi.org/10.1016/j.sapharm.2021.03.009

Nolte, M. T., Shauver, M. J., & Chung, K. C. (2015). Analysis of four recruitment methods for obtaining normative data through a web-based questionnaire: A pilot study. *The Hand, 10*(3), 529–534. https://doi.org/10.1007/s11552-014-9730-y

O'Brien, K. K., Solomon, P., Worthington, C., Ibáñez-Carrasco, F., Baxter, L., Nixon, S. A., Baltzer-Turje, R., Robinson, G., & Zack, E. (2014). Considerations for conducting web-based survey research with people living with human immunodeficiency virus using a community-based participatory approach. *Journal of Medical Internet Research, 16*(3), e3064. https://doi.org/10.2196/JMIR.3064

O'Cathain, A., Murphy, E., & Nicholl, J. (2010). Three techniques for integrating data in mixed methods studies. *BMJ (Online), 341*(7783), 1147–1150. https://doi.org/10.1136/bmj.c4587

Oberauer, K., & Lewandowsky, S. (2019). Addressing the theory crisis in psychology. *Psychonomic Bulletin and Review, 26*(5), 1596–1618. https://doi.org/10.3758/S13423-019-01645-2/FIGURES/6

Olsen, W. K., Haralambos, M., & Holborn, M. (2004). Triangulation in social research: Qualitative and quantitative methods can really be mixed. In W. K. Olsen, M. Haralambos, & M. Holborn (Eds.), *Developments in sociology* (pp. 1–30). Causeway Press.

Papageorgiou, G., Grant, S. W., Takkenberg, J. J. M., & Mokhles, M. M. (2018). Statistical primer: How to deal with missing data in scientific research? *Interactive Cardiovascular and Thoracic Surgery, 27*(2), 153–158. https://doi.org/10.1093/icvts/ivy102

Peugh, J. L., & Enders, C. K. (2004). Missing data in educational research: A review of reporting practices and suggestions for improvement. *Review of Educational Research, 74*(4), 525–556. https://doi.org/10.3102/00346543074004525

Pozzar, R., Hammer, M. J., Underhill-Blazey, M., Wright, A. A., Tulsky, J. A., Hong, F., Gundersen, D. A., & Berry, D. L. (2020). Threats of bots and other bad actors to data quality following research participant recruitment through social media: Cross-sectional questionnaire. *Journal of Medical Internet Research, 22*(10). https://doi.org/10.2196/23021

Roberts, C. (2016). Response styles in surveys: Understanding their causes and mitigating their impact on data quality. In C. Wolf (Ed.), *The SAGE handbook of survey methodology* (pp. 579–596). Sage. https://doi.org/10.4135/9781473957893.N36

Roberts, C., Gilbert, E., Allum, N., & Eisner, L. (2019). Research Synthesis Satisficing in surveys: A systematic review of the literature. *Public Opinion Quarterly, 83*(3), 598–626. https://doi.org/10.1093/POQ/NFZ035

Smith, G. (2008). Does gender influence online survey participation? A record-linkage analysis of university faculty online survey response behavior. In *ERIC Document Reproduction Service No. ED 501717* (Vol. 501717).

Spitzer, R. L., Kroenke, K., Williams, J. B. W., & Löwe, B. (2006). A brief measure for assessing generalized anxiety disorder: The GAD-7. *Archives of Internal Medicine, 166*(10), 1092–1097. https://doi.org/10.1001/archinte.166.10.1092

Tavakol, M., & Dennick, R. (2011). Making sense of Cronbach's alpha. *International Journal of Medical Education, 2*, 53. https://doi.org/10.5116/IJME.4DFB.8DFD

The British Psychological Society. (2021). Code of ethics and conduct. *The British Psychological Society, 21*, 134. https://doi.org/10.1016/s0315-5463(88)70754-3

Tishler, C. L., & Bartholomae, S. (2002). The recruitment of normal healthy volunteers: A review of the literature on the use of financial incentives. *Journal of Clinical Pharmacology, 42*(4), 365–375. https://doi.org/10.1177/00912700222011409

Tourangeau, R., Rips, L. J., & Rasinski, K. (2000). *The psychology of survey response.* Cambridge University Press. https://books.google.co.uk/books?hl=en&lr=&id=bjVYdyXXT3oC&oi=fnd&pg=PR11&dq=Tourangeau+R,+Rips+LJ,+Rasinski+K.+The+psychology+of+survey+response.+Cambridge:+Cambridge+University+Press%3B+2000.&ots=Z-YhOL8CBV&sig=zAD7y0LC8ZXK6vNvv13Vr8BlpVE#v=onepage&q=To

Tremblay, M. C., Dutta, K., & Vandermeer, D. (2010). Using data mining techniques to discover bias patterns in missing data. *Journal of Data and Information Quality, 2*(1), 1. https://doi.org/10.1145/1805286.1805288

UCAS. (2021). *Starting the conversation: UCAS report on student mental health.* UCAS.

van Teijlingen, E., & Hundley, V. (2001). The importance of pilot studies. *Social Research Update, 35.* https://aura.abdn.ac.uk/handle/2164/157

Watts, G. (2020). COVID-19 and the digital divide in the UK. *The Lancet Digital Health, 2*(8), e395–e396. https://doi.org/10.1016/S2589-7500(20)30169-2

World Health Organisation (WHO). (2021). *Suicide.* WHO.

Wright, K. B. (2005). Researching internet-based populations: Advantages and disadvantages of online survey research, online questionnaire authoring software packages, and web survey services. *Journal of Computer-Mediated Communication, 10*(3). https://doi.org/10.1111/J.1083-6101.2005.TB00259.X/4614509

Part III
Mixed Methods Research. Theory and Examples of Integration

Chapter 8
Using Online Surveys Creatively in Counselling and Psychotherapy Research

Alistair McBeath

Learning Goals

After reading this chapter you should be able to:

- Appreciate the potential benefits of a pluralistic approach to research.
- Understand the ways that online surveys can include qualitative content.
- Know how the story completion qualitative approach is used.
- Understand the power of survey skip logic and advanced branching.
- Know how to effectively present survey findings.
- Understand ways of exploring survey data.
- Appreciate the ways in which online surveys can be effectively publicised.

Introduction

Surveys are undoubtedly one of the most common ways to gauge peoples' views on a diverse range of issues and the online survey has now become established as the principal mode of delivery.

They seem to pop up everywhere and are regularly embedded and encountered on the world-wide web. But surveys have also achieved success as a powerful research tool in many contexts including the professions of counselling and psychotherapy. But there has undoubtedly been some reluctance to promote surveys as an effective research method. In this regard it seems clear that some views about surveys as a research method are out of date, tied to rigid views about underlying

A. McBeath (✉)
Metanoia Institute, London, UK
e-mail: Alistair.McBeath@metanoia.ac.uk

© The Author(s), under exclusive license to Springer Nature Switzerland AG 2022
S. Bager-Charleson, A. McBeath (eds.), *Supporting Research in Counselling and Psychotherapy*, https://doi.org/10.1007/978-3-031-13942-0_8

research philosophies and have not kept pace with recent developments in the ability of surveys to harvest qualitative-rich data.

In this chapter the focus is on seeking to emphasise just how powerful online surveys can be as a research tool within the counselling and psychotherapy professions. In this regard there is a clear focus on their ability to be effective in recording and eliciting both potent quantitative and qualitative information and that online surveys can be legitimately analysed using existing qualitative research techniques.

Other topics covered will include how to effectively publicise a survey and how to maximise the impact of a survey through the effective presentation of findings and also some consideration of when and when not to statistically analyse survey data. There is also an introduction to survey logic which is the basis of so-called *intelligent surveys*. For those unfamiliar with online surveys, how to construct a survey and what types of questions can be used a succinct account can be found by McBeath (2020b).

Background

From a historical perspective the use of surveys in psychotherapy and counselling research has not been particularly widespread with the various qualitative research methodologies (e.g. Interpretative Phenomenological Analysis (IPA), Grounded Theory, Narrative Analysis) proving to be far more popular with both novice and experienced researchers. This situation partly reflects what McLeod (2015) described as, 'a substantial degree of resistance to quantitative methods within the counselling and psychotherapy professional community' (p80).

Traditionally, surveys have been viewed as having an underlying epistemological and scientific approach that is incompatible with being able to capture the complexities, challenges and dynamic nuances inherent in the practice of counselling and psychotherapy. However, a growing interest in pluralistic and mixed methods approaches has seen a steady increase in the use of online surveys in counselling and psychotherapy research (e.g. McBeath, 2019; Davey et al., 2019; McEvoy, 2019; McBeath et al., 2020). The rigid view that somehow qualitative and quantitative research approaches are incompatible, echoing the so-called *paradigm wars* (Tashakkori & Teddlie, 1998), is now fading and there is a growing acceptance that both research approaches have a valid place in counselling and psychotherapy research. McLeod (2015) makes a key point in stating that, 'therapy research needs to be pluralistic because good therapy is pluralistic' (p 8).

The increasing use of surveys in counselling and psychotherapy research and the rationale for such an approach can be seen in mixed methods approaches to research. The key point is that qualitative and quantitative methods are complementary rather than competing research approaches. So, it is perfectly legitimate and hugely profitable to let both quantitative and qualitative research approaches provide their own unique window into the lived experience of individuals; this is the key principle that underlies pluralistic and mixed methods approaches to research.

The potential benefits of a pluralistic approach to research have found precise expression from Landrum and Garza (2015)

> We argue that together, quantitative and qualitative approaches are stronger and provide more knowledge and insights about a research topic than either approach alone. While both approaches shed unique light on a particular research topic, we suggest that methodologically pluralistic researchers would be able to approach their interests in such a way as to reveal new insights that neither method nor approach could reveal alone. (p 207)

These words might prove valuable for all who are considering embarking on research within the counselling and psychotherapy professions and to raise awareness that a well-designed online survey can be a valuable and meaningful research tool across a diverse range of phenomena under study.

Online Surveys and Qualitative Data

It is important to realise that there has been an evolution and development of online surveys that seems to have escaped serious review and discussion. Firstly, some recent research in counselling and psychotherapy has reported just how much rich qualitative data can be harvested from a well-designed online survey. An online survey exploring the challenges and opportunities for therapists working remotely during the Covid pandemic is one example (McBeath et al., 2020).

The 335 survey respondents gave a total of 225 free-text comments; these included statements of clarification, brief comments about a range of issues and, in some instances, a paragraph or more containing quite detailed accounts of personal experiences and reflection, amplifying considerably some of the issues highlighted in the survey. The total word count from the 225 free-text comments was 9051. This body of information and knowledge was recognised and treated as a relevant and valuable source of qualitative data and was subject to a Reflexive Thematic Analysis (Braun & Clarke, 2006, 2019) that provided three unambiguously meaningful themes—new challenges, opportunities and adaption issues.

Some online surveys have gone a stage further and specifically included a few qualitative, open-ended questions. Bager-Charleson and McBeath (2021b) used such an approach to explore the supervision experience in psychotherapy doctorates for both research supervisors and supervisees. Simple questions just asking for an account of lived experience provided wonderful vignettes of the research supervision experience that presented a different window of meaning compared to that provided by the quantitative data collected in the survey. Here are four comments from research supervisees that helped a theme to be created around the need for research supervisors to have *good relational skills*.

- She communicated a sense of belief in me and my research topic as well as a passion for the whole research process.
- My supervisor provided balanced encouragement and positivity with challenge in regard to some limitations of the research.

- He demonstrated excellent listening skills and a sense that he was fully behind me and my research.
- When feeling lost and not good enough, getting normalising support from my supervisor helped me to regain confidence.

Asking qualitative questions in an online survey needs to be done with care but the depth of meaning that they can evoke can be powerful and informative about the individual's experience of a particular phenomenon. Here are two responses, one from a research supervisor and from a research supervisee—the question was quite simple,

Can you think of an example where you had a really productive supervision experience?

Research Supervisee
The main help so far was when I found it difficult and daunting to start my proposal and was also worried about being judged by my supervisors as they were experienced. It was the total opposite. They were empathic, non-judgemental, encouraging and gave helpful tips which was exactly what I needed.

Research Supervisor
One student really struggled with her research, and we scheduled weekly but shorter supervision sessions over a period of time; she wanted very close guidance and lots of feedback, and she took it on board and it worked for her.

These responses seem very positive, but some supervisees offered a more gloomy experience of their research experience; here are two examples,

I'm always left feeling my supervisor knows what she knows and that's it. As if she doesn't take time to actively further her own research knowledge

It is not containing for a supervisee to have a supervisor who admits to being "rusty" with regards to their memory or knowledge of the methodology

The inclusion of some qualitative questions in an online survey can be richly rewarding but there has been a further development of *fully qualitative surveys* (Braun et al., 2020). Fully qualitative surveys consist of a series of carefully chosen open-ended questions and their potential value in research has been articulated with these words,

fully qualitative surveys *can* produce the rich and complex accounts of the type of sense-making typically of interest to qualitative researchers—such as participants' subjective experiences, narratives, practices, positionings, and discourses. (Braun & Clarke, 2013)

Here are three examples of fully qualitative survey-based research

- Living with alopecia areata: An online qualitative survey study (Davey et al., 2019)
- Young adults' experiences of orgasm and sexual pleasure (Opperman et al., 2014)
- Exploring therapists' accounts of social class in therapy (McEvoy, 2019)

The diversity and sensitivity of these online survey topics reinforce one particular advantage of online qualitative surveys, namely, that they can evoke responses on very sensitive issues from individuals who otherwise might not have participated in other research approaches, for example face to face interviews and focus groups. As Braun et al. (2020) have noted qualitative online surveys may communicate a felt sense of anonymity that encourages participation from respondents whose voice might otherwise have remained silent.

The three online qualitative surveys noted above can serve to illustrate that qualitative survey data is amenable to a variety of differing analytical approaches and an alignment with differing underlying philosophical assumptions. For example, in the study exploring the experience of living with alopecia the qualitative data were subject to a *Thematic Analysis* (Braun & Clarke, 2006) and underpinned by *a critical realist philosophical framework*. The critical realist position (Bhaskar, 1989) is important as it both recognises an objective reality and also a form of epistemological constructivism and relativism such that our representations of reality are mediated by language, culture and societal variables such as race and gender.

Reading some of the themes from the alopecia study is a powerful experience and the distress associated with some of the themes is potent and painful such as the intense sense of bereavement associated with loss of hair and the fear, even after treatment, that the condition will return.

In contrast the study exploring therapists' account of social class in therapy (McEvoy, 2019) utilised *Thematic Discourse Analysis* (Taylor & Ussher, 2001) to analyse qualitative online survey data and was underpinned by *a social constructivist position* that rejects any positivist notions of an objective reality that can be scientifically revealed. Instead, reality and knowledge are a series of successive approximations mediated by history, language and culture and are essentially subjective.

The analysis of online qualitative survey data by McEvoy (2019) was extremely revealing about therapists' associations with social class and some significant implications for clinical practice emerged. McEvoy (2019) noted this key finding,

> When it came to their own class background, most participants used rhetorical strategies to disavow a middle-class status and distance themselves from middle class privilege. (p 7)

There seems little doubt that online qualitative surveys have more power, sophistication and research legitimacy than is usually portrayed in the literature. As Braun et al. (2020) have noted, '*qualitative* surveys remain a relatively novel and often invisible or side-lined method' (p 1).

A particularly interesting development within qualitative research and one that can be effectively delivered using online surveys is what is known as the *story completion method* (Moller et al., 2021). Here the primary focus is on offering survey respondents the start of a story which is called the *story stem* and basically asking— *what happens next*? So, survey respondents are offered the opportunity to complete a story based on a scenario or a story beginning which has been created by the researcher.

There are only a few published studies using the story completion method (e.g. Shah-Beckley et al., 2018; McPherson, 2022) but it has been enticingly described as, 'The best new method for qualitative data collection you've never even heard of'

(Clarke et al., 2019, p 1). Some of the key advantages of the story completion method include its theoretical flexibility, being resource-light and offering survey respondents an unusual opportunity to offer their own creativity.

The author has explored the use of the story completion method using an online survey which was focused on the views and knowledge of both research students and research supervisors on mixed methods research (McBeath & Bager-Charleson, 2022). In designing the story stem the key focus was to produce a story beginning that would feel relevant and engaging to survey respondents but also one that did not offer too much detail and thus potentially 'over guide' the direction and content of respondents' stories. Here is the story stem that was used,

> *Story Stem*
> Kate is planning her research project for her psychotherapy doctorate. She is interested to explore the issue of compassion fatigue in therapists. She knows that she wants to explore the individual experience of compassion fatigue and so will use some form of qualitative research method. But she also wants to get an idea of how common compassion fatigue is across the profession.
> Kate is going to discuss how to progress her research with her supervisor (What could happen next?—feel free to add what might be seen as a story of what might happen)

The richness of data that came from this story stem was really quite exciting and seemed to have a unique quality of depth; perhaps this outcome confirms the view of Clarke et al. (2017) that story completion has the potential to 'reach the parts that other methods cannot reach' (Pope & Mays, 1995). The story stem on mixed methods research was effectively completed by 39% of the 125 survey respondents; over a third (35%) of the stories completed were in excess of 100 words in length with two in excess of 300 words (McBeath & Bager-Charleson, 2022). A thematic analysis was used to create meaning from the completed stories which was an approach that worked well.

There's little doubt that using the story completion method can deliver highly rich qualitative data that is certainly different in both quality and depth compared to data captured in more conventional self-report methods such as interviews and focus groups. It is an approach ideally suited to online surveys and hopefully it will become a more frequently used approach and will cease to be located in what Gravett (2019) has termed, 'the margins of qualitative research'.

Survey Logic

When designing and using surveys there is a very useful facility called *skip logic*; sometimes the word branching is used. The key concept is that, depending on earlier responses, a survey respondent can be directed to another specific question or part of the survey. In other words, within the sequential list of survey questions it is possible to 'skip' certain questions or parts of the survey according to a respondent's answer to an earlier question or questions. A good example would be a survey respondent who indicates that they do not agree to their data being used in a future research project; so, in effect they are not giving their consent. In this case the respondent would skip to the end of the survey where they might see a short 'thank you' statement.

An example of skip logic is shown in Fig. 8.1 which comes from an online survey designed by the author to explore the experience of research supervision for both supervisors and supervisees (Bager-Charleson & McBeath, 2021b).

The survey was designed so that it could be answered by both research supervisors and supervisees. This is really a 'two-in-one' survey and it relies on skip logic to work. Following on from the initial survey introduction sheet which explains the purpose of the survey respondents are then asked to identify themselves as either research supervisors or supervisees. If a respondent identifies as a research supervisor, they then progress to a following question which asks how long they have been a supervisor. However, if a respondent identifies as a supervisee they skip this question about supervisor experience (green line) and, instead, are asked to identify the type of research degree they are doing.

Skip logic can be extremely useful and can save time and resources. For example, with regard to Fig. 8.1 skip logic allowed a single survey to capture the views of both research supervisors and supervisees. For survey respondents skip logic is invisible. So, in the research supervision survey both supervisors and supervisees answered the first question which had an inbuilt skip rule. Following the first question both supervisors and supervisees had their own sets of questions and then they were both directed to a common set of questions at the end of the survey about gender and potential contact details. So, in this survey both research supervisors and supervisees had their own survey and never saw each other's questions. This is a good example of the 'two-in-one survey'. Imagine that you were given a customer satisfaction survey by an airline and it could be answered in either English or French. This would be a classic 'two-in-one survey' and it's based on survey logic.

Within a clinical setting skip logic could be used in several ways. For example, in a therapy clinic that is seeking to evaluate the experience of clients and their

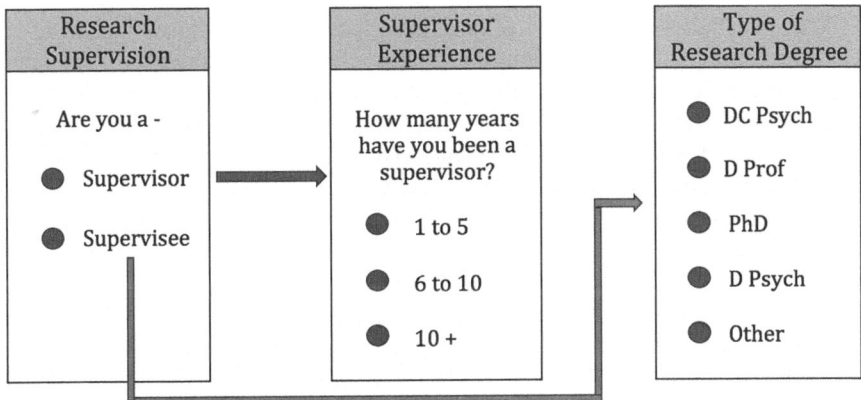

Fig. 8.1 Example of a skip logic question

views on treatment skip logic could be used to differentiate between clients who had either short or long-term therapy and also offer them different sets of survey questions if required.

Advantages of Skip Logic

There are a few important advantages in using survey logic. Already mentioned is the ability to combine two surveys in one so that different types of respondents can have their own tailored experience in a single survey. Another important advantage is that skip logic reduces survey completion time which is a critical factor in securing a good survey response rate. The key factor is that respondents only see survey questions which are relevant to them. If survey respondents find themselves reading redundant questions or questions which they don't feel are relevant to them there is a significantly increased chance that they will not complete the survey. So, skip logic can act to reduce the drop-out rate in surveys whilst, at the same time, allowing researchers the flexibility to reach different types of respondents in a single survey.

Advanced Survey Logic

In designing online surveys there is the potential to utilise the power of what is called *advanced branching*. The key difference between basic skip logic and advanced branching is that skip logic depends on the answers to questions whereas advanced branching can be applied to question answers and a range of other variables. Another key difference is that whereas skip logic depends on the answer to single question responses, advanced branching allows surveys to be customised on the basis of multiple question responses. The use of advanced branching is commonly associated with designing what are termed *intelligent surveys*.

The essential components in advanced branching are *conditions* and *actions*. Here's an example from a fictitious online survey exploring satisfaction with treatment at a community therapy clinic where there is a particular focus on young clients. The survey asks a number of demographic questions related to age, gender and ethnicity. It also asks clients to rate their satisfaction with a number of features of the clinic including satisfaction with therapists.

In this survey it would be possible to set the following conditions and a particular action which selects a specific subset of clients and then offers them a question only for that subset. Here is how it might be expressed.

If a respondent answers question (1) [Age] as *under 16 years of age* AND answers question (4) [Satisfaction with therapist] as *dissatisfied with therapist* then go to [action] question (7) which asks—*How could your therapist have helped you more*? Now, these conditions and the action would offer young dissatisfied clients a specific question which would only be seen by them and provide an opportunity to express how they think their therapist could have helped them more. So, this particular question is hidden from all the survey respondents who don't meet the two conditions stated above.

In using advanced branching, the relationship between conditions is determined by what are called *Boolean operators* and there are two common ones—'AND' is one option, 'OR' is another option.

When using 'AND' to set conditions it means that all conditions must be 'true'. So, in our earlier community therapy clinic only clients who were aged under 16 [condition1] and who were also dissatisfied with their therapist [condition 2] would see a question asking them how their therapist could have helped them more.

Staying with the same example let's consider the use of the Boolean operator 'OR' with one condition being the *age of the client* and a second condition being the *reason for attending the clinic*, for example anxiety and stress. So, consider this sequence; if a client answers question (1) [Age] as *under 16 years of age* and answers question (3) [reason for visiting clinic] as 'depression OR anxiety' then go to question (9) which asks—'Are you currently taking medication for your condition? Now, in this example any client aged under 16 years of age and who was suffering from *either* depression or anxiety would be asked if they were taking medication for their condition. So, here is a slightly different way to select a subset of survey respondents using advanced branching.

It's worth pointing out that skip logic and advanced branching can help to ensure that only the intended sample or subset of survey respondents can complete a survey. Here's an example in which a new fictitious therapy training institute, *Therapy and Research Ltd*, is seeking to obtain ratings of satisfaction for their main taught research course from foreign students. In this case we could use the AND Boolean operator and specify that [condition 1] only students whose email address contains @therapyresearch AND who indicate that [condition 2] they are not from the UK would have their responses validated within the survey. For all other potential respondents any data submitted would be invalidated and therefore would not be counted.

Presenting Survey Findings

Presenting survey findings in an effective and meaningful way is imperative. The critical focus is to find the most effective and impactful way of presenting survey findings. Given the amount of time that has been invested in surveys by respondents there is almost an ethical duty to make sure that survey findings are properly presented.

All the major online survey platforms offer a wide range of graphical presentation options which include pie charts, bar charts, line graphs and even word clouds. But choosing the most effective option requires careful thought and sometimes a specific visually attractive graphical presentation is not necessarily the best option. Consider the pie chart in Fig. 8.2. It shows data for a survey question that asked

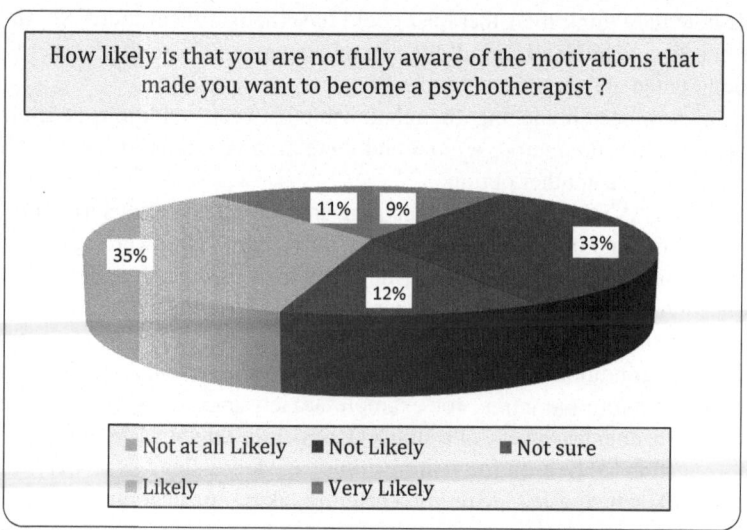

Fig. 8.2 Pie chart—therapists' awareness of their motivations [adapted from McBeath (2019)]

therapists how likely it was that they were not fully aware of the motivations that underpinned their desire to become a psychotherapist (McBeath, 2019). The survey had a large number of respondents, well over 500, and so there was a very solid data set to report.

At a first glance it might be thought that Fig. 8.2 looks quite impressive; there are specific percentages reported, some nice colours for pie chart sections and a meaningful colour-coded chart legend. But is it clear what the main findings actually are? To help answer this question let's take a look at the same data presented in a bar chart in Fig. 8.3.

The comparison between Figs. 8.2 and 8.3 is quite striking. The bar chart presentation clearly has higher impact as it almost immediately allows the main data pattern and findings to be assimilated and understood. In some ways it is a powerful presentation where there is almost a mirror image of percentages at either side of the 'not sure' bar. So, hopefully, this example shows that there needs to be some careful thought in choosing the most effective graphical representation of survey findings. The potential power of graphical presentations can also often make the reporting of statistics and attempts to prove a statistically significant difference within survey findings unnecessary. Let's take a look at Fig. 8.4 where the data presented come from a survey asking psychotherapy doctoral students how important research supervision was to their studies (Bager-Charleson & McBeath, 2021b).

The data pattern shown in Fig. 8.4 seems unambiguously clear and there is certainly no need for a statistical test here. The findings are clear; nearly three-quarters of the students surveyed indicated that research supervision is *extremely important* with a further 19% indicating that research supervision is *important*.

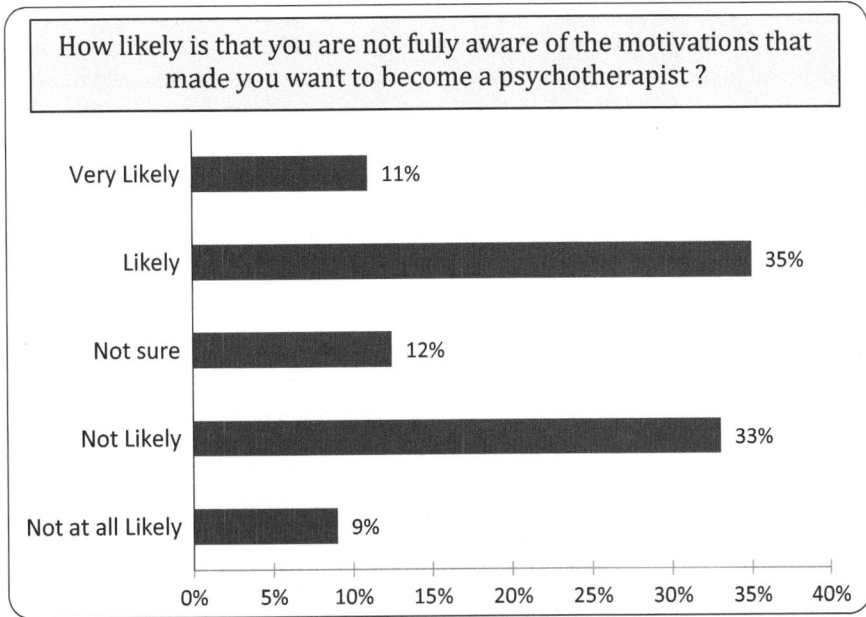

Fig. 8.3 Bar chart—therapists' awareness of their motivations (McBeath, 2019)

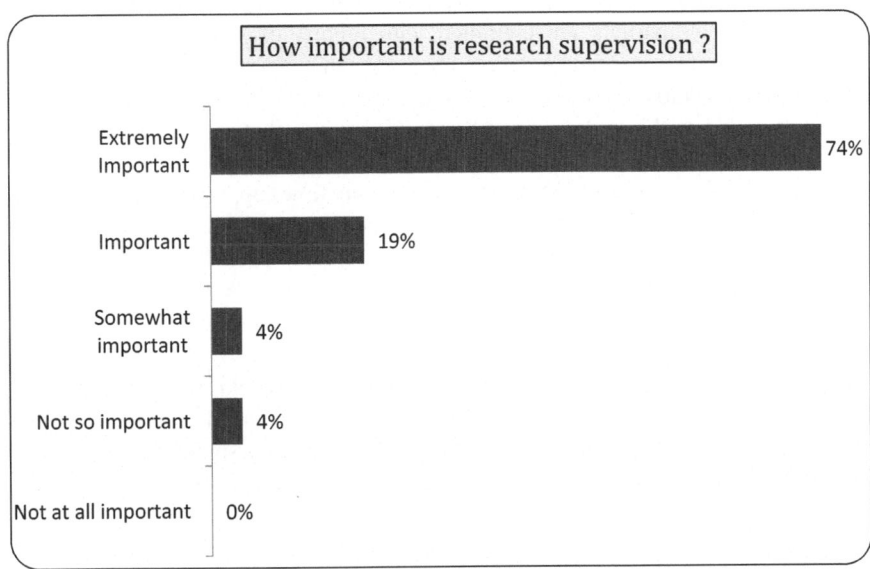

Fig. 8.4 The importance of research supervision to psychotherapy doctoral students

Using graphs without statistics *where data patterns are clear* is to be recommended. In academic journals sometimes the presentation of statistics and the reporting of various levels of statistical significance do not convey added meaning to a readership that might have quite varying levels of statistical knowledge. An overly academic approach to the reporting of survey findings may discourage many readers and make them less interested in what might be very important and relevant survey findings (McBeath et al., 2019).

It's quite common for survey findings to be cloaked in a description of statistical procedures that are unlikely to add additional meaning for readers or indeed might stop them reading further about a survey. Here's an example from a journal paper that was seeking to make comparisons about the efficacy of CBT and 'generic counselling'.

> Using iterative generalised least squares (IGLS) methods, a regression model was developed to identify significant patient variables, before including therapy type, the number of sessions attended and site effect. (Pybis et al., 2017)

Would this paragraph add meaning for those practitioners within the counselling and psychotherapy professions who do not have an advanced knowledge of statistics?

The use of statistics to analyse online surveys can be problematic. All of the various commercial online survey platforms offer a range of statistical tests but their use must be informed by a degree of robust knowledge about statistics. Inevitably statistical tests are underpinned by a range of assumptions that must be considered if any analysis is to be both appropriate and meaningful. Perhaps the most important piece of knowledge to have before using any statistical test or in reading reported statistical results is around the meaning of the phrase—*a statistically significant result*. Academic journals are crammed with reports of statistically significant results but what does it mean? A detailed account can be found by McBeath (2020a) but essentially a statistically significant result is one that is taken to reflect a systematic relationship within a data set or between variables that is not accountable by chance or other extraneous factors.

The use of statistical tests for survey data is sometimes appropriate if there are a set of specific research hypotheses that have been postulated. Statistical tests can basically serve either to support a hypothesis or reject it. An example of using statistical tests with specific research questions comes from an Austrian survey-based study that was focused on the experiences of 1547 therapists using remote therapy delivery during the COVID-19 pandemic (Humer et al., 2020). The study reported 14 research hypotheses such as, 'that psychotherapists would not rate telephone-based therapy to be equal to in-person therapy'. Various statistical tests were applied to the data and the following was reported as a statistically significant result that, 'telephone-based psychotherapy is not totally comparable to in-person psychotherapy'. Another statistically significant result reported was that,

> Psychodynamic and humanistic therapists rated telephone-based psychotherapy more comparably to face-to-face psychotherapy than behavioral therapists.

The study goes on to report several other statistically significant results but there was only a very limited discussion of the clinical implications of the findings obtained. So, was it worth reporting all those statistically significant results? Perhaps

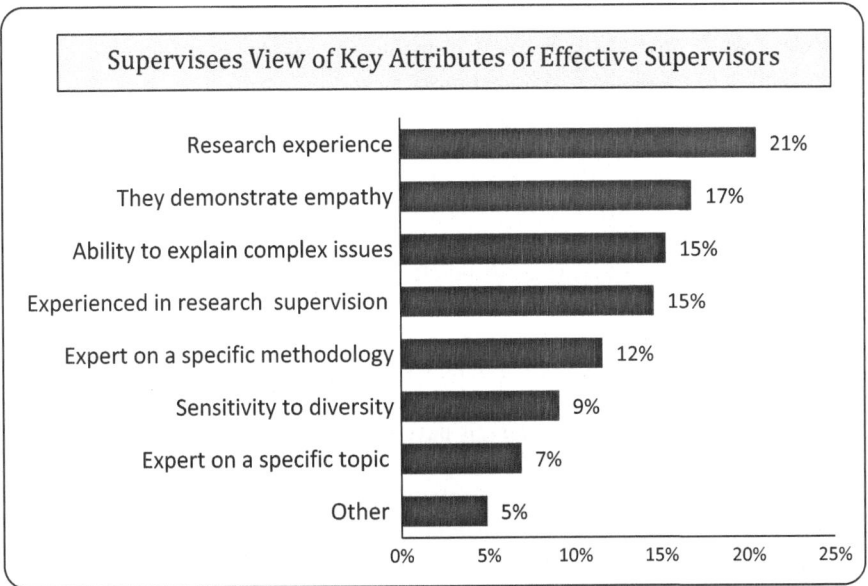

Fig. 8.5 Research supervisees' ratings of the key attributes of effective research supervisors (Bager-Charleson & McBeath, 2021b)

not. So, it's always wise to ask if the meaning and impact of survey findings will be enhanced by the use of statistical tests.

As suggested earlier it's often the case that the impact and importance of online survey findings can find effective expression through the selection of an appropriate graphical representation. The data shown in Fig. 8.5 is a good example which records research supervisees' views on the key attributes of effective research supervisors. The finding that research experience and supervisor empathy were the two most highly rated attributes was both unexpected but revealing. So, empathy was rated ahead of such attributes as expert on a specific methodology; it was the human attribute of empathy that was seen as more important. This particular slide has been used in training presentations to research supervisors and regularly stimulates debate and some surprise at the high rating given to empathy.

Exploring Survey Data

Once you have conducted an online survey and collected a good number of responses there are many ways to explore the data, deepen the research focus and start to ask new research questions. The major online survey platforms offer a good range of tools that allow data to be viewed in different ways. Here is one example that came from an online survey focused on the motivations of psychotherapists (McBeath,

2019); the survey response total is 551. Figure 8.6 shows therapists' responses when they were asked how likely it was that unconscious motivations played a part in them wanting to become a psychotherapist.

Now Fig. 8.6 is quite interesting and clearly there is substantial recognition that unconscious motivations are likely to be involved in choosing to become a therapist. But what happens if you look deeper into the data? One topic of interest was the possibility that the findings shown in Fig. 8.6 might vary by how long a therapist has been practicing. It is quite easy to explore this possibility by the use of data compare rules. The online survey had asked respondents how long they had been a practicing therapist and there was a choice of four time intervals; 1–4 years, 5–8 years, 9–12 years and 12+ years. The next stage was to show the data from the question about unconscious motivations broken down by each of these individual intervals of 'years practicing'. Figure 8.7 shows how this can be done by the use of a *data compare rule* where all of the four intervals have been selected.

When the compare rule shown in Fig. 8.7 was applied the data for the question about unconscious motivations was displayed in the tabulation shown in Table 8.1. The particular format of the data shown in Table 8.1 is called a *crosstabulation* (or crosstabs) which is a way of comparing the data from one variable or question with the data from another.

Although Table 8.1 might look a little bit complex it should be quite easy to understand. So, the grand survey response total of 551 (bottom right) is subdivided

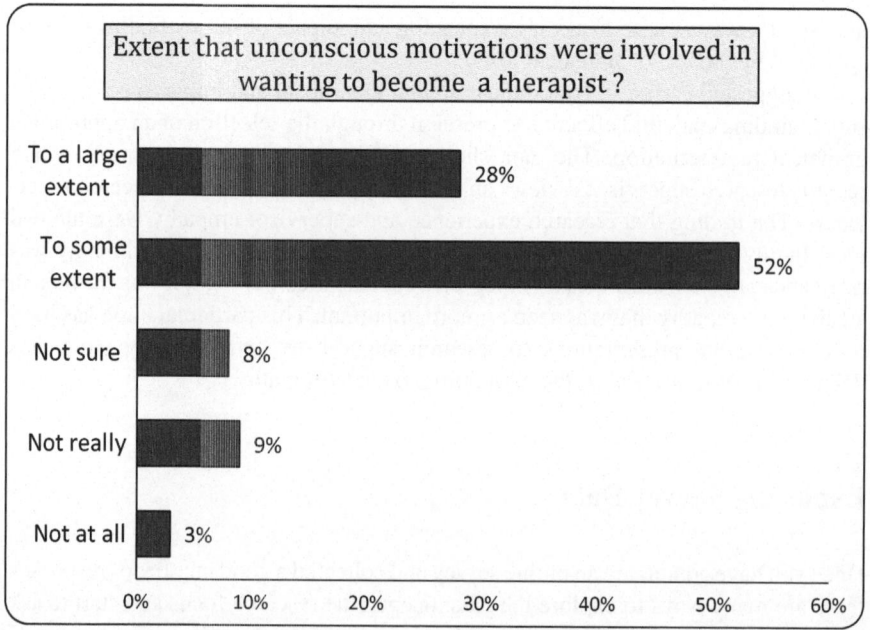

Fig. 8.6 Unconscious motivations to become a therapist (McBeath, 2019)

Fig. 8.7 The use of an online survey data compare rule (SurveyMonkey)

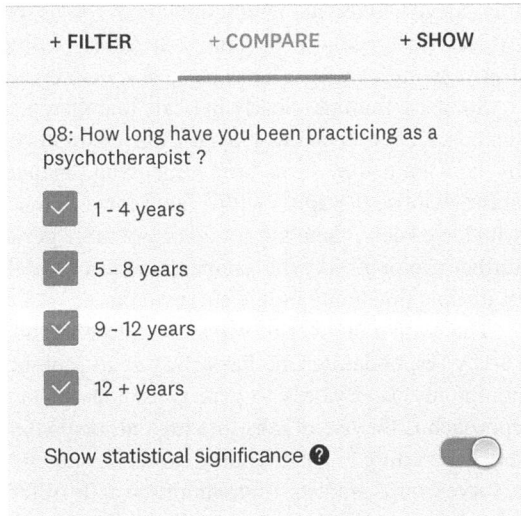

Table 8.1 Crosstabulation—extent to which unconscious motivations were involved in choosing to become a therapist broken down by years practicing

	To a large extent	To some extent	Not sure	Not really	Not At all	Total
1 - 4 years	37 (24%)	83 (55%)	12 (8%)	18 (12%)	2 (1%)	152 (28%)
5 – 8 years	28 (25%)	61 (55%)	10 (9%)	9 (8%)	3 (3%)	111 (20%)
9 – 12 years	23 (24%)	50 (53%)	10 (11%)	7 (7%)	5 (5%)	95 (17%)
12 + years	66 (34%)	94 (49%)	11 (6%)	18 (9%)	4 (2%)	193 (35%)
Total Respondents	154	288	43	52	14	**551**

between the answers to the unconscious motivations question (five columns) and how long therapists have been practicing (four rows).

Within Table 8.1 there are two shaded areas under the column headed *to a large extent* and these are of particular interest. The first shaded area (for 1–4 years) indicates that *significantly fewer* respondents from this interval thought that unconscious motivations played a part (*to a large extent*) in choosing to become a therapist—compared to those respondents in the 12+ years interval. Conversely, the second shaded area (12+ years) indicates that *significantly more* respondents from this category interval thought that unconscious motivations played a part (*to a large extent*) in choosing to become a therapist—compared to those respondents in the 1–4 years interval.

So, these findings clearly indicate that therapists' views about the likelihood that unconscious motivations played a part in them choosing to become a therapist vary by how long they have been practicing. In particular there is a real difference between those therapists with a few years of clinical experience and those therapists who have been practicing for a considerable period of time. This finding facilitated further exploration of the database and is a good illustration of the potential benefits of drilling down into online survey data.

There are a number of ways to explore the qualitative data that are provided by survey respondents. One basic way is to look at the frequency count of the most commonly used words to give some idea of prominent issues. A more powerful approach is the use of tags in which all responses to a specific question can be filtered according to whether they contain a specific word or words. An example from a survey on therapists' motivations was to filter all free-text responses that contained the word 'unconscious' which was of considerable benefit in looking into the data at a deeper level.

Publicising and Marketing Surveys

One of the critical tasks in using a survey in research is to ensure that it is effectively and creatively publicised and marketed. There are a number of different ways to achieve this goal. At a basic level it's possible just to email a hyperlink to a survey. Here's an example from SurveyMonkey.

https://www.surveymonkey.co.uk/r/ZW5B38Q

Although the hyperlink is effective in directing respondents to a survey it has no marketing power and it doesn't tell potential respondents anything about the survey. A more creative way is to customise a survey link using both graphics and a short summary describing the purpose of the survey. Figure 8.8 shows a customised hyperlink from a survey concerned with the challenges and opportunities of therapists working remotely during the Covid pandemic (McBeath et al., 2020).

Figure 8.8 is certainly more eye-catching and informative than just a basic hyperlink. Another effective way to market a survey and to make it accessible is the use of QR codes. Figure 8.9 shows a survey 'flyer' that was sent to a number of psychotherapy and counselling training organisations for distribution to their students. In one case the flyer was posted on a digital student noticeboard and this proved very effective as the QR code could easily be scanned with a mobile phone to gain access to the survey.

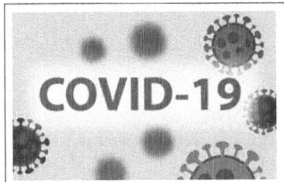

Therapists working remotely during
the coronavirus pandemic

An opportunity for therapists to contribute their views on the challenges and
opportunities of working remotely during the Covid pandemic,

www.surveymonkey.co.uk

Fig. 8.8 Customised survey hyperlink

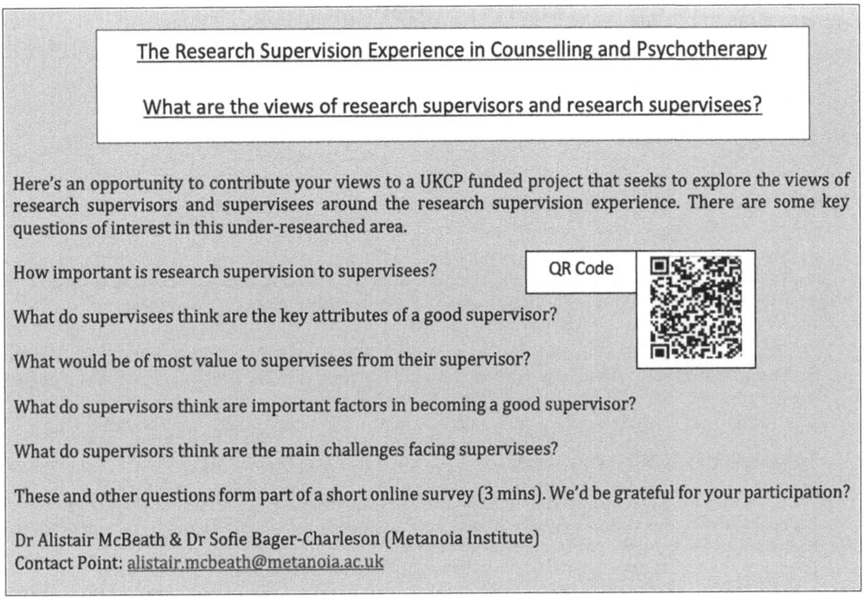

The Research Supervision Experience in Counselling and Psychotherapy

What are the views of research supervisors and research supervisees?

Here's an opportunity to contribute your views to a UKCP funded project that seeks to explore the views of research supervisors and supervisees around the research supervision experience. There are some key questions of interest in this under-researched area.

How important is research supervision to supervisees?

What do supervisees think are the key attributes of a good supervisor?

QR Code

What would be of most value to supervisees from their supervisor?

What do supervisors think are important factors in becoming a good supervisor?

What do supervisors think are the main challenges facing supervisees?

These and other questions form part of a short online survey (3 mins). We'd be grateful for your participation?

Dr Alistair McBeath & Dr Sofie Bager-Charleson (Metanoia Institute)
Contact Point: alistair.mcbeath@metanoia.ac.uk

Fig. 8.9 Survey 'flyer' with QR code

There are more options to market and publicise surveys and the use of social media platforms (e.g. Facebook and LinkedIn) can be very effective. Figure 8.10 shows an embedded customised hyperlink that was posted on a psychotherapy Facebook group.

A final example of publicising surveys is the use of existing psychotherapy organisation websites. As an example, Fig. 8.11 shows a survey link that was embedded in a psychotherapy training institute.

So, there are several ways to publicise a survey. To maximise the exposure of a survey it is recommended that at least more than one of the ways that have been illustrated should be used. There's no point having a great survey if people don't know about it or can't easily access it.

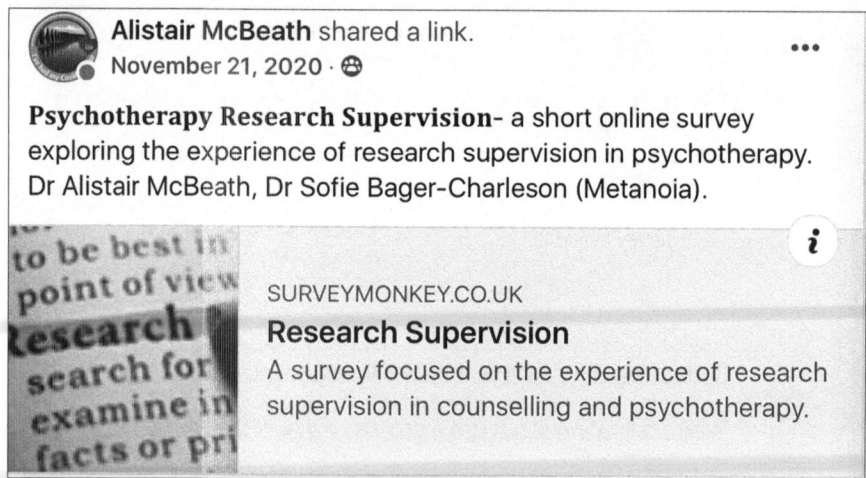

Fig. 8.10 Customised survey hyperlink posted on Facebook

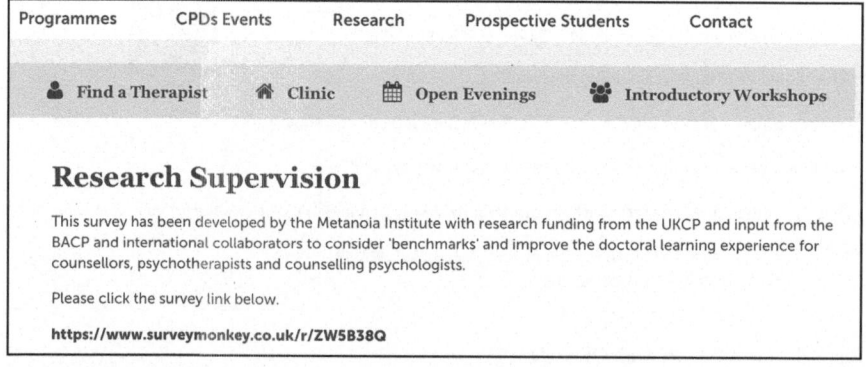

Fig. 8.11 Survey link embedded in a psychotherapy training organisation

Summary and Overview

The use of online surveys is a rapidly expanding research tool within the counselling and psychotherapy professions and one that has considerable power and sophistication in harvesting both quantitative and qualitative data. Online surveys have the potential to reach groups of participants who might not engage in less anonymous research methods and consequently can be focused on very personal and sensitive issues. There have been significant advances in using online surveys and it's clear that they can be a very effective qualitative research method. Using effective online surveys in research can be exciting and offer the researcher a variety of options to present the impact and meaning of their findings. There are also a range of intuitive analysis tools to explore and drill down into inline survey data.

There's probably never been a better time to start exploring the versatility and participant inclusion offered by online surveys. The supporting technology is readily available and easy to use. If used wisely and focused on viable research topics, with due diligence to engaging with research participants, online surveys can deliver a wealth and richness of meaning that can provide new and relevant research to the counselling and psychotherapy professions.

Activity: Design your own survey

What subject do you want to research?
Who do you want to survey—what would be your sample?
Will you need a two-in-one survey design (skip logic)?
Are you testing a hypothesis—and you might need to use statistics?
Would you use qualitative open-ended questions?
What about a story completion stem?
How will you publicise your survey?
How would you effectively present your survey findings?

References

Bager-Charleson, S. & McBeath, A.G. (2021b). Containment, compassion and clarity. Mixed methods research into supervision during doctoral research for psychotherapists and counselling psychologist. *Counselling and Psychotherapy Research*. doi: https://doi.org/10.1002/capr.12498.

Bhaskar, R. (1989). *Reclaiming reality: A critical introduction to contemporary philosophy*. Verso.

Braun, V., & Clarke, V. (2006). Using thematic analysis in psychology. *Qualitative Research in Psychology, 3*(2), 77–101.

Braun, V., & Clarke, V. (2013). *Successful qualitative research: A practical guide for beginners*. Sage.

Braun, V., & Clarke, V. (2019). Reflecting on reflexive thematic analysis. *Qualitative Research in Sport, Exercise and Health, 11*(4), 589–597. https://doi.org/10.1080/2159676X.2019.1628806

Braun, V., Clarke, V., Boulton, E., Davey, L., & McEvoy, C. (2020). The online survey as a qualitative research tool. *International Journal of Social Research Methodology, 24*(1), 1–14. https://doi.org/10.1080/13645579.2020.1805550

Clarke, V., Braun, V., Frith, H., & Moller, N. (2019). Editorial introduction to the special issue: Using story completion methods in qualitative research. *Qualitative Research in Psychology, 16*(1), 1–20. https://doi.org/10.1080/14780887.2018.1536378

Clarke, V., Hayfield, N., Moller, N., & Tischner, I. (2017). Once upon a time … : Story completion methods. In V. Braun, V. Clarke, & D. Gray (Eds.), *Collecting qualitative data: A practical guide to textual, media and virtual techniques* (pp. 45–70). Cambridge University Press.

Davey, L., Clarke, V., & Jenkinson, E. (2019). Living with alopecia areata: An online qualitative survey study. *British Journal of Dermatology, 180*(6), 1377–1389. https://doi.org/10.1111/bjd.17463

Gravett, K. (2019). Story completion: Storying as a method of meaning making and discursive discovery. *International Journal of Qualitative Methods, 18*, 1–8.

Humer, E., Stippl, P., Pieh, C., Pryss, R., & Probst, T. (2020). Experiences of psychotherapists with remote psychotherapy during the COVID-19 Pandemic: Cross-sectional Web-Based Survey Study. *Journal of Medical Internet Research, 22*(11), e20246.

Landrum, B., & Garza, G. (2015). Mending fences: Defining the domains and approaches of quantitative and qualitative research. *Qualitative Psychology, 2*(2), 199–209. https://doi.org/10.1037/qup0000030

McBeath, A. G. (2019). The motivations of psychotherapists: An in-depth survey. *Counselling and Psychotherapy Research, 19*(4), 377–387. https://doi.org/10.1002/capr.12225

McBeath, A. G. (2020a). Doing quantitative research with statistics. In S. Bager-Charleson & A. G. McBeath (Eds.), *Enjoying research in counselling and psychotherapy* (pp. 161–173). Macmillan.

McBeath, A. G. (2020b). Doing qualitative research with a survey. In S. Bager-Charleson & A. G. McBeath (Eds.), *Enjoying research in counselling and psychotherapy* (pp. 175–194). Palgrave Macmillan.

McBeath, A. G., & Bager-Charleson, S. (2022). *Views on mixed methods research within counselling and psychotherapy: An online survey* (manuscript submitted for publication). Metanoia Institute.

McBeath, A. G., du Plock, S., & Bager-Charleson, S. (2020). The challenges and experiences of psychotherapists working remotely during the coronavirus pandemic. *Counselling and Psychotherapy Research, 20*(3), 394–405.

McBeath, A. G., Bager-Charleson, S., & Abarbanel, A. (2019). Therapists and academic writing: "Once upon a time psychotherapy practitioners and researchers were the same people". *European Journal for Qualitative Research in Psychotherapy, 19*, 103–116.

McEvoy, C. (2019). *'Rarely discussed but always present': Exploring therapists' accounts of social class in therapy. D Couns Psych.* University of the West of England.

McLeod, J. (2015). *Doing research in counselling and psychotherapy.* Sage.

McPherson, A.S. (2022). "Are you analysing me?" A story completion exploration of having a friend who is becoming a psychotherapist. *European Journal for Qualitative Research in Psychotherapy*, Vol 12, 64-80.

Moller, N. P., Clarke, V., Braun, V., Tischner, I., & Vossler, A. (2021). Qualitative story completion for counseling psychology research: A creative method to interrogate dominant discourses. *Journal of Counseling Psychology, 68*(3), 286–298. https://doi.org/10.1037/cou0000538

Opperman, E., Braun, V., Clarke, V., & Rogers, C. (2014). "It feels so good it almost hurts": Young adults' experiences of orgasm and sexual pleasure. *The Journal of Sex Research, 51*(5), 503–515. https://doi.org/10.1080/00224499.2012.753982

Pope, C., & Mays, N. (1995). Reaching the parts other methods cannot reach: An introduction to qualitative methods in health and health services research. *British Medical Journal, 311*, 42–45.

Pybis, J., Saxon, D., & Hill., & Barkham, M. (2017). The comparative effectiveness and efficiency of cognitive behaviour therapy and generic counselling in the treatment of depression: Evidence from the 2nd UK National Audit of psychological therapies. *BMC Psychiatry, 17*(1), 215. https://doi.org/10.1186/s12888-017-1370-7

Shah-Beckley, I., Clarke, V., & Thomas, Z. (2018). Therapists' and non-therapists' constructions of heterosex: A qualitative story completion study. *Psychology and Psychotherapy: Theory, Research and Practice.* https://doi.org/10.1111/papt.12203

Tashakkori, A., & Teddlie, C. (1998). *Mixed methodology: Combining qualitative and quantitative approaches.* Sage.

Taylor, G. W., & Ussher, J. M. (2001). Making sense of S & M: A discourse analytic account. *Sexualities, 4*(3), 293–314.

Chapter 9
Mixed Methods Research to Build Bridges

Brittany Landrum and Gilbert Garza

Learning Goals

After reading this chapter, you should be able to:

- Understand the strengths and domains of quantitative and qualitative methods
- Describe the main differences between quantitative and qualitative research methods
- Recognize the complementarity of combining quantitative and qualitative methods
- Have the ability to propose and design a research protocol for a mixed methods study
- Carry out a phenomenological thematic analysis of qualitative data
- Integrate and synthesize qualitative and quantitative findings

Introduction

Mixed methods research is a contested approach, with many theories around how to do it. Holding that 'good fences make good neighbours,' this chapter expands on the domains of quantitative and qualitative research, exploring traditional frontiers between them with new bridges in mind. It offers an overview of some different mixed methods theories and describes practical, step-by-step integrative examples

B. Landrum (✉) • G. Garza
University of Dallas, Irving, TX, USA
e-mail: blandrum@udallas.edu; garza@udallas.edu

© The Author(s), under exclusive license to Springer Nature
Switzerland AG 2022
S. Bager-Charleson, A. McBeath (eds.), *Supporting Research in Counselling and Psychotherapy*, https://doi.org/10.1007/978-3-031-13942-0_9

of designing and conducting mixed methods research with reference to a study exploring the relationship between social media use and anxiety during the pandemic.

What Do You Want to Know?

When undertaking research, we advocate that your research question should guide your choice of methods, rather than methodology dictating what you can and cannot study. We always begin our research with the question: What do you want to know? By being mindful of the knowledge claims and domains of quantitative and qualitative research methods, we can choose our methodology based on what we hope to find in our investigation. If you are seeking to explore relationships between variables, such as how symptoms of anxiety are related to social media usage, a quantitative approach should be adopted. If instead you are interested in what it means to be anxious in light of social media usage, a qualitative approach is indicated. Using mixed methods research allows us to explore both relationships of magnitude between these variables as well as exploring what this experience means.

We have written previously (Landrum & Garza, 2015) about the numerous ways that quantitative and qualitative methods can be 'mixed.' Creswell et al. (2011) identify as best practice three techniques for mixed methods: merging, connecting, and embedding. Merging, when this technique converts and transforms one type of data into another (e.g., transforming qualitative data into numerical counts) in order to compare the two results, and when results from one domain are used to confirm, validate, or refute the other domain, raises serious concerns about violating the unique domains of each approach (Landrum & Garza, 2015). In one of the examples cited by Creswell et al. (2011), Wittink et al.'s (2006) quantitative results did not find any differences in patients' self-reported depression ratings between physicians who rated them as depressed or not. The qualitative results, however, shed light on how patients differed in their feelings toward their doctor. The qualitative results are not in a position to validate or invalidate the quantitative ones (see Landrum & Garza, 2015). Beyond just presenting these two results in the same table, which makes this an example of merging according to Creswell et al. (2011), these two approaches complement each other and point to the limitations of each approach. In exploring whether physician-designation of depression could differentiate patients' self-reports, the quantitative study explores if there is a difference between these two categories. The qualitative study, on the other hand, explores how patients feel about their doctor, providing insights into how the patient experiences their relationship with their physician. Physicians should note well that their initial observations regarding depression are not honed to detect such experiential differences.

Connecting and embedding are techniques that capitalize on the strengths of each approach, respecting the domains and knowledge claims of both methods where the results of each are used to complement and expand on each other. Specifically, connection entails a sequential path where one conducts either a quantitative or a qualitative study, and uses the findings to inform a second study using the other approach. This technique enables the researcher to draw insights from the first study to inform the second which can expand on or augment each other. While both studies share an equal footing when connecting them, embedding, in contrast, designates one approach as the primary one and the second as a supplemental one, where both techniques are used simultaneously. Both of these techniques work so long as the respective knowledge claims and limitations of each are respected. In the embedding example Creswell et al. (2011) cite, Miaskowski et al. (2006–2012) quantitatively explored whether pain was reduced in oncology patients who received an educational intervention. In this primary study, the researchers posed a question of magnitude and appropriately designed a quantitative study to compare two levels of the intervention and a repeated measurement of pain over the course of the study. To complement this study, the researchers also gathered impressions of the intervention from both the nurses and patients involved to shed light on how the intervention was progressing. This secondary qualitative study (conducted at the same time and hence an embedding technique) enabled the researchers to open-endedly explore the experience of the actors involved, potentially expanding on and going beyond the quantitative outcomes that were constrained by the measures surveyed. As Creswell et al. (2011) write, "The results provide evaluation of both the outcomes and process of the intervention" (p. 6) which captures and respects the two domains of both approaches.

In our example of a connection mixed methods study of anxiety and social media use during the COVID-19 pandemic, our first study quantitatively explores whether anxiety and social media use are related, while our second study qualitatively reveals how they are related. This research was conducted over the course of an academic year where we illustrated to our students the methodological techniques of two approaches. In our approach to these two domains, we see the quantitative methods as useful for illuminating relationships between variables, where one variable serves as an antecedent or predictor of the other—what Churchill (2022) calls 'because motives.' Thus, our quantitative study will show that the more one uses social media, the more anxious one is. But even the lack of a perfect correlation here points to other sources of variation and points to the need to explore how one is using social media. Clearly, not everyone who uses social media is anxious nor is social media the only source of anxiety. This quantitative approach does not address the participants' purpose for using social media. The aspirational aims or abiding questions one has in using social media can be explored in a qualitative study. This qualitative study explores what Churchill (2022) calls the 'in-order-to motives.' The value of mixed methods is that the juxtaposition of these two approaches will give us a more complete understanding than either approach on its own.

Step One: Review the Literature

After identifying your area of interest, the first step is to review the relevant literature on your topic. The main goals of this review are to discover what is currently known about the topic and begin problematizing it, by which you identify a point of entry for your own research (see Sandberg and Alvesson (2011) for a discussion of different ways to problematize past research). What questions are raised by past studies and how will your study add to this body of knowledge? Reviewing the literature enables you to gather ideas and inspiration for your own research questions and discern methods appropriate to address them.

In our review of the literature on the topic of anxiety and social media, we found predominantly quantitative studies exploring whether anxiety and other mental health measures increase or decrease with greater media exposure. For example, greater exposure to legacy media (radio, television, and print) was associated with more negative mental health outcomes (McNaughton-Cassill, 2000). However, the extension of these relationships to digital and especially social media has not been consistently replicated. For instance, Roche et al. (2016) found that while TV exposure significantly and positively predicted higher perceived threats, Internet exposure did not. In contrast, Gao et al. (2020) observed a higher probability of meeting criteria for anxiety, depression, and co-morbid anxiety and depression to be associated with higher social media exposure during the COVID-19 pandemic. Likewise, Bendau et al. (2020) found that higher ratings of anxiety and depressive symptoms were associated with higher duration and frequency of social media use during the pandemic. Additionally, Ellis et al. (2020) found that although more time on social media and virtually connecting to friends among adolescents were related to higher reported depression symptomatology, time engaging with family in person was related to less reported depression symptomatology during the COVID-19 pandemic.

Step Two: Problematizing

Our review of the literature revealed that media exposure is related to stress, anxiety, and depression. It suggests that these relationships may possibly extend to electronic, and especially social media. Furthermore, it raises the question of whether mental health may be particularly vulnerable, especially in regard to attempts to maintain connection to broader social networks in the midst of the COVID-19 pandemic. This literature opens the door for a mixed methods study to explore the relationships between anxiety and social media as well as the motivations for using social media during the pandemic.

Step Three: Quantitative Study

We first conducted a quantitative study (Garza, 2020) to test the following hypotheses:

- Social Media Exposure (SME) during COVID will be greater than before;
- SME during COVID and COVID stress will be positively related;
- SME during COVID and anxiety symptomatology will be positively related.

To test our hypotheses, we created a survey that adapted scales from the literature. **SME** was assessed using two questions adapted from Roche et al. (2016) regarding self-reported hours spent per day using social media platforms—one before and one during COVID. **Covid stress** was assessed using the COVID-19 stress scale (Ellis et al., 2020). The scale comprises 8 items on a 1 (not at all) to 4 (very much) response scale, with statements such as, 'To what extent are you worried about how COVID 19 will impact your school year?' Higher scores indicate greater COVID-related stress. **Anxiety** was assessed using the General Anxiety Disorder Scale (GAD-7, Spitzer et al., 2006). The scale comprises 7 items on a 1 (not at all) to 4 (nearly everyday) response scale indicating assessment of statements such as, 'Over the last 2 weeks, how often have you been bothered by the following problems? Trouble relaxing.' Higher scores indicate more anxiety.

Participants were a convenience sample of students ($N = 74$) in introductory psychology courses who were offered extra credit for participating. Fifty-five participants (74.3%) self-identified as female, with the remaining participants self-identifying as male. Two participants did not report a gender. Seventy of the seventy-four participants provided their age ($M = 20.357$, SD = 3.875).

A repeated measures t-test between SME before ($M = 4.324$, SD = 1.924) and during ($M = 4.743$, SD = 2.088) the COVID pandemic revealed that participants reported significantly more SME during the pandemic than before, with a small effect size ($t(73) = -2.566$, $p = 0.012$, $d = -0.298$). Correlation analysis revealed a significant, weak, positive association between SME during COVID and COVID stress ($r(74) = 0.247$, $p = 0.034$). However, there was no significant association between SME during COVID and anxious symptomatology ($r(74) = 0.053$, $p = 0.651$).

Step Four: Qualitative Study

Our quantitative results highlight that increased social media use is associated with COVID stress specifically, but not general anxiety symptoms. These findings point to a relationship between these variables raising the question of one's purposes and goals for using social media. Quantitative results focus on 'because motives,' shedding light on how one set of factors is deterministic or predictive of another set of factors (see Churchill, 2022). Adopting a qualitative perspective, we can add texture to these correlational findings, moving beyond this association and illuminating how one is using, interacting with, and seeking out connections on social media. In sum, a quantitative study shows a relationship of magnitude between variables while a qualitative study can shed light on how it is so. By exploring 'in-order-to motives,' qualitative research explores: What does it mean to be anxious in the age of COVID? How does social media use contribute to this anxiety? What are they anxious about? Our second study explored these qualitative dimensions of our topic.

To gather data, we asked the students who were enrolled in our qualitative research workshop to describe a time when they experienced something COVID related on social media as unsettling. We opted for 'unsettled' instead of 'anxious' or 'stressed' to avoid limiting responses to a preconceived notion of what comprises these clinical terms. By unsettling, we hoped to gather responses that entailed anything that was jarring, upsetting, or distressing.

Activity 9.1

Gathering data from students enables them to be involved in the research process by not only experiencing for themselves what they would ask potential participants, but also to engage empathically with the data (see Wertz, 1985). Below we include the access question (adapted from Garza, 2004) we posed to our students. Read the question below and think about what you would say in response.

Describe a specific situation in which you were engaging with social media about the Covid pandemic and felt upset, rattled, shaken, or unsettled. Describe the situation as completely as possible. Describe this situation like a story with a beginning, middle and end, how you came to be on social media, how this experience affected your understanding of yourself, others and the world as well as your future and possibilities. How did this situation conclude or resolve for you?

To select the data that would be analyzed (see Martin, 1996; Polkinghorne, 1989), we sought descriptions that were about the experience under investigation and included details about their experience. We used this as an opportunity to show the students which responses were off topic, insufficiently detailed, reflective or offered theoretical explanations for why (i.e., because motives) they felt the way they did. After narrowing down the responses, we selected the best ones to follow-up on. Follow-up questions that are open-ended, not leading, and asking for further description were posed to the participants electronically and their responses were integrated into the original data for analysis.

Our analysis of the data draws from Thematic Analysis (Braun & Clarke, 2006) steeped in a phenomenological approach (for more information see: Garza, 2011; Garza & Landrum 2015; Landrum, 2019; Landrum et al., 2017). The first step of our analysis was reading the data to become familiar with it. It may seem obvious, but this first step enables you to dwell with your data, reading it over to get a sense of the whole. Reading and re-reading the data piece is a chance to take stock of your first impressions, get a feel for how it is structured, and find out what happens. This step is a chance to write a summary of the data by asking yourself 'what happened?' It is very important to note that this summary is not the analysis itself, but simply a brief recap of the main events, sort of like a movie trailer or abstract of a paper. What was the data piece about? What took place? Our summary for this datum is: the participant describes herself feeling alienated from and marginalized by others in view of her stance and beliefs regarding the COVID vaccine. As she encounters others with dissonant views on social media, she feels bullied and silenced. Her current place and ability to voice her opinions on social media are contrasted with how she experienced this realm before COVID. By familiarizing yourself with the piece of data and summarizing it, you are then ready to proceed to the next step, which begins the formal analysis (Fig. 9.1).

The second step of our analysis entails identifying *moments* and providing preliminary *codes*. When reading the data in this stage, we are not approaching the data neutrally but rather posing a specific question to the data. This research question, also known as the explication guiding question (von Eckartsberg, 1998), aims to illuminate pieces and parts of the data that answer it. In our example here, our guiding question was: What does it mean to be unsettled? By interrogating the data with this question in mind, we were able to start selecting pieces and parts of the data (i.e., *moments*, see Garza, 2004) that we discerned as pointing to answers to our explication guiding question. This step allows us to break the data into manageable chunks to begin analyzing it. It is important to keep in mind that these moments are not independent pieces that have been severed from the whole corpus but are meaningful in light of their connection with and place in the entire data piece. We would also like to note that not all of the data is relevant to our question, hence the selection of these moments enables us to focus on the parts that give us insight into what it means to be unsettled. We coded these moments (see Braun & Clarke, 2006) with our initial observations of the relevance and meaning we were seeing afforded by our interrogation of the data in view of the guiding question. What light does this piece of data shed on our research interest? For each moment, we wrote down our observations of how this piece elucidated the meaning of being unsettled. These codes are your working notes in preparation for the next step of the analysis and need not be formal or finalized. Our ongoing interrogation of the data continues throughout the analytic process, hence in Figure 10:1, a dual arrow is placed between the second and third steps to show that identifying moments continues until you feel you have addressed the question at hand and arrived at a comprehensive list of moments. Ultimately, a single moment can have multiple codes and thus be used to illustrate multiple themes.

What follows is an example of identifying moments and coding them. The follow-up question and the participant's response are italicized while the moments are bolded.

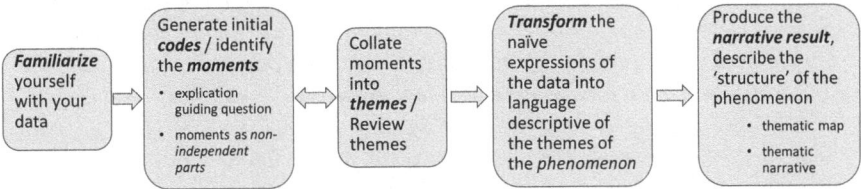

Fig. 9.1 Steps of phenomenological thematic analysis for the qualitative study. Adapted from sources: Garza (2004, 2011), Garza and Landrum (2015), Landrum et al. (2017), Landrum (2019)

Throughout this summer, I found myself on social media fairly consistently. As has been the case for the past 14 months, Instagram, Facebook, Twitter, Snapchat, even TikTok *have been relatively inundated with various theories, rants, and PSAs about all things to do with COVID-19.* I think it is fair to state that the topic of COVID in general raises **negative emotions across the board and on either side of debate.** For myself, **the topic that made me feel the most upset was that of the vaccine, and on a larger scale, the lack of a respectful dialogue about any COVID related topic.** *[Tell me more about this lack of respect. What does this mean to you?]* *By lack of respect, I mean that I've witnessed (from both sides of the debate) a complete dismissal of opinions or chance for conversation if someone doesn't immediately agree with someone else. I've been told that I am stupid and selfish without even being given the chance to explain my thoughts that I have spent time formulating and researching. It is like the second I disagree, my thoughts and opinions have lost value and my dignity as an individual has become lost to them.* In my experience, **my feeds were overrun** with posts and PSAs involving vaccine 'information', that were less information based and more **a source of virtue signaling and fear mongering.**

For each of the moments identified above, we provided an initial list of codes that describe a preliminary take on what we were noticing in this selection of data (Table 9.1).

Activity 9.2

Garza (2004) describes a 'moment' as "an aspect of the data (sentences, words, phrases, even the 'voice' or 'tone' of the data) that cohere about and illuminate a theme of the experience under investigation" (p. 133). We include a passage from a second piece of data below. Read over this passage and identify moments that stand out to you. What are you noticing with respect to meanings of being unsettled? How do these insights vary from the first piece of data?

Well, the night before my birthday I'm scrolling through snapchat and I see two of my friends were at a party, like a pre-pandemic kind of party; no masks, no social distancing, everyone sweaty and gross and breathing all over each other. I was already annoyed that I couldn't do what I originally had wanted to do for my birthday because of covid, so I was even more irritated that my friends didn't care and would put me and the 6 other people I had invited in danger **[Tell me more about what this danger meant to you.].** *What I meant by danger was that I didn't want to get covid and risk my friends getting covid and then worst case scenario happen (like them getting REALLY sick/ hospitalization/ etc). And I know my friends and I probably would be fine if we got it since we're young and we don't have any preexisting health conditions or anything but there's always that "what if." Also, no one likes getting sick in general, it's just not a good time, you feel gross, you're out of work/class for two weeks (or however long recovery is), and you can give it to other people who could have an even worse time than you.* And to find out on social media was absolutely annoying, because if I wasn't casually scrolling through snap, would they even have told me? Probably not.

Table 9.1 An initial list of codes

Moments	Codes
[Social media] have been relatively inundated with various theories, rants, and PSAs about all things to do with COVID-19	Pervasive New world
Negative emotions across the board and on either side of debate	Adversarial Confrontation
The topic that made me feel the most upset was that of the vaccine, and on a larger scale, the lack of a respectful dialogue	Lost peer standing and valued dialogue
A complete dismissal of opinions or chance for conversation if someone doesn't immediately agree with someone else	Adversarial Dismissed Unrecognized
I've been told that I am stupid and selfish without even being given the chance to explain my thoughts that I have spent time formulating and researching	Loss of self Loss of place and standing
The second I disagree, my thoughts and opinions have lost value and my dignity as an individual has become lost to them	Loss of voice and personhood
My feeds were overrun	Adversarial
A source of virtue signaling and fear-mongering	Insincere Untrustworthy Loss of footing in the other's regard

In tandem with the second step, the third step begins to group and combine meaningfully related moments together to form themes. By collating the moments together (see Garza, 2011), we can start to see how various moments throughout the dataset shed light on similar dimensions of meaning. For example, we might notice that a focus on the shared world with others comes up multiple times throughout the data and begin to group those moments together to form a theme that describes how the participant is attuned to the world with others. Drawing upon our phenomenological approach, a good starting place for theme generation is the four corners of the lifeworld: how we meaningfully orient to body/self, others, space, and time (van den Berg, 1972). As one begins to take stock of the moments that have been compiled, one starts to discern how various moments cohere together around similar concerns and dimensions. Each moment might add nuance and detail to how the participant is taking up their experience meaningfully, while the collated moments form themes that capture an overarching concern. For instance, in the participant's focus on how things used to be in the 'before times,' we can group these moments together under a theme about time where each moment in this theme focuses on a specific aspect that the participant longs for (i.e., civil discourse, speaking freely, no sides of the debate, etc.). These moments collectively describe how the participant aims for a world that used to be and the future that she hoped for that did not come to pass. As these themes start to emerge, you can return to the original dataset to verify that all the moments that fit under this theme of temporality have been identified.

After going through the moments and collating them together under collective thematic categories, each theme is then transformed. By transforming the original naive expressions from the data into descriptions of the themes being identified, the researcher is calling specific attention to how the participant is attuned to their world, how they are meaningfully invested in the situation, and how they are participating in the events that unfold. These transformations take the original account given by the participant and begin to describe how one must be attuned to experience the situation as such. In our example, in order for the participant to be unsettled, she must be attuned to a shift taking place where the world as it used to be and the world she currently finds herself in are at odds and not in line with her expectations and hopes. This shift is both unpleasant and unwelcome as the participant becomes attuned to the question of where she fits. This experienced placelessness is unsettling for her as she pines for the comfort and at homeness she felt prior to the pandemic. This fourth step marks the shift from what the participant says to the researcher's overt focus on the meaning structure of the experience.

Below (Table 9.2), we provide an example of the theme 'a world transformed' that includes all the supporting moments from the dataset as well as our transformation of this theme.

Activity 9.3
Below we present another theme with supporting data. Try transforming this theme yourself before reading our transformation.

The last step of the analysis represents the final cumulative synthesis of all the themes identified in the dataset. The previous four steps provide the preliminary background work necessary to write this final description of the results. Considering all the themes together, the researcher writes a narrative that describes the meaning structure of the topic. Your narrative should attempt to describe what it means to have the experience being investigated. There are two levels of analysis that can be described: situated and general (see Giorgi, 1985). In a situated analysis, the narrative describes your topic for a single participant, detailing how one participant experienced the topic. As idiographic, this situated narrative accounts for individual and specific experiences relevant and pertinent to one individual that may or may not be true for everyone experiencing this topic. In a general analysis, the researcher compares and contrasts multiple accounts of the topic to discern which themes are essential to the experience under investigation. The general structure synthesizes the situated narratives to arrive at the themes that must be in place for the experience to unfold and which themes are non-essential and idiographic. These narratives can be accompanied by a thematic map (see Braun & Clarke, 2006) that visually illustrates the findings of your analysis. Graphically, the researcher can present their findings by drawing connections and links between the themes. In the example below, we present our findings as an overarching situated narrative describing what it means to

Table 9.2 The theme 'a world transformed'

Theme: New transformed world/reality. Being unsettled in her world by way of social media during COVID entails an experienced qualitative and discontinuous transformation of the world in which she finds herself.
Transformation: Being unsettled in her world by way of social media during COVID means that she encounters the world in which she finds herself as discontinuously transformed from what she had previously understood. It means she experiences the world as unwelcoming and unresponsive to the previous ways of engaging with it and others in it. This world is characterized by confrontation and adversarial relations with battle lines being drawn with respect to her understandings regarding COVID and the vaccines. For this participant, it means being caught between the possibility of being true to herself or being accepted by others with an understanding that these two aims are not compatible and cannot be simultaneously achieved.
Supporting Data
[Social media] have been relatively inundated with various theories, rants, and PSAs about all things to do with COVID-19
Negative emotions across the board and on either side of debate
The topic that made me feel the most upset was that of the vaccine, and on a larger scale, the lack of a respectful dialogue
I fail to understand the push behind a vaccine
I was frustrated that I felt that I couldn't say what I wanted to even when (seemingly) everyone else could, simply because I hold unpopular opinions.
I felt like there wasn't a channel I could go through to have an honest conversation
Everything has become black and white, right or left, and the perceptions of a group are being applied to individual people.
A loss of the connection that truly matters; dialogue, healthy debate, truth from the media, and real charity
I have either been cut off from relationships or there has been a serious strain placed on relationships
I'm trying to approach the world in an understanding, truth-seeking way rather than being fearful and allowing myself to be shut out of the conversation
Theme: Discrepancy of self for self and for others. Being unsettled in her world by way of social media during COVID entails a lived discrepancy between the way she understands herself to be and the way she understands others to understand herself.
Your Transformation:
Supporting Data
A complete dismissal of opinions or chance for conversation if someone doesn't immediately agree with someone else.
I've been told that I am stupid and selfish without even being given the chance to explain my thoughts that I have spent time formulating and researching.
The second I disagree, my thoughts and opinions have lost value and my dignity as an individual has become lost to them
I was frustrated that I felt that I couldn't say what I wanted to even when (seemingly) everyone else could, simply because I hold unpopular opinions.
Downplaying my opinions for the sake of keeping the peace
And the perceptions of a group are being applied to individual people. What I'm trying to portray is that regardless of my personal leanings, I see myself as a person with my own thoughts and ways of coming to conclusions.

(continued)

Table 9.2 (continued)

Being 'shut out' as I said, I think means to be belittled and not be given the chance to have a voice.
Our Transformation: Being unsettled in her world by way of social media during COVID entails encountering the discrepancy between how she views herself and how she takes others to view her. This discrepancy is lived as meaning that she is less than, other than, or at odds with her own self-understanding in the eyes of others. This unfolds across the horizon of a project to peacefully and respectfully be alongside others. It involves understanding herself to be in the impossible position of both wishing to express her true self while seeing such expression as precluding the possibility of harmonious being alongside others.

be unsettled for one of our participants. In demonstrating this data analytic technique to our students, we chose the same piece of data to analyze independently in our respective sections, which we present below.

> **Activity 9.4**
>
> While this example is using written accounts, qualitative data can include any form of human expression. For instance, our own research has used transcribed oral interviews (Landrum et al., 2017), a TV show (Garza & Landrum, 2015), and archived student emails sent to a professor (Landrum, 2019). Other examples include social media posts (Kugelmann, 2017), diary and journal entries, letters, and even magazines (see Garza, 2007; von Eckartsberg, 1998). What other possible data sources might there be that shed light on our topic of being unsettled?

Situated Thematic Narrative for Garza's Section

The participant's experience of becoming unsettled on the occasion of interacting with social media in the context of the COVID pandemic unfolds as a lived loss, rupture, and dissolution across three domains. Being unsettled means the participant's relationships with and understood place in regard to others, the world and herself are all experientially volatile and fluid in marked contrast to her previous experience.

Regarding others, the participant intends to be alongside others as peer and comrade and aims at a world where this is possible even in the face of disagreement or disparity of opinion. Instead, the others the participant encounters on social media during COVID appear as adversaries, quick to dismiss her and disregard what she takes to be her well-reasoned and thoughtful views. Thus, being unsettled for the participant means feeling denigrated and diminished in the other's eyes, finding in their regard a confrontation with possibilities of herself as selfish, foolish, or otherwise at odds with how she intends to be. Being unsettled means that these encounters also revealed divergent possibilities of the other from who and how she had imagined them to be insofar as the participant finds them, dismissively rejecting her and her voice, seemingly actively dis-placing her from the shared world alongside them at which she aims.

Being unsettled in her world means the participant finds herself bereft of her sought-after and aimed-for place in the world alongside others. It further means the participant finds herself at cross-purposes—on the one hand she aims to be her true self and to find purchase as a peer among others who may disagree in her aimed-at world, but also has come to understand that being her true self and speaking her mind may cost her this very place and this very world. Being unsettled means the participant has come to understand that her pursuit of her aimed at self-in-world is impossible in as much as gaining standing in a shared communal world appears to her to be connected to squelching and denying aspects of herself and her truth.

Being unsettled ultimately means that the participant finds herself to be displaced from a world she understood and aimed at. It means the participant sees the world as it was and as she had hoped it would be as inaccessible from the world in which she finds herself at the moment. It means she experiences the harmonious being alongside she aimed at to be unobtainable and instead to be replaced by a space of confrontation, 'cancellation,' and debasement. For the participant, to be unsettled means to feel the previously understood world in which self and other coexisted as peers and relational ties were clear and one's standing in the other's regard was certain to have dissolved like quicksand underneath her feet and to place her in a kind of no-man's-land where her standing with regard to others and with regard to herself is fractious and disintegrative. For this participant, to be unsettled in her world on the occasion of interacting with social media in the context of the COVID pandemic means that the world as she understood it to have been and aimed for it to be seems hopelessly out of reach and impossible to enact from the world in which she finds herself and that she and others are transformed from peers to adversaries even as she experiences a division within herself and feels compelled to be other than her true self in order to be alongside others in the world in a pale mimicry of the world she had previously aimed at (Fig. 9.2).

Situated Thematic Narrative for Landrum's Section

In being unsettled, the participant experiences a **lived discrepancy** in her expectations of the world, her understanding of others, and her understanding of herself. Disconcertingly, the participant finds the world to be at odds with how she had expected it to be. Finding herself trapped in a world she no longer recognizes, the world is perceived as foreign, hostile, and unwelcoming. She longs to be accepted and embraced both as she had been previously and had expected to be in the future. In this startling rupture, the participant experiences a chasm opening up, as she struggles to find her footing and a place where she belongs. She aims to return to the world she used to know, a world that welcomed her, where she could be her true self without fear of retribution. In feeling rejected, dismissed, and cast aside for her

Thematic Map

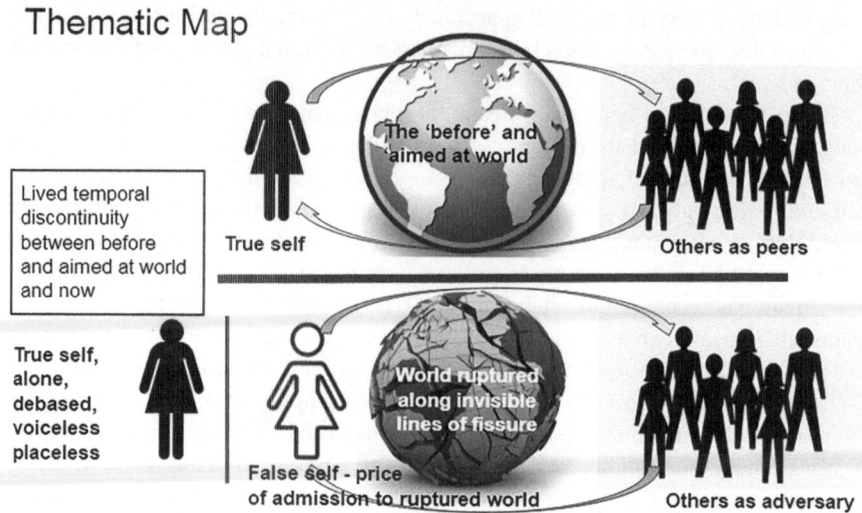

Fig. 9.2 Garza's thematic map

beliefs, the participant seeks to belong, to be accepted, and to be respected by the others she had previously considered herself to be one with. In seeing herself now being cast as the enemy, the participant is attuned to a fissure that divides and separates her from the others who once embraced her. The participant questions how she can return to the world where she could be true to her own understanding of herself. Being unsettled means she feels lost, placeless, and trapped in a world with others she no longer recognizes nor expected or anticipated.

In fighting to **reclaim her standing**—both her longed for place in the world and how she is seen in the eyes of others—the participant sees battle lines being drawn while facing the uncomfortable realization that she is on the wrong side. In her abiding attunement to whose side one is on, the participant yearns for a return to a time when one's beliefs were not cause for contention and rejection, but harmonious dialogue, instead. The world is now an unwelcome, hostile place where the participant feels trapped and placeless. No longer feeling accepted, the participant sees herself as being cast as the enemy, and forced to the outskirts of the social world, an understanding that does not match or mesh with her own. Despite her own attempts to seek connections, converse, and be friendly, the participant feels she has been labeled as an outcast, and in being silenced, she feels unable to stand up for herself in order to correct these perceived misunderstandings. Being unsettled means that her place is uncertain and her standing diminished and demolished.

In feeling forsaken, the participant experiences others and the world as having turned against her, leaving her alone and abandoned. Being unsettled means the participant is focused on what she has lost: a **lived loss** of voice, agency, and relationships/bonds. In her attunement to deprivation, the participant mourns the loss of her valued projects, including being heard, being accepted, being valued. These lived losses occasion feeling hopeless as the participant seeks to recover and restore the world she had previously known. As she contemplates her current situation, she

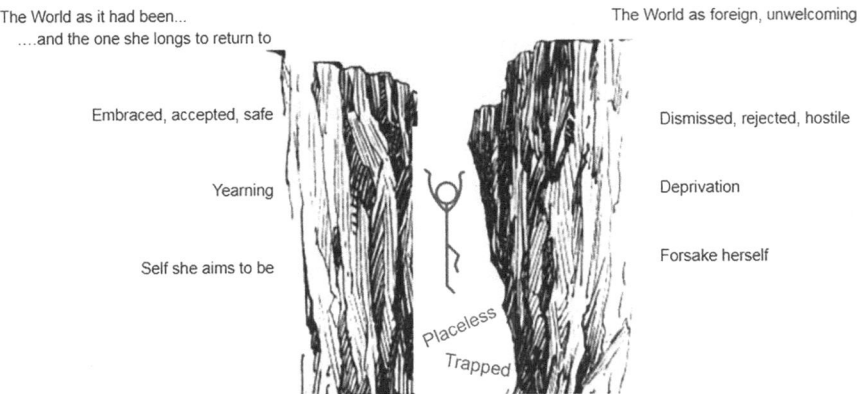

Fig. 9.3 Landrum's thematic map

grapples with an impossible choice to forsake her own sense of who she is by being silent or continue to be an outsider by standing up for what she believes in. Being unsettled means she yearns for the anticipated future that didn't come to pass (Fig. 9.3).

Validity and Reliability in Qualitative Research

Whereas we would expect two independent researchers to arrive at the same quantitative findings if running the same statistical analysis on the same dataset, this is neither expected nor a cause for alarm in qualitative research. As evidenced above, each of us arrived at our own understanding of what it means to be unsettled, yet the two descriptions and maps share a thematic coherence and resonate with each other and the data. Because qualitative research deals in the currency of meaning, exact replication is a faulty goal; rather, meaning emerges in light of the researcher's presence to the data. Hence, replication cannot be the standard. One researcher's insights neither will nor should be the exact same as another's. Your findings are valid so long as you stay true to your method and provide a coherent analysis of the data that illuminates the research question (see Churchill, 2022; Churchill et al., 1998; Garza, 2004; Landrum & Garza, 2015 for a more substantial discussion of reliability and validity in qualitative research).

Step Five: Connection as Complementarity

In our example above, our quantitative research reveals that anxiety and social media use are related. Specifically stress about COVID increases, albeit weakly, with increased social media usage. Thus, the correlation reveals that these two variables go hand in hand, yet this analysis does not shed light on how they are related. Our qualitative research explores how one's aims and goals in using social media are an occasion to feel anxious. Our analysis shows that this participant is particularly concerned with the question of where and how she fits alongside her peers and how her relationships with others will unfold. In view of those concerns, what she discovered on social media is unsettling. Our analysis of additional pieces in the dataset suggests that regardless of one's 'side' with respect to these divisions, the structure of being unsettled through social media during the pandemic remained consistent. Our preliminary general structure suggests that in being unsettled, one adopts an evaluative rubric to know where and with whom one stands. Abiding questions include asking 'Who are others to you and who are you to them?' in light of one's own beliefs as the gauge for how close one is to others. Thus, one is anxious about one's place and closeness to others with respect to beliefs and positions on COVID, which are occasions for fractures and disruptions in a previously shared social world. The qualitative findings neither confirm nor reject the quantitative ones; instead, the two domains are aiming toward different knowledge claims—claims that are neither better than or worse than the other, nor greater than or less than the other. Together, quantitative and qualitative research provides a more complete understanding of what it means to be anxious in the time of COVID. One's choice for methodology should be based on what the researcher wants to know. In our case, we wanted to explore both a magnitude and meaning question.

While the insight from the quantitative study that social media use and anxiety are related, it is perhaps not helpful or beneficial to recommend that one simply stop using social media. Our qualitative research points to an abiding question of where one stands and one's fear about the future are driving one's use of social media. Clinically, the qualitative results highlight one's purpose in using social media and potentially guide the therapeutic process to address these concerns.

Summary

Our chapter has explored the concerns and benefits of mixing quantitative and qualitative methods. Among our key points, we advocate that methods should be chosen based on what the researcher wants to know and past research is to be reviewed in terms of a problem being identified and investigated. Using one of our own examples, we discuss the following steps for quantitative and qualitative research:

Quantitative and Qualitative studies:

- Define your initial interest
- Review the literature
- Establish a problem
- Determine the methodology

Quantitative studies specifically:

- begin with a hypothesis, exploring a because motive where variables are said to be determinative or predictors of each other
- Numerical data are gathered
- Statistical analysis illuminates relationships of magnitude

Qualitative studies specifically:

- begin with an access question, exploring a dimension of meaning to elicit descriptive data.
- Data are interrogated with a guiding question to illuminate in-order-to motives where one focuses on how participants are concerned with, experience, and understand their world
- Qualitative analysis illuminates some dimensions of meaning in the human world

References

Bendau, A., Petzold, M. B., Pyrkosch, L., Mascarell Maricic, L., Betzler, F., Rogoll, J., Große, J., Ströhle, A., & Plag, J. (2020). Associations between covid-19 related media consumption and symptoms of anxiety, depression and covid-19 related fear in the general population in Germany. *European Archives of Psychiatry and Clinical Neuroscience*. https://doi.org/10.1007/s00406-020-01171-6

Braun, V., & Clarke, V. (2006). Using thematic analysis in psychology. *Qualitative Research in Psychology, 3*(2), 77–101. https://doi-org.dbproxy.udallas.edu/10.1191/1478088706qp063oa

Churchill, S. D. (2022). *Essentials of existential phenomenological research*. American Psychological Association.

Churchill, S. D., Lowery, J., McNally, O., & Rao, A. (1998). The question of reliability in interpretive psychological research: A comparison of three phenomenologically- based protocol analyses. In R. Valle (Ed.), *Phenomenological inquiry: Existential and transpersonal dimensions* (pp. 63–85). Plenum Press.

Creswell, J. W., Klasses, A. C., Plano Clark, V. L. & Smith, K. C. (2011). Best practices for mixed methods research in the health sciences. *Office of Behavioral and Social Sciences Research*.

Ellis, W. E., Dumas, T. M., & Forbes, L. M. (2020). Physically isolated but socially connected: Psychological adjustment and stress among adolescents during the initial COVID-19 crisis. *Canadian Journal of Behavioural Science/Revue Canadienne Des Sciences Du Comportement, 52*(3), 177–187. https://doi.org/10.1037/cbs0000215

Gao, J., Zheng, P., Jia, Y., Chen, H., Mao, Y., Chen, S., Wang, Y., Fu, H., & Dai, J. (2020). Mental health problems and social media exposure during COVID-19 outbreak. *PLoS One, 15*(4), e0231924.

Garza, G. (2004). Thematic moment analysis: A didactic application of a procedure for phenomenological analysis of narrative data. *The Humanistic Psychologist, 32*(2), 120–168.

Garza, G. (2007). Varieties of phenomenological research at the university of Dallas: An emerging typology. *Qualitative Research in Psychology, 4*(4), 313–342.

Garza, G. (2011). Thematic collation: An illustrative analysis of the experience of regret. *Qualitative Research in Psychology, 8*(1), 40–65. https://doi.org/10.1080/14780880903490839

Garza, G. (2020). Doom scrolling: Social media, Covid-19 stress, anxiety, and depression. Poster presented at the *2021 Meeting of the Southwestern Psychological Association (SWPA)* in San Antonio, TX.

Garza, G., & Landrum, B. (2015). Meanings of compulsive hoarding: An archival projective life-world approach. *Qualitative Research in Psychology, 12*, 138–161. https://doi.org/10.108 0/14780887.2014.948698

Giorgi, A. (1985). Sketch of a phenomenological method. In A. Giorgi, (Ed.), *Phenomenology and psychological research*, (pp. 8–22). Pittsburgh: Duquesne University Press.

Kugelmann, R. (2017). *Constructing pain: Historical, psychological and critical perspectives.* Routledge.

Landrum, B. (2019). 'See me as I see myself:' A phenomenological analysis of grade bump requests. *Qualitative Research in Education, 8*(3), 315–340. https://doi.org/10.17583/qre.2019.4329

Landrum, B., & Garza, G. (2015). Mending fences: Defining the domains and approaches of quantitative and qualitative research. *Qualitative Psychology, 2*, 199–209.

Landrum, B., Guilbeau, C., & Garza, G. (2017). Why teach? A projective life-world approach to understanding what teaching means for teachers. *Qualitative Research in Education, 6*(3), 327–351. https://doi.org/10.17583/qre.2017.2947

Martin, M. N. (1996). Sampling for qualitative research. *Family Practice, 13*(6), 522–525.

McNaughton-Cassill, M. E. (2000). The news media and psychological distress. *Anxiety, Stress, and Coping, 14*, 193–211.

Miaskowski, C. (2006–2012). Improving cancer pain management through self-care. Research grant funded by the National Cancer Institute and the National Institute of Nursing Research (5R01CA116423).

Polkinghorne, D. E. (1989). Phenomenological research methods. In R. S. Valle & S. Halling (Eds.), *Existential-phenomenological perspectives in psychology* (pp. 41–60). Plenum Press.

Roche, S. P., Pickett, J. T., & Gertz, M. (2016). The scary word of online news? Internet news exposure and public attitudes toward crime and justice. *Journal of Quantitative Criminology, 32*, 215–236. https://doi.org/10.1007/s10940-015-9261-x

Sandberg, J., & Alvesson, M. (2011). Ways of constructing research questions: Gap-spotting or problematization? *Organization, 18*(1), 23–44. https://doi.org/10.1177/1350508410372151

Spitzer, R. L., Kroenke, K., Williams, J. B. W., & Lowe, B. (2006). A brief measure for assessing generalized anxiety disorder. *Archives of Internal Medicine, 166*, 1092–1097.

van den Berg, J. H. (1972). *A different existence: Principles of phenomenological psychopathology.* Duquesne University Press.

von Eckartsberg, R. (1998). Introducing existential-phenomenological psychology. In R. Valle (Ed.), *Phenomenological inquiry in psychology: Existential and transpersonal dimensions* (pp. 3–20). Plenum Press.

Wertz, F. (1985). Method and findings in a phenomenological psychological study of a complex life event: Being criminally victimized. In A. Giorgi (Ed.), *Phenomenology and psychological research* (pp. 155–216). Duquesne University Press.

Wittink, M. N., Barg, F. K., & Gallo, J. J. (2006). Unwritten Rules of Talking to Doctors About Depression: Integrating Qualitative and Quantitative Methods. *Annals of Family Medicine, 4* (4), 302–309. https://doi.org/10.1370/afm.558

Chapter 10
Mixed Methods Research: The Case for the Pragmatic Researcher

Alistair McBeath

Learning Goals

After reading this chapter you should be able to:

- Understand the background and emergence of mixed methods research.
- Appreciate the core principles of Pragmatism and its linkage to mixed methods research.
- Understand the main mixed methods research designs.
- Appreciate the key concept of 'integration' in mixed methods research.
- Understand the rationale and advantages of mixed methods research.

Introduction

This chapter is focused on advocating that mixed methods research (MMR) is a seldom chosen but legitimate and progressive approach to research within counselling and psychotherapy. Historically, there has been a long academic debate where qualitative and quantitative research methods were seen as mutually incompatible and spawned the so-called *paradigm wars* (Tashakkori & Teddlie, 1998). One of the principle arguments made around what Howe (1988) has termed the '*incompatibility hypothesis*' is that qualitative and quantitative research methods are underpinned by conflicting research paradigms and philosophical assumptions or what Creswell and Plano Clark (2007) have usefully termed '*worldviews*'.

A. McBeath (✉)
Metanoia Institute, London, UK
e-mail: Alistair.McBeath@metanoia.ac.uk

© The Author(s), under exclusive license to Springer Nature
Switzerland AG 2022
S. Bager-Charleson, A. McBeath (eds.), *Supporting Research in Counselling and Psychotherapy*, https://doi.org/10.1007/978-3-031-13942-0_10

One of the consequences of the 'incompatibility hypothesis' was the widespread adoption of a *monomethod approach* to research which was based exclusively on choosing either qualitative or quantitative approaches. So, a mixed methods approach was essentially rejected as a valid model of research. The debate about the 'incompatibility hypothesis' was particularly prominent in the 1980s (Gage, 1989), but there was eventually some change in view which was evidenced by the launch of the *Journal of Mixed Methods Research* in 2007. Around the same time Bryman (2006a) considered that, 'the paradigm wars can be considered over' and *'paradigm peace'* had been achieved but he also noted that, 'there are occasional skirmishes as authors occasionally revive old debates' (p. 113). Those old debates continue to resurface from time to time.

The whole quantitative versus qualitative debate rests on a core assumption that certain research paradigms are inextricably linked to specific research methods. However, this view has been challenged and described as a 'fallacy' by Reichardt and Cook (1979) who offered several examples to support their view (e.g. qualitative procedures are not necessarily subjective and quantitative procedures are not necessarily objective). In a similar vein Johnson and Onwuegbuzie (2004) contend that the 'linkage between research paradigm and research methods is neither sacrosanct nor necessary' (p. 9); these authors suggest that quantitative and qualitative methods are best viewed as two poles of a continuum with mixed methods occupying the middle ground. In advocating the benefits of mixed methods Johnson and Onwuegbuzie (2004) emphasised the value of the underlying *methodological pluralism* of mixed methods research which they stated, 'frequently results in superior research (compared to monomethod research)' (p. 14).

Although mixed methods research has gained some real legitimacy it seldom features in research publications within counselling and psychotherapy and, in the author's experience, is hardly ever chosen by doctoral research students. Why this should be is a question worth considering. Perhaps one reason is that mixed methods research requires a demanding skill set and is quite time-consuming (Maarouf, 2019). However, perhaps a more prominent reason is that many of those contemplating doing research in counselling and psychotherapy simply know very little about mixed methods research and therefore continue the historic tradition of choosing either qualitative or quantitative approaches to their research projects. In a recent piece of survey-based research conducted by the author, only 53% of counselling and psychotherapy research students considered that they had knowledge about mixed methods research (McBeath & Bager-Charleson, 2022).

This chapter will seek to emphasise that mixed methods research is legitimate both in theory and practice and can provide an enriched blend of data that is potentially superior to any provided by a monomethod approach to research. Mixed methods research can be seen as a unifying approach within the field of research methods and in combining elements of both qualitative and quantitative approaches it has been referred to as the 'transformative paradigm' (Mertens, 2007; Williams, 2020) and the 'third research paradigm' (Johnson & Onwuegbuzie, 2004). One of the singular advantages of mixed methods research is the fact that it can be aligned with a powerful underlying 'worldview' called *pragmatism* which offers a refreshing and realistic basis with which to reflect on the realities of doing research and how we can acquire knowledge.

Background

Before the advantages offered by mixed methods research can be considered and evaluated it's important to review the history and context from which this approach has emerged. From a historic and purist view debate around qualitative and quantitative approaches has been focused on differences surrounding some key philosophical assumptions and beliefs. In this respect both Ponterotto (2005) and Creswell and Plano Clark (2007) have suggested that the following key domains should be considered; *ontology* (the nature of reality), *epistemology* (the study and acquisition of knowledge), *axiology* (the role of values in research), *rhetoric* (the language used to present research) and *methodology* (the processes and procedures used in research).

From an ontological perspective, quantitative methods have been associated with *realism* which proposes that there is a single external reality that exists beyond our senses that awaits inspection and discovery (this is sometimes called *naïve realism*). In contrast qualitative methods have been associated with *relativism* which proposes that reality is a subjective experience and that there can be multiple realities and each is as valid as any other (Neuman, 2014). From an epistemological perspective there is further polarisation between qualitative and quantitative approaches, especially in how knowledge may be acquired. The assumptions underlying *positivism,* which is associated with quantitative approaches, include *dualism* where the researcher and researched are viewed as independent of each other and *objectivism* which proposes that rigorous scientific method can be applied to research without distortion through bias (Ponterotto, 2005). There is also a *post-positivist* position which grew, in part, from a rejection of the rigidity of positivism and suggests that reality can only be 'imperfectly apprehendable' (Lincoln & Guba, 2000).

The epistemological position associated with qualitative approaches which can be called the *constructivist-interpretivist* position is strikingly different to positivism and post-positivism. Here there is a belief in multiple realities constructed both cognitively and socially rather than an existence of a single fixed objective reality. From a research perspective the *constructivist-interpretivist* position would see the dynamic between the researcher and research participants as central to a process of co-creating knowledge. Perhaps a key point to emphasise is that a *constructivist-interpretivist* researcher would be focussed on the interpretation of meaning rather than the discovery of facts or causal relationships. The contrast between positivism and the constructivist-interpretivist position has significant implications for the position of the researcher and research participants. So does the researcher believe that they are essentially a scientific, and distanced observer of the research process or someone who is immersed in the research process as a co-creator of knowledge with research participants?

A handy way to capture the essential difference between the concepts of ontology and epistemology is to think of these two questions; *does God exist?* is an ontological question about the nature of reality. In contrast—*how would we know that God exists?* is an epistemological question about how we might acquire knowledge about reality and ways of knowing.

Axiology refers to the role of values in the research process, and there are significant differences here between the positivism/post-positivism and constructivist-interpretivist epistemological positions. Essentially, there is no place for values or biases in research from a positivist perspective. As Ponterotto (2005) has emphasised, 'One's values, hopes, expectations, and feelings have no place in scientific inquiry' (p. 131). In contrast the constructivist-interpretivist position holds that it is impossible to isolate the researcher's values and lived experience (*Erlebnis*) from the research process. In this context the researcher would be encouraged to recognise and name their values, biography and biases.

Rhetoric refers to the language used to describe the research process and the presentation of findings is heavily influenced by the researcher's epistemological position. In the positivist/post-positivist domain there is the use of objective, descriptive and emotionally neutral language. The researcher is a detached reporter of scientific facts. In stark contrast the research aligned with a constructivist-interpretivist position will favour language which is personal, emotive and, importantly, acknowledging of the impact of the research experience on the researcher.

A final critical difference between quantitative and qualitative approaches and their respective epistemological positions concerns *methodology* which includes the researcher's approach to research and how it is conducted. From a positivist/post-positivist position the scientific method prevails where hypothesis testing, control of variables and the aggregation of data are paramount; the goal of this approach is to understand relationships between variables (not people) leading to the formation of statistically verified 'facts'. The scientific approach is based on *deductive reasoning* (top-down). The use of random control trials (Stafford, 2020) and large-scale surveys (McBeath, 2019) are two examples of this quantitative-bound approach.

The contrast with the constructivist-interpretivist position is abundantly clear where the researcher is personally immersed in the research process and is a co-creator of meaning with research participants.

The focus is ultimately on the lived experience of individuals and on their meaning-making. This approach follows *inductive reasoning* (bottom-up) where the researcher looks at the experiences and observations from individuals with the aim of finding patterns both within and across qualitative data. Two methods which illustrate this approach are Interpretative Phenomenological Analysis (Pietkiewicz & Smith, 2012) and Narrative Inquiry (Etherington, 2020).

What has been presented is a framework for identifying and considering critical concepts that influence the research process against the backdrop of the historic quantitative versus qualitative debate. A useful summary has been proposed by

Creswell (2003) which will be relevant when we consider mixed methods in greater detail,

> Philosophically, researchers make claims about what is knowledge (ontology), how we know it (epistemology), what values go into it (axiology), how we write about it (rhetoric), and the processes for studying it (methodology). (p 6)

Mixed Methods and Pragmatism

Over the last two decades there has been a recognition that the historic quantitative versus qualitative debate with their respective underlying epistemologies was a stale debate (Howe, 1988), and there has been a growing acceptance of mixed methods research (Biddle & Schafft, 2015; Cameron, 2011; Molina-Azorin, 2016). Cameron and Miller (2007) stated that 'Like the mythology of the phoenix, mixed methods research has arisen out of the ashes of the paradigm wars to become the third methodological movement' (p. 2). Johnson and Onwuegbuzie (2004) make the important point that mixed methods research was not intended to replace quantitative and qualitative approaches but to capitalise on the strengths and minimise the weaknesses of both approaches.

Within mixed methods research there has been a significant alignment with the assumptions and beliefs of pragmatism (Maxcy, 2003; Tashakkori & Teddlie, 2003), and Johnson and Onwuegbuzie (2004) referred to pragmatism as, 'the philosophical partner for mixed methods research' (p 16). So, what are the cornerstone beliefs and claims that underpin pragmatism? Perhaps most important is the fact that pragmatism is not necessarily aligned with any one system of philosophy or reality (Creswell, 2003); there can be multiple realities. Pragmatism allows the researcher to reject the forced dichotomies of positivism/post-positivism and constructivist-interpretivism (Kaushik & Walsh, 2019). The pragmatic researcher focuses on 'what works' to answer research questions rather than making a choice between the positivist/post-positivist and constructivist-interpretivist epistemologies (Brierley, 2017). So, in this sense the pragmatic researcher is freer to make research-based decisions. As Creswell (2003) has noted in relation to pragmatism,

> Individual researchers have a freedom of choice. They are "free" to choose the methods, techniques, and procedures of research that best meet their needs and purposes. (p. 12)

So, the pragmatic researcher avoids being drawn into philosophical argument and debate about the nature of truth and reality; instead, the focus is on the research question, how best to address it and with a focus on real-world issues. A good insight into the relationship of pragmatism to mixed methods research has been provided by Morgan (2007) who looked at three key issues in research and how he thought they could be positioned within qualitative, quantitative and pragmatic approaches; Table 10.1 shows the material for consideration.

The first row in Table 10.1 clearly shows how different a pragmatic approach to research can be compared to traditional approaches. So, the pragmatic approach

Table 10.1 Pragmatic alternatives to key issues in research methodology [adapted from Morgan (2007)]

Key issues	Qualitative approach	Quantitative approach	Pragmatic approach
Connection of theory and data	Induction	Deduction	Abduction
Relationship to research process	Subjectivity	Objectivity	Intersubjective
Inference from data	Context	Generality	Transferability

refuses to be drawn into the dichotomous view that reasoning within research is either deductive or inductive. Instead, the focus is on *abductive reasoning*. Morgan (2007) emphasised,

> a version of *abductive* reasoning that moves back and forth between induction and deduction—first converting observations into theories and then assessing those theories through action. (p. 71)

These words seem to portray more realistically what the thought processing might be in research activity as it seems very unlikely that a researcher's thinking could be exclusively either inductive or deductive.

Looking at the second row in Table 10.1 will reveal another rejection of a false dichotomy by the pragmatic approach to research. So, notions of complete objectivity or complete subjectivity are rejected as being unrealistic. Morgan (2007) chose these words,

> Any practicing researcher has to work back and forth between various frames of reference, and the classic pragmatic emphasis on an *intersubjective* approach captures this duality. (pp. 71–72)

So, again the pragmatic approach to research as proposed by Morgan (2007) seems a more authentic approach.

In the third row of Table 10.1 is a final rejection of dichotomous extremes such that research results are either uniquely specific to a particular context or, in contrast, can be generalised completely. Morgan (2007) references the notion of *transferability*. Here the emphasis is on whether research findings from one setting may be transferred to other contexts. So, it's the value of research findings that is of central importance not whether they are context-specific or generalisable.

Morgan's conception of the potential differences between qualitative and quantitative approaches and a pragmatic approach seems to reveal a significantly different and more authentic way of thinking about research and the process of research. There is no slavish adherence to metaphysical or philosophical dogma. What counts is a 'what works best' approach and a more considered view of how to research real-life issues in real-life situations. This is the unifying view that makes pragmatism the ideal philosophical partner for mixed methods research.

Before considering what mixed methods research looks like and reviewing some of the mixed methods designs, it's worth restating some of the principal components of mixed methods research and pragmatism.

- Pragmatism supports the use of both quantitative and qualitative research methods in the same study and rejects the '*incompatibility hypothesis*'.
- Pragmatism considers the research question as being more important than underlying methods, epistemologies or paradigms.
- Pragmatism rejects the forced choice dichotomies around logic, epistemology and reasoning.
- Pragmatism promotes methodological decisions that are connected to the research question and stages of research.
- Pragmatism rejects *methodolatory* and the privileging of certain research methods (Frost & Bailey-Rodriquez, 2020).

It is these key beliefs that make mixed methods research so different from traditional research approaches and their supporting research philosophies. The pragmatic researcher is not hamstrung by the dominance of theory or philosophy but instead has a freedom of choice that is informed by considerations of the most expedient and effective ways to progress a research question embedded in real-life situations. The pragmatic researcher is indeed pragmatic and, in the author's view, is a more effective researcher.

Mixed Methods Research Designs

In reviewing mixed methods research designs it seems prudent to begin by offering some reasonably robust definition of mixed methods research. One good example comes from Johnson et al. (2007) who reviewed 19 different definitions from leading mixed methods researchers and then offered the following definition,

> Mixed methods research is the type of research in which a researcher or team of researchers combines elements of qualitative and quantitative research approaches (e.g., use of qualitative and quantitative viewpoints, data collection, analysis, inference techniques) for the broad purposes of breadth and depth of understanding and corroboration. (p. 123)

Within the literature many different variants of mixed methods design can be found but they can be reduced to a smaller number of basic design formulations. In constructing a mixed method design the researcher has to make two fundamental decisions. The first is what Creswell and Plano Clark (2007) call the *timing decision* which is to do with whether the researcher wants to run qualitative and quantitative research phases concurrently or sequentially. The second design decision is what Creswell and Plano Clark (2007) have called the *weighting decision*, and this refers to whether qualitative and quantitative research phases will have equal priority in a research study or one will be the dominant research phase and the other will be the auxiliary research phase.

These two decisions can generate nine different mixed method research designs as shown in Fig. 10.1. Looking at the top row shows the design possibilities when qualitative and quantitative research phases are of equal priority or weighting which then leaves the researcher to decide whether they will be run concurrently or

Timing Decision

		Concurrent	Sequential
Weighting Decision	**Equal Status**	QUAL **+** QUAN	QUAL ⟹ QUAN QUAN ⟹ QUAL
	Dominant Status	QUAL **+** quan QUAN **+** qual	QUAL ⟹ quan qual ⟹ QUAN QUAN ⟹ qual quan ⟹ QUAL

Fig. 10.1 Mixed method design matrix with mixed methods designs shown in each of four cells [Adapted from Johnson and Onwuegbuzie (2004)]. *Qual* qualitative, *Quan* quantitative, Rightwards arrow is sequential; Plus sign is concurrent (at the same time); capitals denote dominant approach; lower case denotes auxiliary approach [from Morse (1991)]

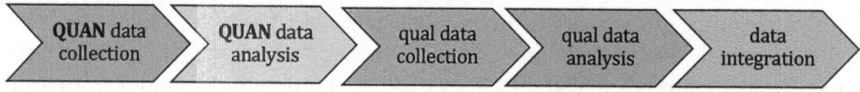

Fig. 10.2 Sequential explanatory mixed methods design with QUAN dominant

sequentially and, if so, in what order. The bottom row is all about the design permutations that follow when a qualitative or quantitative research phase is given priority or more weighting than the other. What then follows are decisions about timing (concurrent or sequential) and the order of the qualitative and quantitative research phases. So, the mixed methods researcher must consider the timing, weighting and mixing of quantitative and qualitative research phases.

Let's look at a real example of a mixed methods research design which can be called the *explanatory sequential design* (Hesse-Biber, 2010) and is shown graphically in Fig. 10.2. This design is probably the most straightforward approach where an initial phase of quantitative data collection and analysis is then followed by a secondary phase of qualitative data collection and analysis. Priority or higher weighting is typically given to the initial quantitative phase with both phases being integrated during the final integration and interpretation of data.

The sequential explanatory design was used in a research study looking at the attitudes of psychotherapists to academic writing (McBeath et al., 2019). The context was a concern that a gap was growing between psychotherapy academics and practitioners and that academic writing might be a divisive factor in this dynamic.

The main research instrument was an online survey which was designed to collect both quantitative and qualitative data. The basic research design was planned to have an initial large-scale survey followed by a secondary phase where qualitative data would be collected from the survey and subject to a *Reflexive Thematic Analysis* (Braun & Clarke, 2019).

The survey was completed by 222 psychotherapists and the quantitative data produced some key findings which included (a) a significant lack of confidence in therapists about academic writing (b) a belief that academic writing seemed detached from the concerns of practitioners and (c) that academic writing should be taught in psychotherapy trainings. Now, it's important to emphasise that this initial phase of quantitative data collection and analysis was done in advance of any focus on qualitative data. The subsequent collection and thematic analysis of qualitative data yielded a powerful enrichment and testimony to the quantitative data where a number of powerful themes were created including—'fear and lack of confidence' and 'lack of knowledge and support'.

As Creswell (2003) has emphasised, the sequential explanatory design is typically used to assist in explaining and interpreting the findings from a preliminary quantitative research phase. The design is also useful for interpreting any unexpected findings from the quantitative phase of the research. A good example of this comes from a study reported by Hesse-Biber (2010) and conducted by Brannen et al. (1994).

The study was focused on the health and family life of teenagers and followed a sequential explanatory design with the quantitative phase being dominant (QUAN) which was followed by an initial ancillary qualitative phase (qual). A self-administered survey was distributed to over 800 London teenagers followed by 142 interviews with teenagers and parents. It's important to note the design used allowed a valid interview sample to be identified.

There were two noteworthy discrepancies between the qualitative and quantitative research phases. In the survey teenagers were more likely to indicate that they looked after their health (rather than their parents) than during interviews. There was also a higher level of drug use reported in the surveys than during interviews. These discrepancies were regarded as important rather than problematic and raised questions about the reliability of findings and a search for explanations to account for the discrepancies. For example, perhaps the relative anonymity of a survey encouraged higher reported drug use by teenagers. But the overarching point was made by Hesse-Biber (2010) who stated that 'this juxtaposition of findings from each dataset allowed the researchers to enhance the validity of their findings' (p 109).

The sequential explanatory design was used by Bager-Charleson & McBeath (2021) to explore the experience of psychotherapy doctoral research supervision for both research supervisors and research supervisees. This study used a large-scale online survey as the initial quantitative research phase (QUAN) from which research participants were sampled and identified for in-depth interviews which made up the following qualitative data collection phase (qual). The qualitative data were subject

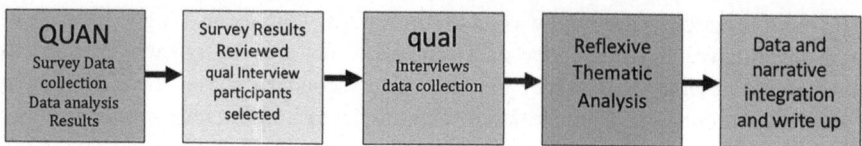

Fig. 10.3 Sequential explanatory design from Bager-Charleson and McBeath (2021)

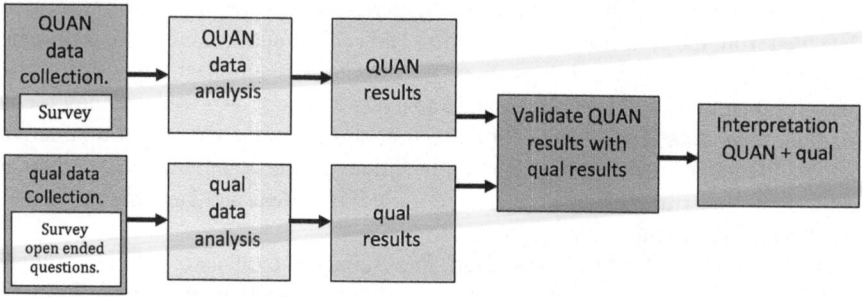

Fig. 10.4 Concurrent triangulation design—validating qualitative data model [adapted from Creswell and Plano Clark (2007)]

to a Reflexive Thematic Analysis (Braun & Clarke, 2019); Fig. 10.3 shows the sequence and constituent phases of the research.

Another sequential mixed methods design is the _exploratory sequential design_ (Hesse-Biber, 2010) which, again, is a two-phase design but the priority or weighting is given to an initial qualitative research phase. This particular approach is suited to explore a phenomenon and also its distribution in selected populations (Morse, 1991). As Creswell and Plano Clark (2007) have noted the exploratory sequential design is also useful in the development of new measurement instruments. For example, the initial qualitative phase could be used to help develop a survey which is then tested in the subsequent quantitative phase.

There are many variants of mixed methods research, but a few can be regarded as major design formulations. The sequential design just discussed is a major design formulation. Another more complex but important model is what can be called the _concurrent triangulation design_ which involves the important concept of _methodological triangulation_ (Denzin, 1978). A schematic representation of the model is shown in Fig. 10.4.

Creswell (2003) has described the reasoning behind the concurrent triangulation design as follows,

> It is selected as the model when the researcher uses two different methods in an attempt to confirm, cross-validate, or corroborate findings within a single study. This model generally uses separate quantitative and qualitative methods as a means to off-set the weaknesses inherent within one method with the strengths of the other method. (p 217)

This account by Creswell (2003) summarises just how useful and powerful mixed methods research can be.

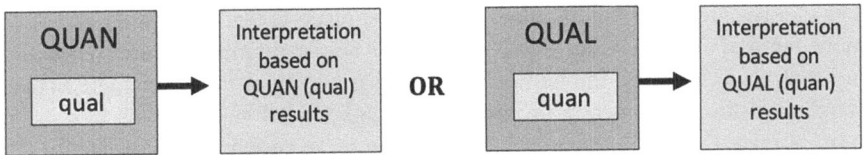

Fig. 10.5 Embedded mixed methods design [adapted from Creswell and Plano Clark (2007)]

In a research context triangulation is a concept borrowed from navigation and is used to explore a viewpoint from multiple perspectives (Cameron & Miller, 2007). Within mixed methods research methodological triangulation is essentially a validation strategy where different methods are used with the aim of confirming findings and also checking that they are not an artefact of any particular method used.

In Fig. 10.4 there are two concurrent phases of data collection portrayed; there is collection of quantitative data from a survey (QUAN) and *at the same time* there is collection of qualitative data from the survey's open-ended questions (qual); in the design QUAN is the dominant approach. The design aims to integrate the results from both concurrent phases of data collection. The outcomes could be a convergence of meaning or, indeed, a lack of convergence which would require reflection and explanation on the part of the researcher (Creswell, 2003).

Another major design formulation in mixed methods research is the *embedded design* which is also sometimes called the *nested design*; Fig. 10.5 shows a typical graphical representation of the embedded design.

In the embedded design there is a primary method (either QUAN or QUAL) which guides the main research study. The secondary method (either quan or qual) is 'embedded' or 'nested' within the dominant method and can be used to ask different research questions. There are a number of variants of the embedded design and they can operate both sequentially and concurrently. An interesting example of an embedded mixed methods design comes from Grocke et al. (2014) who researched whether group music therapy could improve the well-being of individuals with severe mental illness. The research design was essentially an ongoing experiment which collected varied quantitative data (QUAN) but within this research there was also qualitative data collected (qual) about how participants experienced the experimental intervention, namely, group music therapy.

The sequential explanatory design, sequential exploratory design, the triangulation design and the embedded design each have several variants (see Johnson et al., 2007) but they represent the four major design formulations within mixed methods research (Creswell & Plano Clark, 2007).

Integration Within Mixed Methods Research

A key concept that underpins mixed method research is *integration* which refers to processes which allow qualitative and quantitative data to 'come together', to be linked, connected or merged. There are several ways in which the different types of data can be integrated, but the underpinning rationale is that integration can offer more depth of understanding than if quantitative and qualitative data are considered in isolation. Ultimately, the aim of integration is to gain a more complete understanding of the phenomenon of interest. It is this 'added value' which lies at the heart of mixed methods research and why it can be an enriching experience for the committed researcher.

Two interesting forms of integration have been described by O'Cathain et al. (2010). The first is referred to as the *triangulation protocol* where comparisons are made between data sets to explore the coherence of findings. There are three possible outcomes from the triangulation protocol. These are when research findings from qualitative and quantitative data appear to be mutually confirming (convergence), offer additional information on an issue (complementarity) or appear to be contradictory (discrepancy or discordance). O'Cathain et al. (2010) make an important point when data sets do not agree,

> Explicitly looking for disagreements between findings from different methods is an important part of this process. Disagreement is not a sign that something is wrong with a study. Exploration of any apparent "inter-method discrepancy" may lead to a better understanding of the research question. (p 2)

A second approach to data integration is aptly described as *following a thread*. The notion here is to explore a theme or hypothesis across qualitative and quantitative data sets in an iterative manner which sees a 'to and fro' movement between data sets. The author used this approach when researching the experience of doctoral research supervision (Bager-Charleson & McBeath, 2021). A large-scale survey identified that a need for empathy from research supervisors was rated very highly by supervisees. Initially, there was a feeling that this need for empathy was not reflected in the qualitative data but on greater examination it certainly was but was only discovered by 'following a thread' and weaving between the data sets.

Two further important methods of integration are *'data transformation'* and *'integration through narrative'*. Data transformation happens when one type of data is converted into the other and the converted database is then integrated with the data that have not been transformed (Fetters et al., 2013). One way to do this is through *content analysis* where a coding process is applied to qualitative data and the frequency of identified codes is then counted and explored; so, here, qualitative data are being transformed into numerical data. The process of integration through narrative seems intuitively appealing and should probably be an essential requirement from the researcher. O'Cathain et al. (2010) describe a 'weaving approach' which involves writing both qualitative and quantitative findings together on a theme-by-theme or concept-by-concept basis.

There is another important form of integration which doesn't explicitly appear in the literature but can be termed *cognitive integration* and is derived from the author's own research experience. The process really comes from a complete immersion in both qualitative and quantitative data. So, for example, a single qualitative comment can stimulate an examination of the specific quantitative data relating to the author of the comment which, in turn, can invite further re-examination of qualitative data.

In this way a depersonalised quantitative survey database changes its complexion and can yield very individual personalised data. It's no exaggeration to say that the researcher can actually get a sense of who a person is and some of the challenges and experiences they have met in their life. On a conscious level the differentiation between quantitative data and qualitative data becomes forgotten or indeed is merged and what comes into focus is the lived experience of the individual. Cognitive integration can be a moving experience where the researcher is impacted by people rather than data.

The examples of integration that have been highlighted are a selection from a wider pool of variants and research stages (e.g. design, method, data analysis, interpretation). However, the key point to emphasise is that mixed methods requires some tangible process of integration. Without integration qualitative and quantitative data would stand separated, unconnected and unable to contribute to a deeper understanding of a phenomenon under study.

Without utilising different types of data and integrating different types of data there's a risk that an understanding of a phenomenon could be limited, fragmented and incomplete. This situation is characterised by the parable of the six blind men and the elephant (Fig. 10.6) where false conclusions came from limited and unshared information.

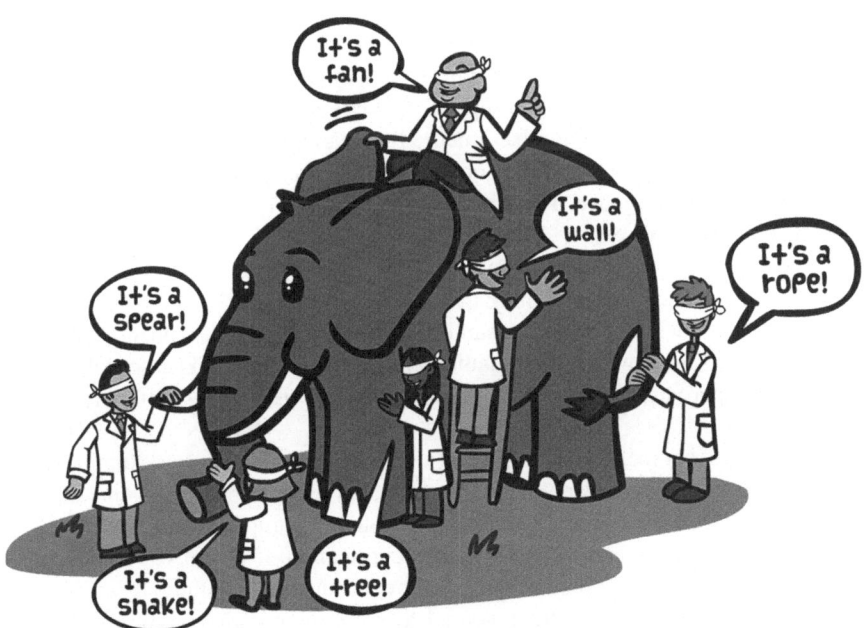

Fig. 10.6 The six blind men and the elephant

Rationale and Advantages of Mixed Methods Research

In using mixed methods it's important that the researcher has a firm grasp of the rationale or justifications that underpin this approach to research. Hesse-Biber (2010) asked the question—why use Mixed Methods? To answer the question, she referred to the works of Greene et al. (1989) who identified five specific justifications or reasons for combining qualitative and quantitative data in mixed methods research. The first reason is *methodological triangulation* which has been mentioned earlier and where the aim is to seek *convergence corroboration and correspondence of findings* from different methods (Bryman, 2006b). A second reason is *complementarity* which, 'seeks elaboration, enhancement, illustration, clarification of the results from one method with the results from another' (Greene et al., 1989, p 259).

A third reason for using mixed methods is *development*, 'which seeks to use the results from one method to help develop or inform the other method' (Greene et al., 1989, p 259). An example would be where an initial set of interviews helped in the development of a survey. Hesse-Biber (2010) refers to 'development' as a 'synergistic effect'. A fourth reason to use mixed methods is *initiation* which, 'seeks the discovery of paradox and contradiction, new perspectives of [sic] frameworks, the recasting of questions or results from one method with questions or results from the other method' (Greene et al., 1989, p 259). Hesse-Biber (2010) makes a valuable point in suggesting that addressing paradox and contradiction of findings might reveal a completely new research question. The fifth and final reason to do mixed methods is *expansion* which, 'seeks to extend the breadth and range of enquiry by using different methods for different inquiry components' Greene et al., 1989, p 259).

The justification framework compiled by Greene et al. (1989) presents some compelling reasons for doing mixed methods research and undoubtedly is focused on striving to find meaning within qualitative and quantitative data regardless of their degree of convergence. There is also an emphasis on seeking out new ways to use mixed methods research.

There are several distinct advantages to using mixed methods. Perhaps most important is the fact that combining qualitative and quantitative approaches facilitates a better understanding of research questions and complex phenomena than either approach alone whilst, at the same time, offsetting the weaknesses inherent in using either approach on its own. So, this is really the win/win basis of mixed methods research.

There are, of course, several important subsidiary advantages. For example, findings from a qualitative research phase can be tested for their potential generalisability in a subsequent quantitative phase. Another example would be where a quantitative research phase promoted the identification of new research questions that could be explored in a subsequent follow-up qualitative study. A very useful feature of mixed methods is the potential to use a quantitative method to help to identify a target sample for qualitative study. Perhaps one of the understated potentials in mixed methods research is the ability to explore contradictory findings which, itself, may lead to further research and the development of new research questions.

For the creative and pragmatic researcher mixed methods offers endless opportunities to promote a deeper and more authentic understanding of complex phenomena based in real-life situations. Underpinned by methodological pluralism a mixed methods approach allows the limiting and dichotomous 'either/or' logic associated with the quantitative versus qualitative debate to be replaced with the much more authentic 'both/and' logic which is more faithful to the complexity and diversity of psychological issues of concern (Cooper & McLeod, 2012). A specific example of the benefits to be offered by methodological pluralism and the use of 'both/and' logic has been offered by Mahalik (2014) regarding research on masculinity.

End Piece

In the introduction it was stated that mixed methods is a seldom chosen research approach within counselling and psychotherapy and especially in the case of doctoral research students and there is some firm evidence of this lack of up-take. In the United States researchers found just 8.4% of empirical articles published in the journal *Counseling Outcome Research and Evaluation* from 2010 to 2017 contained mixed methods (Cade et al., 2018). There was also a report from the same country that mixed methods was the least used research approach in doctoral dissertations (Borders et al., 2015).

As noted previously recent research by the author has revealed that knowledge about mixed methods research is quite limited amongst UK research students in counselling and psychotherapy (McBeath & Bager-Charleson, 2022). A lack of knowledge about mixed methods risks perpetuating two disparate research cultures where the dominant qualitative and quantitative approaches are viewed as competing and incompatible choices. More needs to be done by researchers, educators and trainers to ensure that those within the counselling and psychotherapy professions are made aware of the amazing possibilities that can come from doing mixed methods research.

Summary

This chapter presents an introduction to mixed methods research and seeks to emphasise that the approach offers more potential to reveal a deeper understanding of life experiences than the use of either qualitative or quantitative research methods on their own. The history and emergence of mixed methods research are described and also its potential to be aligned with the world view of pragmatism. The fundamental design variants of mixed methods research are presented with reference to supporting research examples. The rationale and advantages of mixed methods are discussed as is the importance of its underlying methodological pluralism which favours the inclusive logic of 'both/and' as opposed to the dichotomous logic of 'either/or'. The chapter concludes with a call for more information about mixed methods to be made available to those with a research interest within counselling and psychotherapy allowing them to discover the wonderful possibilities that are offered by mixed methods research.

Activity: Design Your Own Mixed Methods Research Project

Activity: Design your own mixed methods research project.

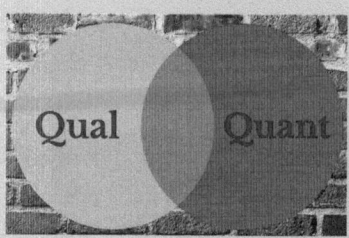

- **What research area do you think would be suitable for a mixed methods approach?**

- **What advantages would a mixed methods approach offer?**

- **What mixed methods research design would you choose?**

- **How would you collect both quantitative and qualitative data?**

- **Do you have the necessary skills to do mixed methods research?**

- **Would you need to collaborate with another researcher?**

- **How would you integrate qualitative and quantitative data?**

- **What research area do you think would be suitable for a mixed methods approach?**
- **What advantages would a mixed methods approach offer?**
- **What mixed methods research design would you choose?**
- **How would you collect both quantitative and qualitative data?**
- **Do you have the necessary skills to do mixed methods research?**
- **Would you need to collaborate with another researcher?**
- **How would you integrate qualitative and quantitative data?**

References

Bager-Charleson, S., & McBeath, A. G. (2021). Containment, compassion and clarity. Mixed methods research into Supervision during Doctoral research for Psychotherapists and Counselling psychologist. *Counselling and Psychotherapy Research*. doi:https://doi.org/10.1002/capr.12498.

Biddle, C., & Schafft, K. A. (2015). Axiology and anomaly in the practice of mixed methods work: Pragmatism, valuation, and the transformative paradigm. *Journal of Mixed Methods Research, 9*, 320–334. https://doi.org/10.1177/1558689814533157

Borders, L. D., Wester, K. L., Fickling, M. J., & Adamson, N. A. (2015). Dissertations in CACREP-accredited doctoral programs: An initial investigation. *The Journal of Counselor Preparation and Supervision, 7*(3). https://doi.org/10.7729/73.1102

Brannen, J., Dodd, K., Oakley, A., & Storey, P. (1994). *Young people, health and family life*. Open University Press.

Braun, V., & Clarke, V. (2019). Reflecting on reflexive thematic analysis. *Qualitative Research in Sport, Exercise and Health, 11*(4), 589–597. https://doi.org/10.1080/2159676X.2019.1628806

Brierley, J. A. (2017). The role of a pragmatist paradigm when adopting mixed methods in behavioural accounting research. *International Journal of Behavioural Accounting and Finance, 6*(2), 140–154.

Bryman, A. (2006a). Integrating quantitative and qualitative research: How is it done? *Qualitative Research, 6*(1), 97–113. https://doi.org/10.1177/1468794106058877

Bryman, A. (2006b). Paradigm Peace and the Implications for Quality. *International Journal of Social Research Methodology: Theory & Practice, 9*(2), 111–126. https://doi.org/10.1080/13645570600595280

Cade, R., Gibson, S., Swan, K., & Nelson, K. (2018). A content analysis of counseling outcome research and evaluation (CORE) from 2010 to 2017. *Counseling Outcome Research and Evaluation, 9*(1), 5–15. https://doi.org/10.1080/21501378.2017.1413643

Cameron, R. (2011). Mixed methods research: The five P's framework. *The Electronic Journal of Business Research Methods, 9*, 96–108. Retrieved from http://www.ejbrm.com/volume9/issue2/p96

Cameron, R., & Miller, P. (2007) Mixed methods research: Phoenix of the paradigm wars. *21st Annual Australian and New Zealand Academy of Management (ANZAM) Conference*, Sydney, December 2007.

Cooper, M., & McLeod, J. (2012). From either/or to both/and: Developing a pluralistic approach to counselling and psychotherapy. *European Journal of Psychotherapy and Counselling*, 1–13.

Creswell, J., & Plano Clark, V. (2007). *Designing and conducting mixed methods research*. Sage.

Creswell, J. W. (2003). *Research design: Qualitative, quantitative, and mixed methods approaches* (2nd ed.). Sage.

Denzin, N. (1978). *The research act: A theoretical introduction to sociological methods* (2nd ed.). McGraw-Hill.

Etherington, K. (2020). Becoming a narrative inquirer. In S. Bager-Charleson & A. G. McBeath (Eds.), *Enjoying research in counselling and psychotherapy* (pp. 71–94). Palgrave Macmillan.

Fetters, M. D., Curry, L. A., & Creswell, J. W. (2013). Achieving integration in mixed methods designs - Principles and practices. *Health Services Research, 48*(6), 2134–2156.

Frost, N., & Bailey-Rodriquez, D. (2020). Doing qualitatively driven mixed methods and pluralistic qualitative research. In S. Bager-Charleson & A. G. McBeath (Eds.), *Enjoying research in counselling and psychotherapy* (pp. 137–160). Palgrave Macmillan.

Gage, N. L. (1989). The paradigm wars and their aftermath: A "historical" sketch of research on teaching since 1989. *Educational Researcher, 18*(7), 4–10. https://doi.org/10.2307/1177163

Greene, J. C., Caracelli, V. J., & Graham, W. F. (1989). Toward a conceptual framework for mixed-method evaluation designs. *Educational Evaluation and Policy Analysis, 11*, 255–274. https://doi.org/10.3102/01623737011003255

Grocke, D., Bloch, S., Castle, D., Thompson, G., Newton, R., Stewart, S., & Gold, C. (2014). Group music therapy for severe mental illness: a randomized embedded-experimental mixed methods study. *Acta Psychiatrica Scandinavica, 130*(2), 144–153. https://doi.org/10.1111/acps.12224

Hesse-Biber, S. N. (2010). *Mixed methods research: Merging theory with practice.* The Guilford Press.

Howe, K. R. (1988). Against the quantitative-qualitative incompatibility thesis or Dogmas Die Hard. *Educational Researcher, 17*(8), 10–16. https://doi.org/10.2307/1175845

Johnson, R. B., & Onwuegbuzie, A. J. (2004). Mixed methods research: A research paradigm whose time has come. *Educational Researcher, 33*, 14–26. https://doi.org/10.3102/0013189X033007014

Johnson, R. B., Onwuegbuzie, A. J., & Turner, L. A. (2007). Toward a definition of mixed methods research. *Journal of Mixed Methods Research, 1*, 112–133. https://doi.org/10.1177/1558689806298224

Kaushik, V., & Walsh, C. A. (2019). Pragmatism as a research paradigm and its implications for social work research. *Social Sciences, 8*(9), 255. https://doi.org/10.3390/socsci8090255

Lincoln, Y. S., & Guba, E. G. (2000). Paradigmatic controversies, contradictions, and emerging confluences. In N. K. Denzin & Y. S. Lincoln (Eds.), *The handbook of qualitative research* (2nd ed., pp. 1065–1122). Sage.

Maarouf, H. (2019). Pragmatism as a supportive paradigm for the mixed research approach: Conceptualizing the ontological, epistemological, and axiological stances of pragmatism. *International Business Research, 12*(9), 1–12. https://doi.org/10.5539/ibr.v12n9p1

Mahalik, J. R. (2014). Both/and, not either/or: A call for methodological pluralism in research on masculinity. *Psychology of Men & Masculinity, 15*(4), 365–368. https://doi.org/10.1037/a0037308

Maxcy, S. J. (2003). Pragmatic threads in mixed method research in the social sciences: The search for multiple modes of inquiry and the end of the philosophy of formalism. In A. Tashakkori & C. Teddlie (Eds.), *Handbook of mixed methods in the social and behavioural sciences* (pp. 51–89). Sage.

McBeath, A. G. (2019). The motivations of psychotherapists: An in-depth survey. *Counselling and Psychotherapy Research, 19*(4), 377–387.

McBeath, A. G., & Bager-Charleson, S. (2022). *Views on mixed methods research in counselling and psychotherapy: An online survey of research students and research supervisors* (Manuscript submitted for publication). Metanoia Institute.

McBeath, A. G., Bager-Charleson, S., & Abarbanel, A. (2019). Therapists and Academic Writing: "Once upon a time psychotherapy practitioners and researchers were the same people". *European Journal for Qualitative Research in Psychotherapy, 19*, 103–116.

Mertens, D. (2007). Transformative paradigm: Mixed methods and social justice. *Journal of Mixed Methods Research, 1*(3), 212–225.

Molina-Azorin, J. F. (2016). Mixed methods research: An opportunity to improve our studies and our research skills. *European Journal of Management and Business Economics, 25*, 37–38. https://doi.org/10.1016/j.redeen.2016.05.001

Morgan, D. L. (2007). Paradigms lost and pragmatism regained: Methodological implications of combining qualitative and quantitative methods. *Journal of Mixed Methods Research, 1*, 48–76. https://doi.org/10.1177/2345678906292462

Morse, J. M. (1991). Approaches to qualitative-quantitative methodological triangulation. *Nursing Research, 40*, 120–123.

Neuman, W. (2014). *Social research methods qualitative and quantitative approaches.* Pearson.

O'Cathain, A., Murphy, E., & Nicholl, J. (2010). Three techniques for integrating data in mixed methods studies. *British Medical Journal, 341*, c4587. Retrieved from https://www.bmj.com/content/341/bmj.c4587

Pietkiewicz, I., & Smith, J. A. (2012). Praktyczny przewodnik interpretacyjnej analizy fenomenologicznej w badaniach jakościowych w psychologii. *Czasopismo Psychologiczne, 18*(2), 361–369.

Ponterotto, J. G. (2005). Qualitative research in counseling psychology: A primer on research paradigms and philosophy of science. *Journal of Counseling Psychology, 52*(2), 126–136. https://doi.org/10.1037/0022-0167.52.2.126

Reichardt, C. S., & Cook, T. D. (1979). Beyond qualitative versus quantitative methods. In T. D. Cook & C. S. Reichardt (Eds.), *Qualitative and quantitative methods in evaluation research* (pp. 7–32). Sage.

Stafford, M. R. (2020). Understanding randomised control trial design in counselling and psychotherapy. In G. McBeath (Ed.), *S. Bager-Charleson & A* (pp. 242–265). Enjoying Research in Counselling and Psychotherapy.

Tashakkori, A., & Teddlie, C. (1998). *Mixed methodology: Combining qualitative and quantitative approaches*. Sage.

Tashakkori, A., & Teddlie, C. (2003). *Handbook of mixed methods in social and behavioral research*. Sage.

Williams, R. T. (2020). The paradigm wars: Is MMR really a solution? *American Journal of Trade and Policy, 7*(3), 79–84. https://doi.org/10.18034/ajtp.v7i3.507

Chapter 11
Dialectical Pluralism in Counseling and Psychotherapy Research

Trés Stefurak, Victoria S. Dixon, and H. Burke Johnson

Learning Goals

After reading this chapter, you should be able to:

- Describe the philosophical foundations of the Dialectical Pluralism (DP) model
- Understand the process the DP model follows regarding pluralistic approaches to formulating research questions and inquiry methods
- Understand the process the DP model follows regarding embedding values of multiple stakeholders into research and evaluation projects
- Describe the philosophical pragmatism reasoning the DP model applies to making decisions about research questions, methods, and analysis.
- Describe the dialectical listening and synthesis process for which DP advocates to embed values into research questions and methods
- Describe specific correctives to the counseling and psychotherapy research process that the DP model prescribes.

T. Stefurak (✉) • H. B. Johnson
Department of Counseling & Instructional Sciences, University of South Alabama, Mobile, AL, USA
e-mail: jstefurak@southalabama.edu; bjohnson@southalabama.edu

V. S. Dixon
Clinical and Counseling Psychology Ph.D. Program, University of South Alabama, Mobile, AL, USA

© The Author(s), under exclusive license to Springer Nature Switzerland AG 2022
S. Bager-Charleson, A. McBeath (eds.), *Supporting Research in Counselling and Psychotherapy*, https://doi.org/10.1007/978-3-031-13942-0_11

Introduction

Dialectical Pluralism (DP) is a process theory and a metaparadigm of research and evaluation put forth originally by Johnson (2012, 2017) and expanded upon in the mental health context by Stefurak et al. (2016, 2018). DP offers an approach to research that ensures the values of all stakeholders surrounding the research are used to guide the development of research questions, methods, and analyses. This is accomplished through the embedding of values in the psychotherapy research, pragmatically linking values to specific research questions and methods, considering a pluralistic range of possible questions and methods when studying psychotherapy. The result is an approach to research that produces findings in which the widest array of stakeholders may find relevance, and which extends the understanding and impact of the research in a manner that both illuminates new knowledge and also expands the impact of such knowledge in terms of addressing social needs.

Overview of Dialectical Pluralism

The goal of Dialectical Pluralism (DP) is to provide a research/evaluation "process theory" as well as a metaparadigm. In any field the concept of a metaparadigm is a collection of ideas that identify the key phenomenon of interest for that discipline and broad statements about the relationships between those phenomena. The process outlined in Dialectical Pluralism is to listen to multiple paradigms, disciplines, values systems, inquiry methodologies, worldviews, cultures, and attempt to find common ground to identify inquiry projects of mutual interest (while acknowledging and maintaining differences in perspective) and to practice deliberative democracy that seeks to conduct inquiry that has points of relevance for all stakeholders and aids all stakeholders. In a sentence DP is a process in which we work together to understand and solve problems, while thriving in our differences and intellectual tensions.

Johnson (2012) outlined the basic ideas in DP for empirical research and program evaluation. Among these were to urge researchers to listen to and integrate multiple paradigms and perspectives. In addition, he urged researchers to combine ideas from competing paradigms and values into a new workable whole for each new inquiry project. The research must also integrate the epistemological and social-political values of the stakeholders surrounding a project into specified methods and goals. This step requires that the researcher attend to the unique values of each stakeholder as well as identify common ground between the seemingly divergent perspectives of stakeholders and ensure the valued means and ends of the project reflect this common ground.

Johnson and Stefurak (2014) point out that DP can be engaged as an intellectual process involving an individual researcher integrating diverging paradigms, and as a group process in which a researcher working with a heterogeneous group of stakeholders is able to arrive at win-win methods, research goals, and findings.

Johnson and Stefurak (2014) cite Rawls' (2001) concept of justice as fairness and its requirement that the voices and perspectives of those with the least power be centered, and to learn from them as research is planned and executed. A distinctive feature of the DP model is the emphasis on interpersonal skills, listening skills, and group processes as integral mechanisms by which research can be conducted in a manner that is "thick" with values and which leads to findings in which all stakeholders can accept.

DP Philosophical Assumptions

DP's philosophical approach makes several important assumptions. These are briefly summarized in the list below and can be read in more depth in

- Axiological, methodological and ontological pluralism
- Synthesis, integration and the "both-and" rather than "either-or" thinking
- Procedural justice and multiple validities justification

DP values pluralism in multiple ways. First, DP recognizes that there are multiple vantage points on reality that are useful and that there are many kinds of realities in the world. DP advocates thinking that includes and transcends subjective, intersubjective, and objective epistemologies. This ontological pluralism extends to how a DP researcher views different disciplines. Disciplines have unique histories, values, biases, and methodological strengths and weaknesses; each contributes a unique and potentially useful perspective, and none are sidelined in this model.

DP's approach to resolving seemingly incompatible different ways of knowing is to focus on the logic of synthesis and dialectical reasoning, for example thesis, antithesis, and synthesis. This requires constructing answers that combine and transcend seemingly contradictory positions, to find the common ground while retaining the unique perspective of a given viewpoint. This leads to research questions, methods, and conclusions that reflect a consensus of the various stakeholders that surround the endeavor.

DP's pluralism extends to axiology in its insistence that the values, including socio-political, epistemological, ethical, and moral perspectives, of all stakeholders involved in research and evaluation be attended to, and for such perspectives to guide the inquiry process from the inception. The goal here is to attain as much agreement as possible through the intentional use of sustained dialogue during which the researcher actively listens for values positions, draws them out, and attempts to find points of values consensus and identify what specific questions and inquiry methods most logically flow from the values positions of the stakeholders.

Activity 11.1

Using dialectical process as an integrative theory for 'mixing' methods rests on the logic of synthesis and dialectical reasoning, e.g. thesis, antithesis and synthesis. A distinctive feature of this is to draw on interpersonal skills, listening skills and group process guided by a genuine interest into different socio-political, epistemological, ethical, and moral perspectives with the view of attain as much agreement as possible.

- **Consider a scenario where qualitative and quantitative researchers may engage in this way. Think of a topic or research question, where listening from both sides with mutual change or 'synthesising' might be useful and constructive.**

When this listening and dialogue process results in a research or evaluation plan that reflects both the unique perspectives of stakeholders, including marginalized stakeholders, and the higher-order synthesis between those perspectives, procedural justice can be thought to have been attained. Rawls' (1971) concept of procedural justice requires that a common standard be invoked and that outcomes of a process are equitable to all parties. DP's focus on dialogue and synthesis at the front end of a research project can produce procedural justice by "packing" the research with the values and curiosities of the stakeholders, including things that transcend their apparent differences, and producing results that are relevant to all parties, as well as results that are of particular interest to subsets of stakeholders.

DP's pluralism, as can likely be seen from the paragraphs above, leads to a diverse methodological pluralism, driven by the values positions of the stakeholders surrounding the research. This methodological pluralism includes the ways in which knowledge/data is conceptualized, but also how knowledge is measured/assessed and analyzed. Methods are judged based on their logical connection to revealing a new understanding of the questions derived from the stakeholders' values and curiosities that drive the research or program evaluation.

The culminating goal of DP is that the researcher arrives at conclusions from diverse forms of data that result in *multiple validities legitimation* (Onwuegbuzie & Johnson, 2006). This requires that each inquiry method has been carefully selected and conducted in a manner that the relevant metrics and standards of validity of a given type are met in a robust manner, and this must be true for every type of inquiry method used in each project. Only by doing this can meta-inferences (Tashakkori & Teddlie, 2006) that integrate these different inquiry methods be made in a manner that is valid and trustworthy, and which forms a new understanding that is more than the sum of its diverse methodological parts. Secondly, if inquiry methods have been selected through intentional early dialogues to ensure that methods flow from values, then this embedding of values within research methods, alongside attention paid to the validity of each constituent method, allows for results of research and evaluation to be trusted and strongly taken up by the stakeholders surrounding the project.

In the subsequent sections of this chapter the process of dialogue and listening, through which the DP researcher maps out shared and divergent values among research stakeholders will be described. From there the rationale for the importance of embedding and making research "thick" with values is discussed, followed by a discussion of how methodological pluralism fuels the infusion of values by allowing multiple ways to investigate phenomenon such as counseling and psychotherapy. Finally, we discuss the deep philosophical pragmatic logic that drives the DP researcher's reasoning and decision-making process. In all these sections we attempt to apply these concepts as squarely as possible to counseling and psychotherapy research, and particularly to contexts where DP's tenets have relevance to contemporary disagreements and research gaps in the counseling and psychotherapy research literature.

Dialectical Listening

At the heart of DP's procedural directives is to "dialogue with difference and with the 'other'" (Johnson & Stefurak, 2014, p. 64). Its vision for psychotherapy research would privilege a democratic process at the outset of an inquiry project, which spends considerable time in intentional dialogue, attended to by the researcher with a specific set of listening and questioning skills that draw out stakeholder desires, values, biases, and passions. In this role the DP researcher upholds values of frankness and transparency, as well as a desire to fully elicit, parse, and integrate diverse perspectives and values, particularly when they are expressed by stakeholders who are in one of many possible ways marginalized or othered in larger social contexts, and particularly when stakeholders vociferously disagree in their worldview and values. DP researcher teams and stakeholders must avoid viewing disagreement as a regrettable necessity, but as a catalyst for putting the team's values into action. No development of research questions and ideas or methods can occur that will ultimately be meaningful to all parties without treading through dissonance (Stefurak et al., 2016). Johnson articulated his vision for the need for a listening method that attends to, but transcends and integrates, opposing polarities:

> The dialectical method of dialog and reasoning is perhaps the oldest in history [..] It keeps returning in history because it offers a way to thoughtfully consider, combine, or synthesize ideas when binary and dualistic logics fail. Its need and time have come again in the areas of methodologies and paradigms … It will keep returning because reality is complex and multifaceted. (Johnson, 2017, p. 158)

In the process of conducting this dialectical method of dialogue, the DP researcher is not the czar of this process, rather one among many participants in a deliberative democratic process. Both research and program evaluation are endeavors in which an investigator can be easily swayed into privileging their own frame of reference, more often in the case of the researcher, or the frame of reference endorsed by those with institutional power, more often in the case of the evaluator. Such tensions must be transparently brought into the dialectical dialogues and final decisions as to the focus and inquiry methods must derive from this democratic and transparent process.

Ensuring a democratic outcome means that the DP researcher pays close attention to how the research team's decision-making is conducted in an intentional manner that represents all relevant perspectives. In the area of psychotherapy research, the omission of important perspectives, particularly the perspective of the client or other disempowered social groups that disproportionately access and depend on this type of care, are frequently omitted. As will be mentioned frequently in this chapter, there is more than a moral justification for this democratic approach to research decisions, rather this philosophy is pragmatic in that the DP research invokes it because doing so produces an experience of procedural justice by stakeholders. This means stakeholders, who have been thoroughly engaged in these decisions, ultimately find the product of the research to be relevant, sensible and something they can accept and utilize. Procedural justice particularly requires the inclusion of stakeholders whose interests are habitually deemphasized and suppressed in each region, nation, or society.

Dialectic Listening in Psychotherapy Practice and Research

The practice of listening intentionally and with a goal to fully include diverse perspectives is foundational to most approaches to counseling and psychotherapy. For this reason, while the DP researcher would bring this emphasis to any research project, this practice of intentional dialectical listening in DP has particular resonance with in the study of psychotherapy. A foundational theoretical approach to listening within therapy is the concept of *reflective listening* developed by the seminal psychotherapy researcher and humanistic psychologist Carl Rogers (1942). Reflective listening inherently involves a dialectical process in which conflicting beliefs within the client's experiences and between the client and therapist are omnipresent. Rogers notes the conflict between the therapist's empathy and positive regard versus the mandate to be congruent, genuine, and honest with the client (Arnold, 2014). Rogers' approach to psychotherapy can serve as a foil to how a DP researcher would approach the dialectical dialogue in the initial stages of research. Both approaches note that the therapist/researcher is inevitably confronted with conflicting data, but also burdened with the need to resolve those contradictions so the client/research team can move forward in a manner that is just and satisfying. Just as Rogers urged restraint for the therapist, who quickly accrues multiple insights into the contradictions within the clients' experiences and thoughts, DP urges researchers to be patient, thoughtful and put in the time required for the early research dialogues to build a democratic foundation for the strategic decisions of what is to be asked by the research project, and how it is to be asked. Just like

Rogerian therapy, with its concerns about therapists being seduced by the allure of overly directive stances, DP holds concerns about the researcher, or other powerful entities, making unilateral decisions about these strategic research directions. A final useful parallel is Rogers' admonition that the therapist serves as a mirror to the client to promote their growth, but also that the therapist should mirror the client's attitude, values, and emotions, not just what the client verbalizes (Arnold, 2014). This is often referred to as advanced empathy, for example, listening to the content of client's verbalizations and inferring broader experiences not explicitly stated, but implied. Similarly, the DP researcher in the early dialogue stages of a research project must listen to the implied values, desires, and biases of stakeholders that may lie behind words and the vagaries of group dynamics. This ability to listen and reflect back to the client these broader attitudes and values is what lays the foundation for future comfort with disclosure in both therapy and research planning.

> **Activity 11.2**
> - Think of some examples where Rogers's principles for 'reflective listening' can be drawn upon in research. Discuss and compare in pairs or group, if possible.

Dialectic Listening and the Potential of Psychotherapy Integration

Within the practice of psychotherapy are recent trends focused on integrating the diverse, and often contradictory, theories and models of counseling into a unified coherent unitary model. This is most often proposed through identification of shared variance and common factors across all or most types of therapy that drive its success. To some degree efforts to create a new, singular paradigm of psychotherapy practice is not necessarily in-line with DP's goals, which are squarely in valuing differences rather than attempting to leave them on the cutting room floor as a sacrifice to a new theory of everything. That said DP's philosophy would support, as part of the multiplicity of perspectives, research projects that seek to pack into its strategies, a clear conception of where the disparate perspectives overlap, integrate, and synthesize.

Anchin (2008) articulates a similar view, quoting William James' observations about the balancing between "the one and the many" (James, 1907, p. 71), to make the point that any effort to unify psychotherapy practice must rely on a balance of research and theory that both finds order and clarity amid the cacophony of divergent models, and also research and theory that reveals the pragmatic utility of such pluralism, given the complexity and breadth of the problems and type of clients that enter the psychotherapy enterprise. Anchin also speaks directly to the role of dialectical thinking and, in particular, the development of a theoretically logical whole rather than psychotherapy remaining mired in technical eclecticism. To accomplish this task, the contrasts and disagreements between psychotherapy models are the fuel to adopting psychotherapy research strategies that are inclusive of the unique perspectives of each model, but which also focus on the shared variance common to all models. DP would avoid any research approaches that insist that only one psychotherapy model or strain of prior findings is worthy of further inquiry, and, instead, would pursue research that accepts that both the specific ingredients and the common factors are valid perspectives on what is occurring in the practice of psychotherapy. This view is aligned with Felice et al.'s (2019) recent literature review and their observation that specific ingredients and common factors are likely correlated with one another, and with temporal variables in treatment, rather than being orthogonal possibilities to explain psychotherapy processes. Most phenomena are comorbid and interrelated and deserve approaches to research that give opportunity for this complexity to be revealed and better understood.

Dialectic Listening and the Evidence-Based Psychotherapy Debate

DPs emphasis on dialectical dialogue has relevance to ongoing debates within psychotherapy research such as the polarities of evidence-based practice and manualized therapy versus more theoretically driven, intuitive, culturally responsive, and non-directive forms of therapy. At its worst this dialectic includes extreme beliefs that exclude the relevance in total for empirical research to inform psychotherapy practice (Zeldow, 2009) on the one hand, and ideas such as that expressed by preeminent child psychologist Alan Kazdin, who asserted that the relationship between the client and therapist "plays no causal role whatsoever" in treatment outcomes (Szalavitz, 2011). In this competition of militant extremes, a synthesis is driven by a desire to conduct psychotherapy that includes the contributions of the polarities, but also explores potential integrated common ground. DP's philosophy in its dialectical dialog phase is that no differences are to be obscured or left behind in the process, but equally important, no potential for integrated common ground is left unexplored.

Fago (2009) offers an approach to this psychotherapy debate that closely mirrors what DP would advocate. Among Fago's suggestions for an integrative research agenda is the prospect of qualitative research or single-case, time-series analysis research with practicing therapists, developing networks of practitioners interested and willing to contribute to psychotherapy research efforts, and disseminating software and tools to help practitioners collect systematic data on their work. Fago goes on to advise providing equal value to research focused on microlevel and macrolevel phenomena, for example, nuanced therapeutic process versus psychotherapy outcomes. Taking square aim at the orthodox positivists in the psychotherapy research realm, Fago urges the field to walk back away from scientism and the potential autocratic and dogmatic use of scientific findings to shut down and close off dialogue with those whose perspectives on psychotherapy research diverge from the behavioral, objectivist and quantitative epistemics. This advice harkens to William James' early advice for the nascent field of American psychology that it remains humble, skeptical of grand and dogmatic theories, and tolerant of pluralistic vantage points on psychological phenomena (Viney & King, 2003). Fago ends this commentary by making a clear argument for the "both-and" that DP also yearns for, noting the necessity of consulting objective indicators of psychotherapy's benefits, limitations and dangers, while also being skeptical of grand theories of psychotherapy often too divorced from systematic observation. In other words, be humble of what we know about psychotherapy, see the pragmatic benefits of consulting multiple perspectives and multiple research paradigms on the matter—resist the allure of monism, hubris, and intellectual zealotry. Fago's commentary is a clear example of a perspective that would align with DP's focus on intentional dialogue, inclusion of differences and leveraging of divergent methods.

Values

The dialectical dialogue, that is, the focus of the previous section has a pragmatic purpose within the DP model—to allow the researcher to embed stakeholder values into research questions, methods, and analysis. These values are ensconced in professional ethical codes as well in the minds of individual mental health professionals who hold aspirational values as to what, at their best, their counseling work should be able to accomplish and why. In addition, those seeking counseling services bring with them a personal set of values that have been demonstrated to be influential on the process of achieving positive outcomes in treatment. While most mental health professions formally or informally endorse some concept of evidence-based practice, equal emphasis is given to the role of client values and preferences. Specifically, the American Psychological Association Council of Representatives adopted a policy statement on evidence-based practice in psychology at their August 2005 meeting that states: "Evidence-based practice in psychology (EBPP) is the integration of the best available research with clinical expertise in the context of patient characteristics, culture, and preferences."

Thus, when DP examines how to infuse values into the research of counseling and psychotherapy, the focus is on both the values of the profession, the values of the individual treatment provider and the values of the client/patient. Other stakeholder values may also prove important, such as those held by a managed care organization, a private non-profit mental health agency, or a public mental health authority that oversees and dispenses mental health treatment or by the values held by a client's family, albeit weighed against supporting the client's autonomy. A final aspect of values in mental health services is the degree to which various stakeholders place a value on social justice by paying attention to contextual and systemic forces, particularly those forces that create differential levels of mental health need and create disparities in access to mental health care. The social justice concerns of the mental health professions focus on how broad-based social systems produce psychopathology and how identity and the experience of oppression create unique challenges in the delivery of counseling and psychotherapy.

Ethical Codes

In the context of research on psychotherapy and counseling, there are two categories of professional values that should be considered: those that are minimum requirements based on the relevant code of ethics and those that are aspirational values that guide what mental health services and mental health professionals "should" be in their ideal forms. For providers of psychotherapy, the American Psychological Association (APA, 2017) endorses five principles that are to guide providers when conducting psychotherapy, teaching, research, counseling, and consulting. Beneficence and non-maleficence ask for providers to protect the rights and welfare of those they for whom they work including all relevant stakeholders. Fidelity and responsibility refer to the moral responsibility providers carry to ensure others in the field are upholding the ethical code. Integrity represents a provider's responsibility to be honest by not engaging in deception or misrepresentation. Justice is perhaps one of the more subjective principles, but, overall, it refers to a provider's responsibility to be fair and impartial, a concept that is upheld well by the DP framework.

Other professional organizations have set forth distinct ethical codes as well, though outlining each is beyond the purpose or scope of this chapter. The primary implication of these ethics' codes, from a DP perspective, is that their precepts serve as minimum and non-negotiable standards for what matters in counseling research and what research must guard against producing in terms of its impact on the client. Broadly speaking, ethics codes in the mental health professions point toward the need for research to shed light on how much a given counseling intervention does "good" for the client and doesn't do "harm." This means that research questions must target things like symptom relief, long-term well-being, and flourishing as phenomena that should follow receiving counseling. In addition, these ethical mandates may mean that valued-embedded counseling research should also target the process of counseling and the degree to which client privacy, preference, values, and autonomy were upheld, independent of the results derived. Lastly, ethical mandates in these professions would suggest that counseling research must actively assess and attend to the prospect that clients not only do not benefit from services but also may be actively harmed. Research findings suggest that between 3 and 10% of psychotherapy clients become worse after receiving treatment (Lilienfeld, 2007; Boisvert & Faust, 2003; Mohr, 1995; Strupp et al., 1977), particularly in the treatments that target high-risk groups such as substance abuse (Ilgen & Moos, 2005). These are all examples of minimum ethical values that a DP approach to counseling research would attend to as these are values deeply embedded and obligatory in the mental health professions.

The primary critique the DP model would have of psychotherapy research in this vein is that its guiding values are often not explicitly stated and may not be robustly discussed as the research is planned. Rather, as is the case with most quantitative social science, initial discussions focus on logical-empirical hypotheses. While the qualitative psychotherapy literature more often states values commitments up front, both forms of psychotherapy research may not directly assess how values are operating in the process of the psychotherapy experiences they are studying. In other words, it's one thing to conceptually discuss values and allow them to shape research strategies, but the gold standard from a DP perspective would be that psychotherapy research also includes values among providers, clients and others who surround the enterprise, as a target of inquiry.

Therapist Values

Values also exist at the individual level, held within both clients and providers. Provider individual values have been the subject of much academic discussion, particularly in the realm of counseling and psychotherapy. The values of providers affect diagnoses, goals, and the overall process of therapy (Tjeltveit, 1999). Bergin writes that values influence every phase of psychotherapy and are essentially inseparable from the therapeutic process and suggests that providers move from implicit to explicit, openly being used to guide and evaluate change (1984).

Counseling research that does not follow a planning process that attends to research stakeholder values are not in-line with DP, but in addition research that does not account for the values/biases of the counselor/therapist that impact the process of psychotherapy delivery would also not be in-line with DP. The model advocates for the strongest attending to values in all aspects of researchers as well as the values held by the targets of research, for example, therapists in this case.

Client Values

DP calls for researchers to fully dialogue with and infuse within research the values of as many stakeholders as possible that surround inquiry projects. In the case of psychotherapy research, this would include the clients being served and studied. Research needs to account for situations in which client and therapist values are in conflict and how this impacts the process and outcomes of therapy. In research on components of cultural competency related to religious and spiritual beliefs, Owens and colleagues found that perceptions of a therapist's level of cultural humility were positively associated with treatment outcomes (2014). Echoing this finding, but not specific to religious/spiritual components of multicultural competency, a meta-analysis on client preferences found that clients whose preferences for treatment (i.e. shared decision-making) were valued had significantly higher levels of satisfaction, completion rates and better clinical outcomes. In other words, the degree to which the clients felt as though their values were understood and integrated into treatment predicted the efficacy of therapy. DP fully supports efforts to better measure client and therapist values and account for these as important moderators and mediators of treatment. In addition to objective measurement of client values in psychotherapy, the addition of qualitative data approaches to assessing such values would be strongly in-line with DP's philosophy.

Psychotherapy research that fails to account for client values may miss important opportunities to impact those who may someday need treatment or are considering seeking counseling, to the degree psychotherapy research makes its way into media and public consciousness. Research that speaks to client values and their role in the intervention process, if disseminated broadly in an effective manner, could serve an important public health role in terms of educating potential consumers of counseling and psychotherapy as to how their personal values are or should be involved in treatment. More generally, much of the disconnect between practice and science in counseling and psychotherapy may be improved by a more overt inquiry into and inclusion of the counselor/therapist values in research examining counseling process and outcome.

Social Justice Values

In the field of counseling, social justice has been cited as a broad value since its inception (Fouad et al. 2006). The importance of this value has changed over time, even more so in the field of psychology. Dr. Martin Luther King Jr.'s criticism of social scientists' inaction in response to the brutality of racial segregation at the 1967 APA Annual Convention became a catalyst for what we would later refer to as the Social Justice Movement. Heightened emphasis on systems-level change and addressing the disparities which under-privileged groups face has developed into a primary value of both counseling and psychology fields (DeBlaere et al., 2019; Vasquez, 2012). Those who provide mental health services are called to actively gain multicultural competence, recognize the impacts of oppression, and seek social justice through social action. Endorsement of this value influences each role a provider plays from individual therapy to research efforts. Through adopting a multicultural lens, providers can identify their own values as well as those of their clients' and ensure that treatment aligns with the client's values.

A degree of pluralism is required to practice in this manner, as the provider must be able to respect the viewpoints and lived experiences of those whom they serve, not relying on their own interpretations of reality. While DP clearly advocates taking a pluralistic and dialectical attitude to gathering the perspectives of the researchers and the stakeholders surrounding research, it also argues that stakeholders include individuals that sit outside the target of research. In the case of psychotherapy research this includes the communities, particularly socially and politically marginalized communities, who may be most in need of mental health services.

Research that can integrate the perspectives of larger groups of individuals in society who have not yet sought counseling could yield results that further the goal of research conducted from a DP perspective, which is to produce research findings that can have the broadest pragmatic impact. This is best accomplished if pluralistic research methodologies are brought to bear that provide a multifaceted view of how psychotherapy operates on the individual, how it impacts broad groups of people, and in what social spaces its prospects for aid are poorly understood or inaccessible. If the core of the approach is transformational, then the values of the stakeholders, again broadly speaking, and researchers alike serve as metaphorical lighthouses, guiding discussion and subsequent decisions on how to approach scientific inquiry, and telling us something about where psychotherapy practice fails, misses groups of people, or serves to propagate injustices and status quos that are counter to the values of those who pursue its practice.

Pluralism

Inherent in DP's emphasis on conducting research that is deeply embedded in the values of the stakeholders is an assumption that the researcher can listen to divergent perspectives simultaneously and find value in each perspective. We have already outlined the dialectical listening approach that is required if psychotherapy researchers are to infuse values into research, but none of this speaks to whether a researcher is aware of, and open to, a true diversity of perspectives. Thus, a strong philosophical pluralism is required to conduct research in this manner that is worthy of additional elaboration. Beyond the specific admonitions of the DP model, the field of counseling research and practice has, itself, struggled with a debate between monomethod versus pluralistic approaches to both the practice of psychotherapy (Norcross et al., 2016) and the conduct of psychotherapy process and outcome research (Slife & Gantt, 1999).

Pluralism in Counseling and Psychotherapy Research

Multiple authors have called for methodological pluralism in counseling research (Sliffe & Gantt, 1999) in terms of both a technical plurality of inquiry methods and a philosophical plurality of methodological conceptualization. This push is based, in part, on the recognition that even using traditional positivistic scientific methods is not a values-free endeavor. In most discussions within the counseling research literature this contest of methods breaks down into the traditional qualitative versus quantitative dichotomy. DP calls for leveraging both unique advantages of each, but also to fulfill the goal of mixed methods research in terms of triangulating diverse inquiry methods to create an understanding of counseling process and outcome that could not be achieved through any monomethod used in isolation.

A common example of this is counseling research is the desire by both scientists studying mental health services and mental health organization administrators to know that a given intervention method works, broadly speaking, which sits alongside the potential reality that a counseling method works only for some clients in some circumstances. In addition, knowing "that" a counseling method works, we also need to know "for whom, in what respects, to what extent, in what contexts," and "how a given counseling method works" (Pawson & Tilley, 1997). Inherent in this set of questions is a requirement for pluralism, even if this simply takes the form of quantitative research that looks robustly at moderators and mediators of psychotherapy outcomes. To the extent the current literature has not studied such complexities sufficiently, such a critique would fall within the *scientific realism* philosophical camp, that argues research should reveal the underlying causal variables that drive an outcome, such as client recovery at the end of counseling. DP would argue that to fully realize such an expanded vision a plurality of inquiry methods must be entertained. For example, often the level of measurement instrumentation is not yet developed to allow for an objective, questionnaire-driven, approach to measuring a given counseling process variable. In cases where no reliable objective method is available, phenomenological methods may be useful. An approach to psychotherapy research that insists on only an objectivist and quantitative approach is limited in its ability to fully assess the complexities of its target and may also be limited in its ability to meet DP's requirement that research be able to investigate the full range of factors that flow from stakeholder values.

DP's position would be that any inquiry method that allows for full exploration of the valued means and end states held by the stakeholders surrounding the research is potentially useful, including methods that are not within the realm of positivistic science. Qualitative data in general, and as a surrogate method in situations where no reliable objectivist approach is available, can shed important light on counseling process in particular. A common scenario in counseling research is that we have available objective data that points toward an outcome for a given counseling intervention that is superior to a control group but may not have clear data on why that outcome was achieved. Methods like memoing and journaling on the part of the client and provider during the counseling process can help offer guiding themes, from which later objective hypotheses and provisional explanatory theories can be developed, as to what occurred in the counseling process that drove the result that has been observed. Key to DP's pluralism is that both quantitative and qualitative approaches are valued, and their relative worth is measured by the ability a given method must provide results that satisfy the values positions of the stakeholders surrounding the research.

Nowhere is that diversity of stakeholders clearer than in the case of counseling, in which the client, the counselor, the organization within which the counselor operates, the client's family, and the larger community may all have distinct perspectives and values positions on questions about the efficacy and process of effective counseling. As previously discussed, rarely does counseling research account for this diverse set of values perspectives. Pluralism within DP is in service of procedural justice for these stakeholders and to increase the chance that research results are consumable and likely to be "taken up" by all stakeholders, as the research methods are closely aligned with these diverse values positions, and particularly designed to reflect the common ground among those values positions.

Shifting counseling research in this direction may help improve the often-lamented case in which mental health intervention researchers know a great deal about "what works," but this knowledge all too rarely is translated into practice or found to be present among broad-based understanding of what constitutes effective counseling among members of the public. If counseling research was conducted with the insistence on accounting for values in the design of research, leading to a pluralism of research methods connected to those values, this may increase the pragmatic likelihood that various stakeholders will find such research relevant, palatable, and presented in the "language" of their own values.

Pluralism and Psychotherapy Outcome Research

A strong example of the potential utility of the DP approach to counseling research is the so-called Dodo Bird Verdict and the common factors approach to interpreting existing findings in the counseling process and outcome research. This general finding is that when multiple types of counseling methods are studied, there is a tendency for all to be superior to control, but not necessarily superior to one another. A major theoretical conclusion drawn from such findings is that the success of counseling is primarily due to "common factors" or "common ingredients" that are shared by all forms of counseling (Luborsky et al., 1975; Wampold & Imel, 2015). Prior reviews have found that between 30% and 70% of the outcome variance in counseling is due to these common factors rather than the specific nature of the counseling intervention used (Imel & Wampold, 2008). This finding has been challenged by research showing the superiority of singular counseling methods, most commonly Cognitive-Behavioral Therapy (Tolin, 2010). More recently the Dodo Bird Verdict has been challenged by evidence that the "specific ingredients" of a given counseling method are correlated with common factors, and that research should evolve to examine the interaction between the two and how they evolve over time in treatment, and other more complex statistical analytic approaches that would allow the interplay between these two factors to be better understood (Felice et al., 2019).

Pragmatism and Psychotherapy Research

DP advocates a commitment to philosophical pragmatism in evaluating what research questions should matter and what methods should be selected in research. DP's pragmatism flows directly from its values-centered and pluralistic commitments. Decisions about research questions should be based on the degree to which they practically further the goals of those surrounding the research and research methods should logically flow from those values and conceptually be valid and sufficient to yield answers that would be meaningful to all stakeholders. In many ways pragmatism remains a strong underlying, though often less explicitly stated, assumption of counseling and psychotherapy research. As societal shifts toward accountability and evidence-based practice gained steam since the late 1980s, the practice of psychotherapy has been increasingly judged by its pragmatic "fruits," for example its capacity to produce symptom reduction and long-term quality of life improvements. Additionally, the practice of psychotherapy has been increasingly titrated and subjected to cost-control forces through the advent of managed care practices in both the public and private sectors of healthcare. These forces have led to a focus on psychotherapy outcomes, and often outcomes that may be limited in scope, such as short-term symptom reduction, at the expense of more complex, longer-term outcomes and more focus on the complex processes at work during psychotherapy. DP's vision would push psychotherapy research to embrace both these proximal pragmatic correlates of treatment and the complex, pluralistic myriad of processes and outcomes that may be obscured by an overly circumscribed set of priorities that surround psychotherapy practice.

There are two broad approaches to holding psychotherapy practice to a pragmatic rubric of its associated benefits. First is the dominant paradigm of evidence-based practice. As previously mentioned, this paradigm argues for a synthesis of the best available evidence, responsiveness to client preferences and the application of clinical expertise. Regarding the best available evidence component of this model, objective, traditional scientific approaches, such as randomized clinical trials and meta-analyses of such trials, are viewed as the "gold standard" of evidence. Utilizing such methodological stances may serve the values and interests of multiple parties that surround mental health practice. Rigorous traditional scientific methods produce results that maximize internal validity, rigorous control of confounding variables and which maximize the capacity to make causal inferences. These products of such research are of interest to the institutions and financial concerns that fund mental health services in that they speak to what counseling methods are most likely to work and reduce the ongoing need for care. They also serve the interest of providers of care in that such evidence can bring legitimacy and efficiency to practice. Finally, such evidence is of potential interest to consumers of mental health services to the degree they provide a guide to what types of counseling are effective for a given mental health problem.

In addition to the evidence-based practice approach to counseling research, there is a parallel concept of practice-based evidence (PBE) (Barkham & Mellor-Clark,

2003). PBE privileges counseling results observed "in the wild" occurring organically and naturally in real-world mental health delivery settings. PBE focuses on capturing what works through a bottom-up approach to research. PBE is not program evaluation, but rather gathering data on counseling process and impact in such settings, but in a broad and generalizable manner (e.g., psychotherapy practice data across a region or nation rather than at the level of an individual program or agency). PBE is distinct from EBP in that the former doesn't prescribe a particular approach to be implemented, but rather studies the approaches naturalistically being deployed in search of organically produced clinical success. Of great appeal from a DP perspective is the capacity to combine and synthesize both EBP and PBE approaches to studying and improving counseling practice.

Many providers adhere to philosophical and theoretical values which are potentially incongruent with more traditional scientific methods and epistemics. An example of such provider theoretical values is beliefs regarding humanistic and existential approaches to treatment. Such perspectives would strongly privilege the phenomenological nature of participating in counseling more than or as much as the objective outcomes associated with counseling. Providers working from this theoretical perspective may also value more esoteric indicators of recovery and healing that go well beyond short-term functional and adaptive improvements observed for the client. Changes in target constructs such as client identity, client overall lifestyle and client beliefs about broad concerns such as death, meaning and their own purpose and potential may be cited as chief values-driven pragmatic concerns for such providers.

Ultimately, the values and preferences of the client are what ethically drive how the fruits of counseling are judged. Outcomes achieved by counseling that were not desired or valued by the client are difficult to claim as evidence of psychotherapy's success if utilizing a pragmatic rubric. Client's goals are pragmatically, and from an ethical and values perspective, typically privileged to a high degree by counseling practitioners, but not as consistently by those seeking to study and understand how counseling works and what it produces for clients. DP would strongly argue that client values are of deep importance in conceptualizing counseling research and should be more actively integrated into what questions are posed and what inquiry methods are used. To this end qualitative methods may play an important role if client values and perspectives on the usefulness of counseling outcomes are to be more squarely targeted by counseling research. A failure to apply whatever methods of inquiry may be used to better understand the client experience in this regard, means that counseling research could end up primarily serving the concerns of the institutions and individual providers surrounding its practice, rather than serving the concerns of the consumer of psychotherapy.

A final point to make in terms of framing how DP's commitment to pragmatism may impact how counseling research is shaped is the aforementioned rising importance of contextual and social justice questions around how counseling is conceptualized, delivered and evaluated. By privileging client values and experiences of counseling, researchers would inevitably learn more about how clients are best empowered and experience respect and dignity in treatment, alongside what objective research methods can tell researchers about the more functional and adaptive impacts of intervention. To fully conduct counseling research in a manner that fully takes up a social justice perspective, though, even more pluralistic research questions and methods must be undertaken. For example, research into individual client experiences and outcomes from counseling is insufficient to answer questions about collective and community-wide impact of mental health services. Similarly, individual-level analysis of the nature of problems clients bring to treatment cannot shed much light on the contextual and broad forces that shape and create such problems. Lastly, individual-focused qualitative and quantitative research methods can shed limited light on the collective values and preferences and the relevant subgroupings that clients inhabit that shape their values. Research methods that include community-level analysis and engagement can allow a much broader understanding of why clients bring the concerns and values to treatment that they do, and what the broader impact of counseling may be on the community. Such questions are not necessarily of concern to the institutions surrounding counseling delivery, the providers or even the individual clients. Thus, community-level data and analytics are often not undertaken as stakeholders surrounding the research may not demand them. As funders of research increasingly are demanding a better understanding of how intervention methods translate to real-world settings and to what degree interventions are scalable to community and regional levels of implementation, the need for such analysis of broad data is rising. DP's approach would privilege obtaining findings relevant to the widest set of stakeholders possible, and findings that would widen the dialogue and lead to increasingly relevant research with the highest chance for pragmatic impact on the individuals and groups who seek and potentially benefit from counseling.

Summary

In this chapter the basic tenets of Dialectical Pluralism (DP) as a process theory of how conducting research should proceed, and as a metaparadigm of what methods and targets a given area of research should comprise were reviewed. In brief DP argues for researchers to adopt a dialectical listening process at the outset of treatment with all stakeholders. Through application of this intentional listening, the researcher ascertains and integrates the unique and shared values of stakeholders surrounding the research into the research questions, methods, and analysis. To accomplish this task the research must adopt the related philosophical stances of pluralism and pragmatism. The infusion of values into research is linked to a pragmatic goal of making research as relevant as possible to all those who sit in and around the enterprise, and pluralism is required to be able to conceptualize and access all the various perspectives of stakeholders and the diversity of inquiry methods required to assess those perspectives in the research that flows from them.

When applying the DP lens to the study of counseling and psychotherapy several conclusions were discussed. First, dialectical listening is closely aligned with the listening process within psychotherapy practice and within existing efforts to integrate the diverse approaches to psychotherapy. Dialectical listening and reasoning are necessary to avoid the bipolar "either/or" entrenchment that has sometimes occurred in psychotherapy practice and research. Values are inconsistently embedded in psychotherapy research, and values of provider, client and the larger society in regard to psychotherapy are neglected in research. If psychotherapy research is to address social justice concerns it will need to broaden its targets beyond the dyadic space between provider and client and do more to privilege the values of the client in therapy involved in a therapy study, and the individual who is not yet a client, but soon will be. Psychotherapy research methods must include both objective and subjective methods of inquiry to full investigate the full range of values-driven research questions. Lastly, pragmatism as an overarching philosophical frame may help psychotherapy research methods better address the practical demands of its various stakeholders' questions about the nature and worth of treatment. Avoiding the pitfall of only privileging certain values and perspectives may mean that psychotherapy research may end up having limited relevance to its full range of stakeholders.

Summary

To accomplish the task of ensuring psychotherapy research reflects the diverse values of the stakeholders surrounding it, the DP researcher must adopt a dialectical reasoning and listening approach to guide initial discussion in a research project, a pluralistic view of reality and psychotherapy research methods and a philosophical pragmatism that guides the linking of stakeholder values and research tactics. DP has several critiques and recommendations for psychotherapy research that may help the field produce a richer, more multifaceted, and socially relevant set of findings regarding counseling and psychotherapy's processes and outcomes.

References

American Psychological Association. (2017). *Ethical principles of psychologists and code of conduct* (2002, amended effective June 1, 2010, and January 1, 2017). https://www.apa.org/ethics/code/ethics-code-2017.pdf
Anchin, J. C. (2008). Pursuing a unifying paradigm for psychotherapy: Tasks, dialectical considerations, and biopsychosocial system metatheory. *Journal of Psychotherapy Integration, 18*(3), 310–349.
Arnold, K. (2014). Behind the mirror: Reflective listening and its Tain in the work of Carl Rogers. *The Humanistic Psychologist, 42*, 354–369. https://doi.org/10.1080/08873267.2014.913247

Barkham, M., & Mellor-Clark, J. (2003). Bridging evidence-based practice and practice-based evidence: Developing a rigorous and relevant knowledge for the psychological therapies. *Clinical Psychology and Psychotherapy, 10*, 319–327.

Bergin, A. E. (1984). Proposed values for guiding and evaluating counseling and psychotherapy. *Counseling and Values, 29*(2), 99–116.

Boisvert, C. M., & Faust, D. (2003). Leading researchers' consensus on psychotherapy research findings: Implications for the teaching and conduct of psychotherapy. *Professional Psychology: Research and Practice, 34*, 508–513.

DeBlaere, C., Singh, A. A., Wilcox, M. M., Cokley, K. O., Delgado-Romero, E. A., Scalise, D. A., & Shawahin, L. (2019). Social justice in counseling psychology: Then, now, and looking forward. *The Counseling Psychologist, 47*(6), 938–962.

Fago, D. P. (2009). Comment: The evidence-based treatment debate: Toward a dialectical rapproachement. *Psychotherapy Theory, Research, Practice, Training, 46*(1), 15–18.

Felice, G. D., Guiliani, A., Halfon, S., Andreassi, S., Paoloni, G., & Orsucci, F. F. (2019). The misleading Dodo Bird verdict: How much of the outcome variance is explained by common and specific factors? *New Ideas in Psychology, 54*, 50–55.

Fouad, N. A., Gerstein, L. H., & Toporek, R. L. (2006). Social justice and counseling psychology in context. In R. L. Toporek, L. H. Gerstein, N. A. Fouad, G. Roysircar, & T. Israel (Eds.), *Social justice in counseling psychology: Leadership, vision and action* (pp. 1–16). Sage.

Ilgen, M., & Moos, R. (2005). Deterioration following alcohol-use disorder treatment in Project MATCH. *Journal of Studies on Alcohol, 66*, 517–525.

Imel, Z. E., & Wampold, B. E. (2008). The importance of treatment and the science of common factors in psychotherapy. *Handbook of Counseling Psychology, 4*, 249–266.

James, W. (1907). Pragmatism: A new name for some old ways of thinking. In D. Olin (Ed.), *William James: Pragmatism, in focus* (pp. 13–142). Routledge.

Johnson, R. B. (2012). Dialectical pluralism and mixed research. *American Behavioral Scientist, 56*(6), 751–754.

Johnson, R. B. (2017). Dialectical pluralism: A metaparadigm whose time has come. *Journal of Mixed Methods Research, 11*(2), 156–173.

Johnson, R. B., & Stefurak, T. (2014). Dialectical Pluralism: A metaparadigm and process philosophy for 'dynamically combining' important differences. *QMiP Bulletin, 17*, 63–69. https://doi.org/10.1177/1558689815607692

King, M. L. (1967, April 4). *Beyond Vietnam: A time to break silence*. Speech delivered at Riverside Church, New York City. Retrieved from https://www.americanrhetoric.com/speeches/mlkatimetobreaksilence.htm

Lilienfeld, S. O. (2007). Psychological treatments that cause harm. *Perspectives on Psychological Science, 2*(1), 53–70.

Luborsky, L., Singer, B., & Luborsky, L. (1975). Comparative studies of psychotherapies: Is it true that everyone has won and all must have prizes? *Archives of General Psychiatry, 32*(8), 995–1008.

Mohr, D. C. (1995). Negative outcome in psychotherapy: A critical review. *Clinical Psychology: Science and Practice, 2*, 1–27.

Oliver, Lindhiem Charles B., Bennett Christopher J., Trentacosta Caitlin, McLear. (2014). Client preferences affect treatment satisfaction completion and clinical outcome: A meta-analysis. *Clinical Psychology Review, 34*(6), 506–517. S0272735814000944. https://doi.org/10.1016/j.cpr.2014.06.002

Onwuegbuzie, A. J., & Johnson, R. B. (2006). The "validity" issue in mixed methods research. *Research in the Schools, 13*(1), 48–63.

Norcross, J. C., Goldfriend, M. R., & Arigo, D. (2016). Integrative theories. In J. C. Norcross, G. R. VandenBos, D. K. Freedheim, & B. O. Olatunji (Eds.), *APA handbook of clinical psychology: Theory and research* (pp. 303–332). American Psychological Association. https://doi.org/10.1037/14773-011

Pawson, R., & Tilley, N. (1997). An introduction to scientific realist evaluation. In E. Chelimsky & W. R. Shadish (Eds.), *Evaluation for the 21st century: A handbook* (pp. 405–418). Sage. https://doi.org/10.4135/9781483348896.n29

Rawls, J. (1971). *A theory of justice*. The Belknap Press of Harvard University Press.

Rawls, J. (2001). *Justice as fairness: A restatement*. Harvard University.

Rogers, C. R. (1942). *Counseling and psychotherapy: Newer concepts in practice*. Houghton Mifflin.

Slife, B. D., & Gantt, E. E. (1999). Methodological pluralism: A framework for psychotherapy research. *Journal of Clinical Psychology, 55*(12), 1453–1465.

Stefurak, T., Johnson, R. B., & Shatto, E. (2016). Mixed methods and dialectical pluralism. In L. A. Jason & D. S. Glenwick (Eds.), *Handbook of methodological approaches to community-based research: qualitative, quantitative, and mixed methods* (pp. 345–360). Oxford Press.

Stefurak, T., Johnson, R. B., Shatto, E., & Jones, K. (2018). Developing and evaluating social programs using dialectical pluralism: Three case studies of youth placed at risk. *International Journal of Multiple Research Approaches, 10*(1), 235–250. https://doi.org/10.29034/ijmra.v10n1a15

Strupp, H. H., Hadley, S. W., & Gomez-Schwartz, B. (1977). *Psychotherapy for better or worse: The problem of negative effects*. Wiley.

Szalavitz, M. (2011, September 13). Q & A: A Yale psychologist calls for radical change in therapy. *Time*. https://healthland.time.com/2011/09/13/qa-a-yale-psychologist-calls-for-the-end-of-individual-psychotherapy/

Tashakkori, A., & Teddlie, C. (2006, April). Validity issues in mixed methods research: Calling for an integrative framework. Paper presented at the *Annual Meeting of the American Educational Research Association*, San Francisco, CA.

Tjeltveit, A. (1999). *Ethics and values in psychotherapy*. Routledge.

Tolin, D. F. (2010). Is cognitive-behavioral therapy more effective than other therapies?: A meta-analytic review. *Clinical Psychology Review, 30*(6), 710–720.

Vasquez, M. J. (2012). Psychology and social justice: Why we do what we do. *American Psychologist, 67*(5), 337.

Viney, W., & King, D. B. (2003). *A history of psychology ideas and context* (3rd ed.). Allyn and Bacon.

Wampold, B. E., & Imel, Z. E. (2015). *The great psychotherapy debate: The evidence for what makes psychotherapy work* (2nd ed.). Routledge/Taylor & Francis Group.

Zeldow, P. B. (2009). In defense of clinical judgment, credentialed clinicians, and reflective practice. *Psychotherapy: Theory, Research, Practice, Training, 46*(1), 1–10.

Chapter 12
Taking Qualitatively Driven Mixed Methods Research Further

Nollaig Frost, Maria Dempsey, and Sarah Foley

Learning Goals

After reading this chapter you should be able to:

- Understand what the qualitatively-driven mixed methods approach is and how it differs from traditional mixed methods research
- Describe the values, underlying philosophy, and epistemological principles of qualitatively-driven mixed methods research
- Know about different designs that can be used in qualitatively-driven mixed methods research
- Have considered when and how qualitatively driven mixed methods research is appropriate and useful to counselling and psychotherapy research
- Have learnt about how to do qualitatively driven mixed methods research, and the challenges and benefits of doing so
- Be aware of the ways in which ethics, quality and the writing up of qualitatively-driven mixed methods research can be thought about and addressed

Introduction

- Brief narrative outline of key points of the chapter

N. Frost (✉) • M. Dempsey • S. Foley
School of Applied Psychology, University College Cork, Cork, Ireland
e-mail: nollaig.frost@ucc.ie; M.Dempsey@ucc.ie; sarah.foley@ucc.ie

© The Author(s), under exclusive license to Springer Nature
Switzerland AG 2022
S. Bager-Charleson, A. McBeath (eds.), *Supporting Research in Counselling and Psychotherapy*, https://doi.org/10.1007/978-3-031-13942-0_12

Qualitatively Driven Mixed Methods

Mixed methods research combines at least two methods in systematic approaches that bring different perspectives to the exploration of a topic (Bailey-Rodriguez, 2021). The research methods can be either all quantitative, all qualitative, or, more usually, both quantitative and qualitative (Morse & Niehaus, 2009). The focus of this chapter will be primarily on combining qualitative and quantitative methods in a qualitatively-driven way. For more on combining qualitative methods with each other, see Chap. 8 in '*Enjoying Research in Counselling and Psychotherapy*' (Frost & Bailey-Rodriguez, 2021 in Bager-Charleson & McBeath, 2021).

The value of combining methods is in providing insight to phenomena and human experience that is multi-dimensional, less limited and more complete than that obtained using a single method (Cresswell & Clark, 2007; Mason, 2006; Morse & Chung, 2003). Mixing can take place at three levels: the data gathering stage, the data analysis stage and the interpretation stage. Therefore the approach mixes worldviews and is concerned with how they can be understood (Moran-Ellis et al., 2006). Until recently qualitative method(s) were used with quantitative methods primarily to confirm and enrich results reached through quantitative methods. They were also used to 'humanise' objective research or to act as a pilot to a larger quantitative study (Todd et al., 2004). In the last decade or so, however, *qualitatively-driven* mixed methods research has emerged as a way of placing human experience and the acceptance of multiple realities (rather than a quest for a universal truth), at the forefront of research. This approach prioritises experience and seeks to uncover subjugated knowledge not accessible through quantitatively driven approaches (Frost and Shaw, 2015). The overarching research question is always a qualitative one and the methodology, rather than the individual methods, determines how best to address it (Hesse-Biber, 2010). In contrast to the more traditional mixed methods approaches, the core is qualitatively-driven and the quantitative methods take on a secondary role, asking a sub-question or set of sub-questions that assist in the elaboration or clarification of the overall qualitative research question(s) (Hesse-Biber et al., 2015).

Why Use Qualitatively Driven Mixed Methods?

Qualitatively-driven mixed methods research offers ways of exploring the multi-dimensionality of human experience (Mason, 2006; Frost et al., 2010, 2011) by foregrounding subjective insight and understanding. It responds iteratively to emerging findings, meaning that unexpected insights, apparent 'outliers' and otherwise subjugated knowledge can be recognised and further explored. By prioritising the existence of multiple realities, qualitatively-driven mixed methods approaches allow for different experiences of the same process to be explored on multiple levels. This can be particularly useful when seeking to understand process, experience and outcome of psychotherapy and counselling because it allows for multi-perspectival exploration of client and therapist experiences and meaning-making. It takes into account context, measurement, micro and macro insight, and public and private knowledge, and uses the quantitative method(s) to extend, generalise or identify aspects of these (Hesse-Biber et al., 2015; Frost & Shaw, 2015; Bailey-Rodriguez, 2021).

Research Example: Nielsen, C. (2019). *Post mortem consciousness: views of psychotherapists and their influence on the work with clients*, unpublished doctoral thesis. The study asked 'How do the views of therapists about life after death inform their work with clients? Formal and informal networks of therapists, as well as word of mouth recruitment at conferences and requests for participation made through journal article publication, were used to develop a large sample of participants. Each was sent a survey comprising open and closed questions in order to elicit demographic data and narrative responses to questions about beliefs in life after death. Descriptive statistical analysis and thematic analysis were carried out on the results to identify a subset of therapists who defined themselves as spiritual, who had at least ten years of practice experience and who were aged over 50 years. The latter criterion was included because it is thought that in the second half of life thoughts are more likely to be directed towards death and what is likely to come afterwards. Twelve individual semi-structured interviews were conducted to elicit accounts of experience of working as a spiritual therapist who had belief sin some kind of post mortem consciousness. The data were analysed using IPA. Amongst the findings was that despite their experience the subject of death was rarely raised in the therapeutic environment, even though all the therapists stated their aim that it be a place where clients could bring their deepest concerns, either overtly or covertly. Reasons for this reluctance seemed to be because of therapist fears for their credibility, and of challenges to their ethical conduct if they discussed it in the context of some sort of afterlife.

It is also the case that qualitatively-driven mixed methods research commands a reflexive approach across the research so that the qualitatively driven mixed methods researcher considers their own role in and impact on the research throughout the process. This is valuable when, for example, practitioner-researchers are conducting research into practice they may be also carrying out themselves.

Combining qualitative methods with other qualitative methods, in a qualitatively-driven approach, termed pluralistic qualitative research, allows for researchers to explore before and after experiences, by for example interviewing participants before an intervention or other experience, and using the findings to generate a post-experience' interview schedule for use with another group who have already experienced the intervention. This saves time and possible loss of participants and can be useful in exploring many counselling and psychotherapy services.

Combining qualitative and quantitative methods means combining paradigms, and with them, different worldviews, in the same research study. Although at first consideration this may seem like a challenge, it is a key underpinning of this approach and in the next section we consider what it means to combine paradigms.

Mixing Paradigms in Qualitatively Driven Mixed Methods Research

A research paradigm comprises the philosophical position, methodology, method and theoretical framework. Broadly, a quantitative paradigm is often positivist, assuming the existence of an external, universal reality, and uses measurements, and tests to confirm or disconfirm that reality. A qualitative paradigm is interpretivist, assumes the existence of multiple, subjective realities and combines systematic analysis of accounts and expressions of experience with subjective researcher engagement to construct explanations and understandings of meaning-making. Both paradigms theorise the research with theories relevant to the topic and focus of interest (Frost, 2021).

Mixing methods within different paradigms means bringing different worldviews and philosophical assumptions to the research. These may be ontological assumptions about what exists in the world and epistemological assumptions about how knowledge about it is accessed and generated. A positivist ontology assumes there is only one reality and that it can be uncovered through hypothetical-deductive approaches to data analysis, whilst social constructionist underpinnings assume that realities are created through interaction with the world and therefore that many exist and are created through interactions. At first glance then it would seem impossible to combine these in inquiry into the same topic. However, in mixed methods research, ways in which this can be done assume the apparent divides in understanding and exploration can be transcended (Frost & Shaw, 2015). Researchers are encouraged to be open to what different perspectives can bring to understanding the data (Bryman, 2007). In qualitatively-driven mixed methods research they are required to acknowledge the complexity, changes and unpredictability of human experience, developing the research in response to the data. The approach promotes deep listening between the researcher and the participants in order to get at 'deeper and more genuine expressions of beliefs and values that emerge through dialogue [and] foster a more accurate description of views held' (Howe, 2004, p. 54). Additionally, qualitatively-driven approaches tend to be open to new information which is less confirmatory and more exploratory and theory-generating (Hesse-Biber et al., 2015).

It has been argued that the different philosophies underlying each of the paradigms mean that they cannot be combined. Historically, such criticisms set the paradigms in competition with each other in a 'paradigm war' (Oakley, 1998). Since then, however, in a tentative 'paradigm peace' (Bryman, 2006), questions about methodological opposition have become increasingly regarded as moot and enable other questions to be asked. These might be about quality criteria and evaluation for example (Bryman, 2006). The aim of mixed methods research is more to encourage selection of the best paradigm(s), theoretical frameworks, and methodologies to address the research questions rather than focussing on using particular methods. Conflict between the methods is minimal as both play a role in generalising, confirming, extending or detailing the research at the levels of data collection, analysis or interpretation.

Although debate continues about the 'rules' of mixed methods research (Morse, 2016), it is an approach that is well established, and recognised by funders.

How to Do Qualitatively Driven Mixed Methods Research

Qualitatively-Driven Mixed Methods Research Designs

The design of a qualitatively-driven mixed methods study will, like all research, be driven by the research question. It will of course be a qualitative question, and the methods selected will be those deemed the most appropriate to address it. Similarly, the decisions about whether to employ the methods sequentially or simultaneously will be informed by this. Whilst a number of designs have been outlined by researchers such as Hesse-Biber (e.g. 2010) and Bailey-Rodriguez (e.g. 2021) the iterative nature of qualitatively orientated research means the list will always be a developing one. Furthermore, researchers may find that designs at the outset of a planned qualitatively-driven study will adapt and change as findings and new foci of interest develop during the research process. In this section we describe some designs and illustrate them with examples of when and why they might be used.

Perhaps one of the simplest qualitatively driven mixed methods designs is the 'Qualitatively-Driven Nested/Embedded' (Hesse-Biber, 2010; Hesse-Biber et al. 2015) design in which data and its analysis are mixed. Semi-structured interview schedules are developed with closed questions embedded within a list of open guide questions. The aim is to gather detailed accounts alongside useful 'facts' (such as demographics, timelines, geographical distances or family size) which can be used in the analysis to identify groups and commonalities found through the qualitative analysis. This may be useful in counselling and psychotherapy research when exploring subjective outcomes of, for example, bereavement counselling. Interview schedules may include closed questions about counselling orientation experienced by clients, and these can then be gathered to gain insight to differences in experience within different forms of practice.

A 'Sequential Exploratory' design aims to enhance generalisability from qualitative studies. As its name suggests, it uses the quantitative method to explore more widely areas identified by the qualitative method. It can be useful therefore when, for example, conducting research in a particular counselling setting. The initial qualitative study highlights areas for further quantitative knowledge to be gathered from different settings. Qualitative interviews or other methods of gathering qualitative data are used to generate the quantitative study.

A 'Sequential Explanatory' design uses an initial quantitative approach to inform ongoing purposive sampling and qualitative methods of data gathering such as semi-structured interviews and focus groups to gain insight into subjective understanding. It can be useful in counselling and psychotherapy research to explore issues such as how therapists are perceived or expectations about what counselling or psychotherapy is.

Variations on the approaches outlined above mean that qualitatively driven mixed methods research designs can be as complex as the research requires. In response to findings, sequential use of qualitative and quantitative methods can extend to inclusion of document analysis or visual methods as well as surveys, questionnaires, interviews and focus groups to elicit information that helps to identify foci for the next stages of the research. Similarly, additional phases of qualitative or quantitative research can be carried out. It is essential to have a rationale for the inclusion of each method or additional phase, and its role and status in the research, so that the overall qualitative research question remains to the fore and is clearly addressed through sub-questions addressed by each method. The sub-questions addressed by the quantitative method(s) remain auxiliary, working to support the research process in addressing the overarching question.

It is worth noting that notations about mixed methods research often includes capitalising the dominant method. In qualitatively-driven mixed methods research you will see references to QUAL-quant (in which a subsequent secondary quantitative element is used in order to generalise or test theoretical ideas generated by the initial qualitative element), quant-QUAL (in which a secondary quantitative element is employed first to enhance the subsequent dominant qualitative findings by identifying a representative sample), qual-QUAL (in which a subsequent qualitative method is brought to supplement a dominant qualitative perspective) and QUAL-QUAL (in which several qualitative methods are used with equal status in the same study to generate multi-layered insight to an experience or phenomenon).

Ethical Considerations in Qualitatively Driven Mixed Methods Research

Before moving on to consider some of the practical and analytical aspects of qualitatively driven mixed methods research, it is important to discuss ethical considerations particular to this approach. Its combining of both objective (quantitative) and subjective (qualitative) elements means that it will ask participants in different ways for information, and that the researcher is seen as being both outside the research and central to it. In ensuring that the highest possible ethical standards have been reached, therefore, the qualitatively-driven mixed methods researcher needs to consider their own role as well as that of the participants. It is always the case too that research carried out as a member of an institution (whether it is a university, training institute or clinical practice setting) requires researchers to obtain approval from the Ethical Review Board of that institution before starting any of the fieldwork for the research.

The different approaches to research that mixed methods brings means that it is particularly important to be clear with participants about what is expected of them. Qualitative research asks participants to provide accounts or other expressions of experience, and researchers must remain aware that this may be about distressing events or that this may be the first time that participants have talked in detail about them. A qualitative researcher works to build rapport with participants, creating a non-judgemental and open environment for interactive discussion. The quantitative researcher on the other hand may be seeking to remain as neutral as possible when eliciting data, and is more likely to be asking participants to carry out tests, provide rankings and ratings or to answer closed questions. Broadly, they seek to remain as witnesses to the data elicitation and gathering phase of the study. This means that the mixed methods researcher, who may be seeking to recruit a subset of participants from a wider sample as part of the research design, or to include participants who have taken part in the first qualitative phase of the study into the second quantitative phase, has to consider how to adjust their role, and consider their impact, accordingly. The qualitatively-driven mixed methods researcher, however, will be reflexive across the study and therefore will have a greater 'presence' in both elements of it. Furthermore, it is important that they fully inform potential participants of what they will be asked to do and what will be done with the data they provide.

It is important too to remember that the data is taken away for analysis in which the qualitatively-driven mixed methods researcher is looking for meanings using methods and approaches that participants may or may have been told about or know about (how often do you tell participants what method of analysis you will be using?). As the researcher you may well be laying claim to accessing meanings about participants or their experiences that they themselves cannot or have not accessed. The need to be aware of the potential power of the researcher, and the potential for abuse of this power in the decisions you make as a researcher about how to look for meanings, how to interpret them and how to present them to a wider audience is of key ethical concern.

Positive approaches to ethics mean thinking about the ways in which psychologists can do better in helping those they work or research with (Knapp et al. 2017). Positive ethics strives to maximise the participation in the development of research, and asks researchers to treat participants as 'moral agents' with intrinsic worth and helpful perspectives, instead of simply being the means by which investigators can reach their research goals (Fisher, 2000, cited in Knapp & VandeCreek, 2006, p. 13). This approach is particularly useful n qualitatively-driven mixed methods research because it retains the qualitative perspective in seeking to include participants' views as a possible conceptual framework, alongside that of the analyst. Positive ethics treats confidentiality as a process of striving to enhance trust throughout the research process, and again this can be a helpful heuristic in qualitatively-driven mixed methods research. It promotes thinking and acting ethically as an ongoing process that goes beyond the one-off contractual obligation to ask participants to sign consent forms at the beginning of the study.

Clearly, ethical issues are not restricted to the design stage of a study but are important considerations throughout the research process (Kvale, 1996). Qualitatively-driven mixed methods research, where enhanced awareness of reflexive engagement with the process is foregrounded, gives an opportunity to increase the quality of the study as well as the wellbeing of the researchers and the participants. Attention to and ongoing review of these aspects of the ethics of a study, if carried out meaningfully, can be a further strength of this approach.

Chapter 8 in the book that accompanies this one, '*Enjoying Research in Psychotherapy and Counselling*', describes other ways of thinking about ethics in mixed methods research. These include Kvale's Five Ethical Questions (1996) that ask about the benefits of the study, how informed consent is ensured, how confidentiality is assured, what the consequences of conducting the study are and the researcher role in it, and the proposal of an ethical chain which connects ethical procedures and practices by linking Procedural ethics, Ethical positions, Ethics in Practice and Writing about Ethics (Palmer, 2017). Both Kvale and Palmer promote 'considering ethics at every step' (Palmer, 2017). The frameworks they provide are useful in suggesting ways of doing this when each step may vary from the previous in its approach to knowledge generation and in the role of the researcher. Both work well in conjunction with a positive ethics stance used in qualitatively-driven mixed methods research.

Recruiting Participants and Gathering Data

Qualitative research usually requires small sample sizes in order to allow for the in-depth, detailed and often time-consuming analysis to be conducted. Conversely, most quantitative research requires a large number of participants in order to be representative and generalisable. How then do qualitatively-driven mixed methods researchers determine participant recruitment strategies? These will of course be determined to a large part by the study design, as well as by the purpose and focus of the study. As we have seen in the section on Research Design above, it is not always the case that the qualitative element of the research is carried out first in qualitatively-driven mixed methods research. It is important therefore to be clear about the research design, or at least the first stage of the design, given that the qualitatively-driven approach allows for changes as the research proceeds. Ways of recruiting large numbers of participants will vary widely to those of recruiting a small sample. It may be that to recruit for a quantitative element of the study, researchers will need to use techniques most likely to reach a large audience through, for example, social media, membership of regulatory bodies such as the BACP, and networks of service providers. When recruiting for qualitative elements of the study, word of mouth and snowballing strategies can sometimes be sufficient to recruit enough participants.

At the data gathering stage a subset of participants from a large sample gathered for a quantitative method can be selected for a subsequent qualitative study. This may be to extend the generalisation of the findings from the qualitative study to a wider population, to define a population of interest within a larger quantitative study that had not been anticipated at the outset of the research and/or to identify a representative sample. Mixing at the data analysis stage is done to address one overarching research question (Mason, 2006) and can transcend differences in the outcomes of the two different perspectives or offer a rich, multi-layered view of the same topic of inquiry view of the same topic of interest.

Analysing Qualitatively Driven Mixed Methods Research Data

It is clear that in order to conduct qualitatively-driven mixed methods research that uses both qualitative and quantitative methods, it is necessary for the researcher/analyst to have skills, or access to skills, in both quantitative and qualitative data analysis. If they do not, it is important that they seek additional researchers with the appropriate expertise or further training for themselves. Whilst there is debate about whether a mixed methods study allows for each element to stand alone, or not (see e.g. Hesse-Biber, 2015; Morse, 2016), it is of no debate that the quality of the data collection, analysis and interpretation of each element in the study has to be of the same quality as it would be if the approach was a single method one. In addition, if one method is regarded as auxiliary to the other, decisions have to be made about how its analysis is integrated with the analyses reached by other methods in the study. Questions such as whether its role is to enrich, supplement or guide the next stage of the research must be asked, and answered, very clearly by the researcher.

When thinking about this during the design and analysis stage, it can be helpful to understand using different methods as a 'methods assemblage' (Law, 2004, cited in Gabb, 2009). This means considering the relationship between knowledge generated by quantitative research that seeks to identify a verifiable reality, and knowledge generated by qualitative methods about the unique perspectives on lived experience with which individuals make sense of themselves and their lives. The 'assemblage' approach creates an openness to the analysis findings, and questions certainties created by using particular methods.

Integration during the analysis phase of a study allows researchers to identify and use the strengths of both the quantitative and the qualitative data, and to ensure meaningful outcomes. Without integration the mixed methods study risks becoming two stand-alone studies—one qualitative and one quantitative (Morse 2016).

Mixing at the analysis stage allows for outliers to be individual case studies, for comparison of different data sources, and to support exploratory, predictive, or confirmatory statistical analyses (Bazeley, 2012). Bazeley identified five useful types of integrative strategies that particularly focus on data analysis which can be adapted to be relevant to qualitatively-driven mixed methods research when they allow for iterative and interactive data analysis (Fetters et al., 2013). The strategies are summarised in Table 12.1.

Table 12.1 Data analysis integration strategies [adapted from Bazeley (2012)]

One form of data informs design and analysis of another	Initial qualitative interviews are conducted and the findings of these inform the development of subsequent surveys and semi-structured interviews. Outcomes of each are compared with each other in relation to the research question. Final conclusions are made based either on the qualitative data only or on convergence between the qualitative and quantitative findings. The qualitative analyses can shape the interpretation of the quantitative analyses and how they are applied to make meaning.
Multiple components of data analysis are integrated during analysis	Qualitative data can be independently coded and then organised according to quantitative variables such as demographics. Variations in this approach allow for a homogenous group to be interviewed and the findings of this used to develop a survey that can be administered to different groups. The survey results determine whether the initial findings can be generalised beyond it. Additional sources of knowledge such as existing theories about the topic can also be utilised to interpret and make meanings of the survey findings.
Data transformation in which more than one strategy for analysis is integrated	1. Quantitative dependent and independent variables are used to create a framework with which to analyse qualitative data. QUAL data can stand independently and/or inform Quan analysis (e.g. QUAL findings may inform which statistical analyses are conducted or used to draw final conclusions). multiple sources of knowledge can drive analysis, and 2. Quantitative findings are used to develop codes to analyse qualitative data Both are deductive strategies using a starting framework rather than developing a framework from the analysis of the data but are relevant to qualitatively-driven mixed methods because the qualitative data can stand independently or be used to inform the quantitative analysis, multiple sources of knowledge can be used to drive the analysis and 'thick' descriptions of participant experiences and contexts can be retained when drawing inferences. Therefore, the focus of analysis remains on mechanisms underlying quantitative patterns rather than on the patterns themselves (Love & Corr, 2022).
Integration of results from analysis of more than one analysis of one data set	Similar to pluralistic qualitative analysis in which different qualitative methods are mixed and each analysed to build multi-layered, insight to the same experience or phenomena (Frost, 2021).
Inherent mixing in which the same data source produces qualitative and quantitative data	Qualitative data collection, such as interviews that intersperse closed questions with open-ended guide questions (Hesse-Biber, 2010).

Ensuring Quality: Quality Criteria for Qualitative and Quantitative Research

With the different aims and approaches to qualitative and quantitative research, it is clear that each has different quality criteria. Whilst both approaches share a commitment to ensuring the highest possible standards in their use, the ways these are assessed differ. Quantitative research methods, with their quest for dis/confirmation of hypotheses, replicability and generalisability, seek to identify variables, rigour and robustness in the research process. The researcher seeks not to influence the research process and the audit trail makes clear the roles that different elements of the methods play so that other researchers can test the process and seek to falsify the research results. Qualitative research, on the other hand, seeks out participants' unique perspectives on their experiences by gathering data in ways that enable agency and choice about what to describe and express. Qualitative researchers aim to remain open to meanings in the data in the analysis process, not to bring assumptions and biases to it and to understand their role in creating meanings with participants through interaction, analysis and interpretation. Indeed, participants in qualitative research are increasingly referred to as co-researchers in respect of this, as well as in efforts to recognise and flatten the power hierarchy inherent in research conduct. Quality criteria, therefore, are more concerned with the trustworthiness, and transparency of the research process as well as with the reflexivity of the researcher and the role this plays in the process.

When bringing qualitative and quantitative research methods together in mixed methods research, therefore, there is often a wide range of criteria that need to be respected. Each method needs to be able to stand alone but, importantly, be integrated in a way that is meaningful and persuasive. In practice this means ensuring that the status of each method brought to the research is made clear, and its role in the process justified. All methods need to be transparent in their role in addressing the research question(s), either by clearly relating to the overarching question or to sub-questions designed to contribute to it.

Applying Quality Criteria to Qualitatively-Driven Mixed Methods Research

Qualitatively-driven mixed methods researchers are encouraged to pursue good practice by drawing on guiding principles of qualitative research quality. These include ensuring the research contributes to wider knowledge, is transparent and systematic in its data collection, analysis and interpretation, and makes claims that are credible, grounded in the data and plausible in relation to the evidence generated by the research (Ritchie et al., 2003). Being clear about the different epistemologies within the study enables different questions about the quality of each analysis to be asked (Madill et al., 2018; Willig, 2013). Such questions might include:

- To what extent does the study capture what is really going on? How reliable is the knowledge generated? (for a realist position as in some versions of grounded theory)
- What is the quality of the accounts? Is the discursive construction internally coherent, theoretically sophisticated and persuasive? (for a constructionist epistemological position as in some discursive methods)
- How has the study demonstrated the researcher's influence on the research? (for social constructionist epistemological positions as in narrative analysis, and some versions of thematic analysis, and of grounded theory)

These questions provide useful starting points for determining quality, but it is more important to be clear about the limitations and status of the knowledge claims being made as an outcome of using different methods. This means being reflexively engaged with the different epistemological positions as each method is used.

Reflexive engagement is a cornerstone of good qualitative research, and qualitatively-driven research has this to the fore throughout the process. Quality checks on each analysis and their synthesis will include careful documentation of the process and decisions made, and discussions and reviews with any other researchers involved (e.g. Yardley & Bishop, 2008). The qualitatively-driven mixed methods approach heightens opportunities for transparency because of its focus on both the choice and use of individual methods and on the combination of the analyses.

It is good practice in qualitative research for researchers to keep reflexive journals in which they can consider their influence on the research process. When research is conducted by a team the journals are sometimes used (with permission) to study the experience of each researcher to understand how this shaped their contribution to the study (see e.g. Dempsey et al., 2019). Another way of accessing the experience of the researcher is to carry out semi-structured interviews with them. These might highlight aspects that researchers are unable or unwilling to write down, may provoke further reflection and may illuminate contradictions between what is written and what is said (see e.g. Frost et al., 2011). Combining the ways of eliciting data from researchers allows for a complex insight to the reflexive processes, and enhances understanding of how these many have shaped the research (Frost, 2021).

Writing Up

Writing up research is an essential part of the process. Not only does it present the research to an audience but it is also a way to reflect on the analysis and interpretation carried out in previous stages. Conversely, writing up may be done in stages itself so that, for example, the Literature Review and Methodology chapters or sections may be written whilst still recruiting participants or collecting data. If this is the case it will always be necessary to revisit the earlier written sections to check them for completeness and accuracy as well as to ensure that the write-up as a whole is coherent.

Writing up all forms of research includes expected and inherent expectations of the potential audience, whether it is for a student assessment, doctoral thesis, journal article or funder's report. When writing up quantitative research it is important to identify Dependent and Independent variables and often requires graphs and charts to show results. Qualitative research, on the other hand, is often written up narratively in the first person, showing clearly the researcher's role in the process, and where and how decisions have been made in it. In all forms of research, rationale for the selected method(s) is essential to show why they were selected as the best ways to address the research question, and how they were employed. It follows therefore that writing up mixed methods research presents additional challenges of incorporating all of these elements as well as those pertinent to the integration of the methods and/or their findings. When writing up qualitatively-driven mixed methods research, it is essential to retain and demonstrate the reflexive engagement that the researcher has with the research across all the methods they are using.

In the next section we will consider ways of addressing some of these challenges so that the research is presented as clearly as possible with attention shown to the important criteria.

A Starting Point

Whatever audience the research write-up is being directed to, it is essential for the researcher to be clear about the message they want to convey and to aim to meet the expectations of potential readers. For qualitatively-driven mixed methods researchers, this often means making clear why the qualitatively-driven approach has been chosen, what the (qualitatively driven) research question(s) is/are, the choice and use of methods, and their status in relation to each other. When presenting the analysis it is important to show not only the outcomes of each method used but also how they are integrated to address the overarching research question. For the qualitatively-driven mixed methods researcher there is also a need to demonstrate reflexive awareness permeating the study and how this informed, influenced and impacted on it.

One of the greatest challenges of including all these elements is adhering to word count whilst also ensuring sufficient depth of information. It is not enough to simply list the methods used, and essential to describe their status, role and how they are integrated. Analyses by each should be clearly illustrated. Often easier said than done, approaches to this can include tables to provide an overview, having sub sections on each method, or a more substantial section that describes all the methods used, and/or scans of drawings or other visual artefacts used in the analysis. There are many ways of presenting quotes as evidence (see Frost, 2021 for more on this) but it is important to ensure that each earns its place and is not simply part of a list. The depth of information will depend on the required style of the write-up—less detail in some sections for a journal article than for student projects or theses, and tailored to whether it is a 'methodology' paper or a topic focussed one. Similarly, reflexivity can be threaded throughout the write-up or included as a separate section. In this case it is important to demonstrate how the methods and outcomes have been qualitatively driven and the researcher role in this. We will consider this in more detail in the next section.

Writing Up and Reflexivity in Qualitatively-Driven Mixed Methods Research

The new Journal Article Reporting Standards for Qualitative Research (JARS-Qual) issued by the American Psychological Association includes a section titled 'Researcher Description' in which The Guidance to Reviewers notes that:

> Researchers differ in the extensiveness of reflexive self-description in reports. It may not be possible for authors to estimate the depth of description desired by reviewers without guidance. (Levitt et al., 2018)

This leaves decisions primarily to researchers, and individual assessment and journal guidelines about how much and in what way to include reflexivity. However, given that making the researcher visible is an essential component of qualitative research (Lazard & McAvoy, 2020), it is therefore key to writing up qualitatively-driven mixed methods research. Including reflexivity in writing up does not mean that researchers have to disclose high levels of personal information but rather to make clear their engagement with the research process and subjective influences they think they may have brought to it. Considering context from the perspective of both researcher and researched, and descriptions of motivations for decisions, not only show reflexive awareness but makes transparent the research process (Shaw et al., 2019).

One obvious way to address this is by writing in the first person to remind the reader of the researcher's presence, and their awareness of it. Not typically done when writing up quantitative methods, this can be extended in ways that show how the researcher chose and used all the methods. The administration of questionnaires, surveys and tests may require the researcher to be a witness to rather than central to the process but it is also the case that in writing up the process the researcher can reflect on how this more objective status was achieved and challenged and how they think this informed the research process.

It is important in qualitative research that decision points and outcomes are clear in the write-up and in qualitatively-driven mixed methods research this is extended to the choice and use of quantitative methods (Frost, 2016). The readers of the research must be equipped with sufficient information to be persuaded that the research question was kept at the forefront of each decision and how the decision-making process was informed by the researcher's knowledge, experience and critical evaluation of the research. If the research design is an evolving one where analysis by another method suggested addition of a new method to ask further questions of the data, showing reflexive awareness in the writing up means including detail about each decision-making point. For this reason, some qualitatively-driven mixed methods researchers prefer to provide a summary section with the key decisions in the main body of the text and include an Appendix with a longer Reflexive Statement to describe and evaluate details of the subjective and additional decisions behind the key moments in the research process (see e.g. Dixon-Woods et al., 2004). For example, researchers may choose to discuss the impact of delays or interruptions to the research in a longer Appendix than in the main body where the key information might be about how the research moved forward after such delays rather than the reason for the delays.

Owing to the range of methodological skills and the approaches taken in qualitatively-driven mixed methods research, researchers sometimes work collaboratively with participants as co-researchers and with other researchers. This can offer a valuable opportunity to develop a new reflexive understanding of the research in its writing up. It draws together individual subjective engagements with differing methodological, epistemological and ontological perspectives, and helps to further understand how they have contributed individually and collectively to the research process. Demonstrating this can lie in skilful crafting of accounts, inclusion of supplementary material and/or innovative presentation of the research.

Challenges and Benefits of This Approach to Counselling and Psychotherapy Research

Qualitatively-driven mixed methods research offers valuable ways of accessing insight to counselling and psychotherapy processes and outcomes. Its emphasis on context and subjective experience allows for the uniqueness of meaning-making by individuals to be combined with evaluation and assessment in ways that retain the complexity of the experiences. This is as useful to understanding counsellors and therapists' experiences as those of clients. The chapter has shown a variety of ways in which it can be done, and the range of findings that can be reached. It's responsiveness as an approach means that it can be tailored to individual and group interests and can be adapted for use by different stakeholders working together. In addition, it can be an approach that is attractive to potential funders because of its ability to inquire in detail into subgroups as well as be more generalisable than qualitative research alone. It is an approach that can be used by researchers working alone if they have the appropriate skills and knowledge, and by groups of researchers with different interests or seeking different perspectives on an area of interest.

As with all mixed methods research, qualitatively-driven mixed methods research requires planning and often more time than single method research approaches. Whilst this can be a challenge to researchers working to deadlines, it also offers opportunities to anticipate and factor in resources for dealing with challenges such as recruitment, or different forms of data analysis. The writing up too can be challenging in meeting journal and student assessment limitations but with the increase in use of this approach comes an increasing number of journals open to receiving qualitatively-driven mixed methods research. An obvious one is the Journal of Mixed Methods, which has a methodological focus, but many qualitative research journals and Counselling and Psychotherapy journals are open to this form of research too.

We have discussed the importance of being clear that the status of the quantitative method(s) brought to the research is secondary to that of the qualitative methods. This may mean that researchers more commonly drawn to using it are more qualitatively orientated than quantitative. It has been found that when combining paradigms and methods, researchers can have a bias towards their preferred one (Bryman, 2007), and it can be challenging to address this. Recognising this is an important step in conducting the research so that it can be addressed but it is also useful to remember that the methods must be chosen in relation to the research question and their contribution to addressing it. Holding this in mind enhances the likelihood that each is used in the most appropriate way and that its findings are reported appropriately and in accordance with the stated status.

Supervision and peer review of qualitatively-driven qualitative research can also present a challenge. Although the situation is changing, it is often the case that supervisors have a leaning towards an expert knowledge of one paradigm or the other. Similarly with peer reviewers who may know more about qualitative or quantitative research than their use together and in a qualitatively-driven way. Being as clear as possible in why and how the approach is being used, showing why it is the best approach for the focus of inquiry, and making as transparent as possible what was done, helps readers and assessors to evaluate it. Supervisors are often willing to learn with you, and clearly explained innovative approaches are of interest to a wide range of journal editors. The emphasis is on you as a qualitatively-driven mixed methods researcher to have knowledge and confidence in what you are doing, and taking up a role to inform others as to its value and use in counselling and psychotherapy research.

Chapter Summary

This chapter has discussed how and why qualitatively-driven mixed methods research is useful in counselling and psychotherapy research. It has discussed the foregrounding of the subjective, reflexive stance of qualitative research and how the different philosophical underpinnings of mixed methods research can be considered whilst prioritising qualitative research questions. It has shown how to design studies so that the quantitative methods used are auxiliary to the qualitative methods, and described different ways of integrating the findings. Practical considerations such as participant recruitment have been discussed along with the importance of maintaining reflexive awareness across the research process. The necessity of ensuring quality in the use of each method as well as in the integration of findings has been discussed along with ethical considerations important to the qualitatively-driven mixed methods researcher and participants. Following a discussion of ways of writing -up, some challenges and benefits of this approach to research in counselling and psychotherapy complete the chapter.

References

Bager-Charleson, S., & McBeath, A. (2021). Enjoying Research in Counselling and Psychotherapy: Qualitative. *Quantitative and Mixed Method Research*. Palgrave Macmillan.

Bailey-Rodriguez, D. (2021). Qualitatively driven mixed-methods approaches to counselling and psychotherapy research. *Counselling and Psychotherapy Research, 21*(1), 143–153.

Bazeley, P. (2012). Integrative analysis strategies for mixed data sources. *American Behavioral Scientist, 56*(6), 814–828.

Bryman, A. (2006). Integrating quantitative and qualitative research: How is it done? *Qualitative Research, 6*(1), 97–113.

Bryman, A. (2007). Barriers to integrating quantitative and qualitative research. *Journal of Mixed Methods Research, 1*(1), 8–22.

Cresswell, J. W., & Clark, V. P. (2007). *Designing and conducting mixed methods research*. Sage.

Dempsey, M., Foley, S., Frost, N., Murphy, R., Willis, N., Robinson, S., Dunn Galvin, A., Veale, A., Linehan, C., Pantidi, N., & McCarthy, J. (2019). Am I lazy, a drama queen or depressed? A pluralistic analysis of participant and researcher data when analysing accounts of depression posted to an Ireland-based website. *Qualitative Research in Psychology*, 1–21. https://doi.org/10.1080/14780887.2019.1677833

Dixon-Woods, M., Shaw, R. L., Agarwal, S., & Smith, J. A. (2004). The problem of appraising qualitative research. *BMJ Quality & Safety, 13*(3), 223–225..

Fetters, M. D., Curry, L. A., & Creswell, J. W. (2013). Achieving integration in mixed methods designs—principles and practices. *Health Services Research, 48*(6pt2), 2134–2156.

Fisher, C. B. (2000). *Relational ethics in psychological research: One feminist's journey*.

Frost, N. (2016). *Practising research: Why you're always part of the research process even when you think you're not*. Palgrave Macmillan.

Frost, N. (2021). *Qualitative research methods in psychology: combining core approaches 2e*. McGraw-Hill Education (UK).

Frost, N., & Bailey-Rodriguez, D. (2021). Doing qualitatively driven mixed methods and pluralistic qualitative research. In *Enjoying research in counselling and psychotherapy* (pp. 137–160). Palgrave Macmillan.

Frost, N. A, & Shaw, R. L. (2015). Evolving mixed and multi method approaches for psychology. In S. N. Hesse-Biber & R. B. Johnson (Eds.), *The Oxford handbook of mixed and multi method research* (pp. 375–392). Oxford Library of Psychology. Oxford University Press.

Frost, N. A., Holt, A., Shinebourne, P., Esin, C., Nolas, S. M., Mehdizadeh, L., & Brooks-Gordon, B. (2011). Collective findings, individual interpretations: An illustration of a pluralistic approach to qualitative data analysis. *Qualitative Research in Psychology, 8*(1), 93–113.

Frost, N., Nolas, S. M., Brooks-Gordon, B., Esin, C., Holt, A., Mehdizadeh, L., & Shinebourne, P. (2010). Pluralism in qualitative research: The impact of different researchers and qualitative approaches on the analysis of qualitative data. *Qualitative Research, 10*(4), 441–460.

Hesse-Biber, S. (2010). Qualitative approaches to mixed methods practice. *Qualitative Inquiry, 16*(6), 455–468.

Hesse-Biber, S. (2015). Mixed methods research: The "thing-ness" problem. *Qualitative Health Research, 25*(6), 775–788.

Hesse-Biber, S. N., Bailey-Rodriguez, D., & Frost, N. (2015). A qualitatively driven approach to multimethod and mixed methods research. In S. N. Hesse-Biber & R. B. Johnson (Eds.), *The Oxford handbook of multimethod and mixed methods research inquiry*. Oxford University Press.

Howe. (2004). A critique of experimentalism. *Qualitative Inquiry, 10*(1), 42–61.

Knapp, S. J., & VandeCreek, L. D. (2006). Multiple relationships and professional boundaries. In S. J. Knapp & L. D. VandeCreek (Eds.), *Practical ethics for psychologists: A positive approach* (pp. 75–97). American Psychological Association. https://doi.org/10.1037/11331-006

Knapp, S. J., VandeCreek, L. D., & Fingerhut, R. (2017). *Practical ethics for psychologists: A positive approach* (pp. 257–271). American Psychological Association.

Kvale, S. (1996). The 1000-page question. *Qualitative inquiry, 2*(3), 275–284.

Palmer, C. (2017). Ethics in sport and exercise research. In B. M. Smith & A. C. Sparkes (Eds.), *Routledge handbook of qualitative research in sport and exercise*. Routledge.

Law, J. (2004). *After method: Mess in social science research*. Routledge. cited in Gabb, J. (2009). Researching family relationships: A qualitative mixed methods approach. *Methodological Innovations Online, 4*(2), 37–52.

Lazard, L., & McAvoy, J. (2020). Doing reflexivity in psychological research: What's the point? What's the practice? *Qualitative Research in Psychology, 17*(2), 159–177.

Levitt, H. M., Bamberg, M., Creswell, J. W., Frost, D. M., Josselson, R., & Suárez-Orozco, C. (2018). Journal article reporting standards for qualitative primary, qualitative meta-analytic, and mixed methods research in psychology: The APA Publications and Communications Board task force report. *American Psychologist, 73*(1), 26.

Love, H. R., & Corr, C. (2022). Integrating without quantitizing: two examples of deductive analysis strategies within qualitatively driven mixed methods research. *Journal of Mixed Methods Research, 16*(1), 64–87.

Madill, A., Flowers, P., Frost, N., & Locke, A. (2018). A meta-methodology to enhance pluralist qualitative research: One man's use of socio-sexual media and midlife adjustment to HIV. *Psychology and Health, 33*(10), 1209–1228.

Moran-Ellis, J., Alexander, V. D., Cronin, A., Dickinson, M., Fielding, J., Sleney, J., & Thomas, H. (2006). Triangulation and integration: Processes, claims and implications. *Qualitative Research, 6*(1), 45–59.

Mason, J. (2006). Mixing methods in a qualitatively driven way. *Qualitative Research, 6*(1), 9–25.

Morse, J. M. (2016). *Mixed method design: Principles and procedures*. Routledge.

Morse, J. M., & Chung, S. E. (2003). Toward holism: The significance of methodological pluralism. *International Journal of Qualitative Methods, 2*(3), 13–20.

Morse, J. M. & Niehaus, L. (2009). Mixed Method Design: Principles and procedures. In *Forum qualitative sozialforschung/Forum: Qualitative social research* (Vol. 12, No. 1).

Nielsen, C. (2019). *Post mortem consciousness: views of psychotherapists and their influence on the work with clients*, unpublished doctoral thesis.

Oakley, A. (1998). Gender, methodology and people's ways of knowing: Some problems with feminism and the paradigm debate in social science. *Sociology, 32*(4), 707–731.

Ritchie, J., Spencer, L., & O'Connor, W. (2003). Carrying out qualitative analysis. *Qualitative research practice: A guide for social science students and researchers*, 219–62.

Shaw, R. L., Bishop, F. L., Horwood, J., Chilcot, J., & Arden, M. (2019). Enhancing the quality and transparency of qualitative research methods in health psychology. *British Journal of Health Psychology, 24*(4), 739–745.

Todd, Z., Nerlich, B., McKeown, S., & Clarke, D. D. (2004). *Mixing methods in psychology: The integration of qualitative and quantitative methods in theory and practice*. Psychology Press.

Yardley, L., & Bishop, F. (2008). Mixing qualitative and quantitative methods: A pragmatic approach. *The Sage handbook of qualitative research in psychology* (pp. 352–370).

Willig, C. (2013). *Introducing qualitative research in psychology*. McGraw-Hill Education (UK).

Chapter 13
Mixed Methods When Researching Sensitive Topics

Jean-Marc Dewaele, Louise Rolland, Sally Cook, and Beverley Costa

Learning Goals

After reading this chapter you should be able to:

- Have an understanding of mixed methods;
- Realise that there is an infinite number of ways to carry out research depending on the researchers' interests, personalities and the context in which participants are recruited;
- Develop awareness that doing research in this field is an embodied experience— working with real people on sensitive issues that can affect them as well as you, the researcher;
- Recognise that there is no such thing as a "perfect" research design but that it is crucial to make it as good as possible and not rush into the research;
- Glimpse the joy of researchers when they realise that the effort has paid off and that their study contributed in a small but significant way to the field as well as to social justice.

Introduction

Yotam Ottolenghi obtained a Master's degree in Comparative Literature and Philosophy, lived in Tel Aviv and Jerusalem, thinking about himself as an academic with a love of cooking and a passion for vegetables. After some years, he decided to switch career and moved to London to become a celebrated chef, owner of several

J.-M. Dewaele (✉) • L. Rolland • S. Cook • B. Costa
Birkbeck, University of London, London, UK
e-mail: j.dewaele@bbk.ac.uk; lrolla01@mail.bbk.ac.uk; beverley@pasaloproject.org

S. Bager-Charleson, A. McBeath (eds.), *Supporting Research in Counselling and Psychotherapy*, https://doi.org/10.1007/978-3-031-13942-0_13

restaurants and author of award-winning cookbooks. One may naïvely think that there are only so many ways to cook food (broiling, grilling, roasting, baking, sauté-ing, poaching, simmering, boiling, steaming, braising and stewing). Ottolenghi showed that using fresh ingredients and combining different methods and approaches can lead to delicious, original dishes. He explained that "a well-made salad must have a certain uniformity; it should make perfect sense for those ingredients to share a bowl" (Ottolenghi, 2012). The parallels with doing research are striking. Researchers need to come up with original findings, collecting data in all shapes and sizes and combining a variety of methods and approaches to find the optimal way of carrying out their analyses. Academic success is reflected in publications in good journals and subsequent citations. There is also one crucial difference between Ottolenghi in his kitchen and researchers in their offices: the latter are not allowed "to cook something up".

As will be demonstrated in the two case studies presented in this chapter, good mixed methods research is not just a matter of choosing the right methods. It requires an appropriate alignment of ontology, epistemological stance and methodological choices (McBeath & Bager-Charleson, 2020). The researcher also needs an acute awareness of the sensitivity of the data elicited from participants who may have suf-fered terrible trauma in the past. A good researcher thus needs a combination of scientific knowledge and skills but also social skills and extreme caution when deal-ing with vulnerable participants. Once the data have been collected, they need to be carefully analysed and turned into an original story that follows academic conven-tions. The reader of that story needs to be fully captivated by it, just as the customer of an Ottolenghi restaurant needs to remain in culinary heaven until the arrival of the herbal tea at the end of the meal.

Definitions of mixed methods vary in their scope. The term often refers to the use of both quantitative and qualitative methods within a single study (Creswell & Plano Clark, 2011), guided by what each approach can offer in response to the research questions. Both types of data can be mixed "concurrently by combining them (or merging them), sequentially by having one build on the other, or embed-ding one within the other" (Creswell & Plano Clark, 2011, p. 5). Mixed methods can also go beyond the QUANT-QUAL binary to encompass any "systematic way of using at least two research methods in order to answer a single over-arching research question" (Frost & Bailey-Rodriguez, 2020, p. 140), regardless of the type of data used in each one. The advantages of mixed methods have been compared to those of binocular vision, allowing researchers to observe phenomena in three rather than two dimensions (Dewaele, 2019). In Case study 1, Sally describes a qualitative pluralistic approach, combining and integrating an Interpretative Phenomenological Analysis (IPA) study with strategies from ethnography. In Case study 2, Louise adopts an exploratory sequential design where an initial quantitative phase was fol-lowed by a qualitative phase in order to offer explanations for the statistical findings (McBeath & Bager-Charleson, 2020).

Mixing methods may prove daunting because of the combination of skills needed by the researcher, but is achievable with appropriate support. We have previously written about how much we have each learnt through cross-disciplinary collaboration (Dewaele & Costa, 2014). Here, Beverley, a psychotherapist, explains how working with Jean-Marc, an applied linguist, introduced her to the benefits of mixed methods research (Dewaele & Costa, 2014: 29–30):

> In psychotherapy, we focus on attending to individuals' voices and their subjective experiences. We are also aware of the impossibility of taking a neutral stance. Our very presence in the encounter shapes it in some way. This would incline me more towards qualitative methods, such as grounded theory, which value the meaning which can be generated from in-depth interviews with a small number of participants [...] Nevertheless I have developed an appreciation for the credibility which greater numbers of respondents, achievable through quantitative methods, can bring to one's research findings, especially in an under-researched area such as the experiences of multilinguals in therapy.

In this chapter, we contrast a qualitative- versus quantitative-driven Mixed Methods model used in psychotherapy research (see also Costa & Dewaele, 2012; Priest, 2020). The case examples focus on multilingualism in psychotherapy but are more broadly relevant, and especially suitable for recruiting and researching with vulnerable participants such as refugees on sensitive topics. The crucial insight at the heart of all this work is that the languages of multilinguals vary in emotional resonance, with later learnt languages typically feeling more detached and disembodied (Dewaele, 2013, 2023; Dewaele et al., 2021; Marcos, 1976, Pavlenko, 2005, 2012). As a consequence, multilinguals may switch languages strategically in order to zoom in or out of highly emotional topics (Costa & Dewaele, 2012; Dewaele & Costa, 2013).

At this point, we hand the floor to Sally and Louise, who will present their work using the first-person pronoun, as they reflect on their individual research journeys.

Case Study 1: Combining Qualitative Approaches in Sensitive Research (Sally Rachel Cook)

Introduction to Case Study 1

My study explored the meanings asylum seekers and refugees, survivors of torture and other human rights violations, ascribe to using a later-learned language, English (ELX), in their healing journey, within a unique therapeutic community, Room to Heal (RtH), based in London. The primary function of the community is to offer a mental health service for asylum seekers and refugees. In common with a traditional therapeutic model of treatment (Kennard, 1998), emphasis was on community building and utilising community as a healing force. All therapy sessions offered by the community, both individual and group, were held in English. Participants shared common experiences characterised, for example, by feelings of the ELX being a liberating tool that empowered them and enabled them to bear witness to their trauma. The ELX also allowed some people to express their same-sex love more easily and be more self-accepting (Cook & Dewaele, 2022) and contributed to the (re)invention and performance of a "new" self. I adopted Pavlenko's (2005) view that multilinguals are people who use a later-learned language (LX) outside of the learning context, and whose LX proficiency may range from minimal to maximal. Moreover, I do not view multilingualism as a state but rather as an ongoing, dynamic process. Multilinguals' languages differ in emotional resonance which can change over time and switches from one language to another can lead to a feeling of being a different person in a different language as language is often a marker of identity (Dewaele, 2013, 2016; Panicacci & Dewaele, 2017; Pavlenko, 2012).

Behind the Scenes of the Research Questions

About a year before I embarked on my doctorate, I had started to volunteer at RtH. I worked there twice a week. Along with another volunteer, we developed the meals and cooking programme within the community. Tuesdays I cooked lunch there, Fridays I helped members cook supper. Friday supper took place in a North London community garden. Even in the winter community members and staff would eat outside in the beauty of the garden. We would eat and chat, sometimes sing together and someone would play a guitar.

My research interests emerged in tandem with my experience of volunteering in this very unique therapeutic community. I saw how it was positively helping people whose lives had been shattered by torture and exile. I became increasingly curious to know about what it was like for the members to experience using a later-learned language, English, in their healing journey within the community. I had come across a growing body of innovative interdisciplinary research in the literature (Bager-Charleson et al., 2017; Costa & Dewaele, 2012, 2019; Dewaele & Costa, 2013, Rolland et al., 2017) which showed the importance of considering the role of multi-lingualism in the therapeutic context. However, few studies examined the lived language experiences of refugees (Dewaele & Costa, 2013), and there were none which examined the language experiences of asylum seekers and refugees belonging to a therapeutic community.

A casual conversation with two refugees while chopping vegetables together for the Friday supper in the garden turned to their language preferences in the therapy. Both said they were quite happy to be using English rather than their first language (L1). They felt freer in English and more able to talk about difficult, emotionally charged experiences despite the fact that they may not be fully fluent in it. In that moment in the conversation, the young woman stopped what she was doing and turned to me and said "I don't like talking about what happened to me in my language. In every word I speak I can feel my shame …" That night I slept on this conversation. The next morning, I thought of the main research question which was to guide my research process:

> Can a (later-learned language) LX contribute to the healing and reparative space offered by a therapeutic community for survivors of torture?

In order to address this main question, I formulated four other research questions, serving as guidelines, in two broad areas of inquiry: 1) the main experiential features concerning the acquisition and use of the ELX and 2) the specific context of RtH. In essence, I wanted to explore if using the ELX has any therapeutic value.

Defining the Mixed Method Research Design: IPA and Ethnography

To answer the research questions, I decided to follow a qualitatively-driven mixed methods design which combined and integrated two qualitative approaches (see Maggs-Rapport, 2000; Morse, 2009, 2017). I combined and integrated IPA and ethnography. Morse and Niehaus (2009) define such research as consisting of one complete project (called the core component) and strategies from a different method used as a supplementary component (conducted simultaneously or sequentially to the core component). In this study, the core component and theoretical drive is IPA, whereas, the supplemental component (which was conducted simultaneously) consisted of my immersion in the field. Morse and Niehaus (2009) define the point of interface between the core and supplemental component as "the position in which the two methods join" (p. 25). In this study the core and the supplemental strategies came together in two positions: the analytical point of interface and the writing up of the report. For example, in the writing up of the report the findings from the phenomenological interviews were integrated and the chapter on the context of RtH led to a detailed and "rich" description of it. I chose IPA, which is rooted in phenomenology, hermeneutics and idiography (Smith et al., 2009: 11–40), in order to explore the lived language experiences of my participants. First, for its consistency with my research aims of gaining an understanding of what it is like to experience acquiring and using an LX, from the perspective of the individual involved. Second, for its idiographic commitment to the detailed analysis of personal experience case-by-case, so that in the final report, "the experience of each individual still has presence" (Smith, 2017: 303). Third, the interpretive aspect of IPA positions meaning-making within a person's personal and social context. Finally, the growing body of research using IPA[1] within the human, social and health sciences (Smith et al., 2009: 1) demonstrated its value to me. The first IPA papers I had come across moved me (e.g. Bramley & Eatough, 2005; Rhodes & Smith, 2010). The studies allowed me to put my feet into the shoes of people with life experiences very different from my own and place these experiences in their wider social contexts. That's what I wished to do with my research.

---

[1] For an inspiring, moving and deeper understanding of the use of IPA in a research journey, in particular, in counselling and psychotherapy research, see John Barton's chapter (Barton, 2020: 51–71).

Langdridge (2007) argues that the addition of a supplemental component, in the form of an ethnographic approach, can help to mitigate the researcher being an outsider and enable the researcher to build a rapport with the participants and elicit richer data. This was very much the case when researching survivors of torture. Torture devastates the capacity for a normal life and the capacity for trust. It shatters a person's sense of self and trust in others and destroys a person's capacity for trust and relationship (Campbell, 2007: 629). Ethnographic sensibility (McGranahan, 2015) allowed me to go beyond what face-to-face encounters and interview settings alone could have given me. The emotional engagement with the organisation and my participants helped me to glean the meanings they attributed to their language experiences and to understand them in the context of their everyday lives (see Yanow, 2006).

The regular contact I had with the refugees and asylum seekers allowed me to encounter experience as directly as possible and immerse myself in their life world. It meant the connections with my participants became strong. They knew and trusted me. I cared for my participants and they cared about me. I was genuinely interested in the phenomena I was exploring and the people who could shed light on it. In sum, regarding research on refugees and asylum seekers, the use of qualitative and ethnographic approaches improves understanding of the richness and complexity of the refugee experience (Hinchman & Hinchman, 1997).

Ethical Considerations

Fieldwork involved taking into consideration both "formalised ethics" and "everyday ethics" which Silverman (2003) defines as the ethical considerations which are involved in building field relationships and concern "crafting a persona and identity that will mutually engage both the researcher and the people, without doing damage to either" and it is about "the continual need for choices everyday" (ibid.: 127–128). My presence at RtH, both as a volunteer and researcher, involved my acting towards all community members in accordance with the community's expectations and principles, which included, for example, respect for the human rights and dignity of its members, open non-hierarchical communication between staff and members. In essence, this meant my being open about my research and my objectives.

Access and Insights from the Field

Access negotiations were long and difficult. The members of RtH are vulnerable, marginalised people and the policy of the organisation is to protect them from anything which could prove potentially harmful, disruptive or inconvenient to their lives within the community. However, my understanding of the community as a volunteer gave me insight into how to approach access negotiations. For example, I suggested to the Directors and staff, that I would be as inclusive as possible with potential participants. I had made this suggestion to be in line with the ethos of the community, which attempts to encourage the free flow of information, democratic decision making, and acknowledges the potential contribution of each member.

Participants and Inclusivity

After negotiating and securing formal access, it was necessary to negotiate informal access with the members of RtH, the participants in this study. It was their acceptance of me as a researcher, and consent to the research as much as the organisation's which determined the scope and quality of the data and therefore the final product. Again, in line with the philosophy behind "everyday ethics", I was clear and open with them about my research intentions and what participating involved. After a Tuesday lunch I gave a talk to members and staff and handed out an information sheet. During my talk I used every day, not academic language, to introduce the topic to my audience. The talk stirred up a lot of interest and questions. Many had not heard of multilingualism. One member was surprised and happy to find out she could consider herself multilingual. It gave her a fresh new term with which to describe and think about herself. The response to my call for participants was positive. Eventually, 15 people came forward, which exceeded the numbers recommended in an IPA study (normally between 4 and 10). I accepted all 15 people, for the ethical consideration of inclusivity and the pragmatic consideration of generating a wide range of accounts. This number could have raised practical and interpretive issues because of the lack of homogeneity (Smith et al., 2009). In fact, the 15 research participants were a heterogeneous group in terms of gender, country of origin, age, religion, the languages they spoke and the circumstances in which they were forced to seek asylum (e.g., persecution for political reasons, because of their sexuality or because they were trafficked), the years they had been using English and their educational backgrounds. However, the participants had the following fundamental things in common. They were all:

- Survivors of torture and organised violence (including human trafficking)
- Members of RtH
- Trying to create a new life for themselves in the UK context of a hostile asylum system
- Proficient in LX English (with varying levels of proficiency).

Interview Style and Being in the Field

Josselson (2013) states that a "good interview results from the emotional and psychological interaction between researcher and participant" (p. 15). Having already an established relationship, within the confines of RtH, with the interviewees, my approach to the interview was consequently friendly, authentic and empathic. In my heart, the participants of my study were "sacred", and I tried to ensure their well-being came before any theoretical or methodological concerns. The research interview was conceptualised in line with Carl Rogers' (1945) humanistic, empathic approach which valorises the respondent's private experiences, narratives, opinions, beliefs and attitudes (cited in Leavy, 2014: 281).

Reflexivity, Emotional Reflexivity and Self-Care

Reflexivity relates to the researcher's consideration of their influence on the research process and knowledge produced (Nightingale & Cromby, 1999). I kept a reflective research journal throughout the research process. Furthermore, I discovered in the case of "sensitive investigations", that qualitative research can profoundly affect the researcher (Cutcliffe, 2003). It was impossible not to be touched and moved and to keep myself distant from my participants' life stories. I was tightly connected to them because of the regular contact. For both the field notes and interviews, I engaged in what Jackson et al. (2013: 9) refer to as "emotional reflexivity". This involved monitoring my emotional reactions during the interviews and later when analysing the data. Keeping a reflective journal helped me to remain aware and reflect on my feelings and thoughts. Furthermore, written reflections with an embodied reflexivity were made during the analysis phase. These reflections helped the development of the analysis since free writing can be a research method in itself (Bager-Charleson & Kasap, 2017). It served to "access emotions, thoughts and feelings beyond obvious conscious reflections" (ibid.: 195).

Analysis

I identified two levels of themes: superordinate and subordinate. The three superordinate themes were "Challenging", "Moving On" and "Empowering" (Cook, 2019). Here I focus on "Bringing suffering into words", which is a subordinate theme found in the superordinate theme "Empowering". It is a significant theme—all of the 15 participants shared this experience—that the perceived detachment effect of the ELX, within the therapeutic alliance, empowered them to disclose their horrific, past experiences.

One of the participants, Brontes, explained how the perceived detachment in his ELX helped him speak out. His torture occurred in Luganda (L1) and Swahili (L2). He prefers not to talk about his torture in his L1 as it reawakens the horror far too vividly for him:

as I said, expressing myself in English about the things which happened to me which are horrible—I think I cut out—that there is not much emotion towards it if I am speaking in

English but if I was speaking in Luganda there would be a lot of emotional attachment towards it.

The distancing effect of the ELX empowered him to express and examine a difficult life experience:

I can say things in English, and you don't feel it—it doesn't hit you. It's like telling a story which didn't exist but if I say it in Luganda

His ability to speak out was also facilitated by his relationship with his therapist:

I knew he was on my side. If I am speaking to someone about myself and I know they are on my side that's what matters [...]—he can defend me, so I can tell him about myself and he hasn't judged me- so that helps a lot.

The findings confirm the LX "detachment effect" (Dewaele & Costa, 2013; Dewaele et al., 2021; Marcos, 1976; Pavlenko, 2012) which can facilitate talk about difficult and traumatic experiences. In the therapeutic context the language of detachment can become the language of enablement, when dealing with heavily charged emotional material (Byford, 2015). Awareness of the effects of multilingualism in the context of therapy is important. In Brontes' case just as his ELX enabled him to disclose his torture, use of his L1 could help him "fully grasp and face" (Burck, 2011: 334) what happened to him.

Conclusion of Case Study 1

IPA allowed me to concentrate on the phenomenon under review, whilst the ethnographic perspective enabled the phenomenon to be considered in terms of the participant group and their cultural background (the "culture" of RtH). In sum, being in the field flowed into every stage of the research process: from access to analysis and writing up. My own lived experience of the community not only helped trust develop between myself and my participants, it also enriched my interpretation of the data.

Case Study 2: Quantitative-Driven Mixed Methods Research (Louise Rolland)

Introduction

In the following case study, I cast a methodological lens on an interdisciplinary research project which investigated the language practices of multilingual adults in one-to-one psychotherapy and counselling (Rolland et al., 2017, 2021; Rolland, 2019). As a person who grew up with two home languages—English and French—I had become interested in studying multilingualism and training as a researcher in applied linguistics. For my doctoral research, I chose to explore the psychotherapy setting in connection with my own experiences as a client and inspired by Jean-Marc and Beverley's cross-disciplinary collaboration (Costa & Dewaele, 2012; Dewaele & Costa, 2013).

Specifically, I will discuss how a qualitative study can help to explain the results of an earlier, quantitative-driven study. This way of mixing methods has been called an explanatory sequential design (Creswell & Plano Clark, 2011). I first designed a survey to capture how language(s) were discussed and used in psychotherapy (past or ongoing), and possible implications for the therapeutic relationship. The aim of this first phase was to reach a broad international sample in order to compare experiences and identify any patterns around how bilingual clients and their therapists approached language in psychotherapy, expanding on the earlier study conducted by my supervisors (Dewaele & Costa, 2013).

The survey items contained mainly closed items, however several were complemented by open-ended items eliciting qualitative data. The web survey was shared in early 2016 through snowball sampling in a non-clinical population— using professional and personal networks—as well as targeted advertising (e.g. university poster boards), inviting anyone with experience of therapy to participate anonymously. On completion, participants could opt into providing an email address in order to receive information about participating in an interview. I subsequently interviewed five participants (selected from those who expressed an interest), in order to explore points of interest emerging from the analysis of survey responses. I discuss the merits of this particular sequential approach from both ethical and methodological perspectives below, providing data excerpts for illustration.

Survey Phase

The survey, which received 109 valid responses from an international sample, contained ten sections: participants provided background information before describing instances of language disclosure and negotiation, the language(s) used in therapy and their motivation for any language switching, perceived therapeutic implications of these patterns and a standard measure of perceived therapeutic empathy (Barrett-Lennard, 1962). Several items combined quantitative and qualitative sub-items in order to first gauge the frequency or type of activity before participants described it or provided an explanation in their own words (see Rolland et al., 2017, 2021). Indeed, free fields can elicit rich data including examples of client language switching (Dewaele and Costa, 2013). Gathering initial data via a survey enabled me to reach a broad sample of clients with a variety of therapy experiences—from the country of therapy to the length of their therapy—and with language practices ranging from exclusively monolingual to regular language switching, in a confidential, self-selecting manner.

Interview Phase

The aim of this qualitative follow-up phase was to shed further light on survey responses. Thus, participants were necessarily drawn from the interview sample (Creswell & Plano Clark, 2011). As a first step, I analysed the questionnaires and "examine[d] the results to see which ones [were] unclear or unexpected and required[d] further information" (op. cit., p. 186). This would inform my decisions about supplementary research questions, who to interview and what to focus on in the interview.

Analysing the Survey

I analysed the survey data using statistical analyses (using SPSS) for quantitative fields and coding qualitative fields (in Microsoft Excel) according to the principles of Thematic Analysis (Braun & Clarke, 2013). With mixed methods items, qualitative codes can be reviewed for each sub-group to see if different themes are present. For example, I asked participants whether they had discussed which languages or dialects could be used in therapy sessions with their therapist (Rolland et al., 2021). Participants could then expand on their "yes" or "no" response in a free field. I filtered these responses according to the closed item response before analysing each of the two sets of free text separately. This enabled me to identify themes relating to what such conversations covered (ranging from agreeing a main therapy language among two shared languages and acknowledging the possibility of switching to merely confirming that a single shared language was adequate for therapy), or how participants felt when there had been no such discussion (ranging from not seeing a need for it, to a feeling of not being consulted). These analyses provided preliminary answers to some of the research questions, but also raised more questions (see below). Forty-seven respondents indicated interest in information about the interview phase, which I turn to below.

Sampling from Survey Participants

One reason for this mixed methods design was the non-clinical route chosen (see Dewaele & Costa, 2014), since the project was part of a degree in applied linguistics. Given the possibly sensitive nature of discussing psychotherapy experiences, the sequential design allowed me to introduce ethical checks before selecting potential interviewees from the survey sample. It also facilitated purposive sampling along criteria of interest, as determined by the preliminary data analyses as well as methodological considerations outlined below.

Anonymity and Informed Consent

At the end of the survey, I invited respondents to opt in if they would like to receive "information about participating in a short research interview". They could then supply an email address for contact. This allowed respondents to remain anonymous if only participating in the first stage (unless they wished to receive a study summary) and to familiarise themselves with the study topics ahead of participating in the second stage. This was intended to facilitate informed consent (see Finlay, 2020) for the interviews.

Explaining what the study involves for participants is particularly important when the topic for discussion may be sensitive and participants may be vulnerable. In a stand-alone interview study, participants would not have had prior experience of how it felt to be asked about the language(s) they spoke in psychotherapy, and whether this triggered difficult memories for them.

On the other hand, remote administration of the survey meant that I could not offer support to participants if they were in distress. To mitigate this, I provided information about mental health helplines in several countries. The survey had also been reviewed by a service user advisory group and tweaked following several suggestions. Finally, data protection is an important consideration when surveying online (see McBeath, 2020).

Purposive Sampling

As mentioned, this design also allows for purposive sampling. The interview criteria used in this case study were determined by ethical considerations, preliminary data analyses and methodological considerations (inc. about researching with multilingual participants).

Firstly, as a safeguarding measure, I screened out all those who rated their problems as "disabling" or "severe" following therapy. The use of self-reports, whilst not a clinical mental health assessment, relies on the fact that people are a key source of expertise on themselves (Parker, 2007). Any incoherent accounts by respondents would also have constituted a red flag. I excluded participants who were personal acquaintances, as well as clients who had had fewer than four sessions with their therapist or whose therapy took place more than five years earlier.

I grouped the remaining 29 interested respondents (out of an original 47) according to key features from the questionnaire data, such as whether or not they had used more than one language in therapy, had experiences with more than one therapist and were in ongoing therapy. The choices I made in response to research questions are detailed in the next section. In total, I carried out five interviews after contacting six potential participants (the total being constrained by the scale of a doctoral study), following an iterative process to address the various areas identified as interesting to pursue. The interview guide for each interviewee was adapted not only according to their survey responses but also to the content of the previous interview, which generated sub-questions and prompts within the overall interview protocol (which is published in Rolland et al., 2019). Although informed by grounded theory (Braun & Clarke, 2013; Burck, 2005), sampling did not aspire to theoretical saturation given the diversity of practices and experiences under investigation.

An additional methodological—and ethical—sampling criterion was sharing more than one language with a participant. When researching with multilingual participants—a high likelihood in diverse populations even when the research does not target multilinguals—it is important to think about the constraints which the interview language may place on the interviewee. Indeed, even if they are highly fluent, multilinguals may recall and retell memories or express emotions quite differently according to which language they are using (see Rolland et al., 2019). There is also the risk of exacerbating a power imbalance if interviewing someone in what is your first language but a foreign language for them (see Connell et al., 2016).

Given my own Franco-British background, this meant selecting a French participant for at least one of the interviews, if possible. This strategy, in addition to allowing me to be flexible about interviewing in French, English or both, according to the participant's preference (see Rolland et al., 2019; Rolland, in prep.), enabled us to explore what it meant to be bilingual in therapy within a bilingual research interview environment. As both the participant and researcher made numerous switches, some of the ways in which the participant used her languages were becoming apparent even as the participant described her language choices in therapy to me.

Explaining Quantitative Data: Explanatory Sequential Design

Questionnaire analyses shed light on participants' language practices in psychotherapy (see Rolland et al., 2017, 2019 for key results). Some findings were surprising.

For example, just over a third of respondents reported no language switching at all, even though many spoke or had private thoughts in more than one language daily. Intrigued, and without clear answers from an earlier survey item enquiring about inhibition regarding code-switching, I formulated a new research question about this. In this way, the absence of code-switching became a sampling criterion with equal weight to the presence of code-switching, so that both phenomena could be investigated in interviews. In fact, less is known about this whereas other studies explore what motivates client code-switching (e.g. Dewaele & Costa, 2013; Pérez-Rojas et al., 2019).

Overall, my use of sampling criteria was constrained by the self-selection process of volunteering for interview. Where this is not necessary, the more systematic approach of interviewing all those fitting a specific profile, such as "participants in the top 10% of depression scores" (Creswell & Plano Clark, 2011, p. 187), can be adopted.

Conducting Interviews on Sensitive Topics: Safeguarding and Self-Care

The five interviewees were all women; two had spoken predominantly in their first language (French or Spanish) in therapy, while the other three had used their second language (English). I was conscious that discussing language practices might bring up sensitive topics relating to their psychotherapy sessions. Whilst I was careful not to ask about their reasons for accessing therapy, recalling the language of conversations with their therapists—and therefore the conversations themselves—could bring these matters to the surface for participants.

I prepared for participant distress by including cues in my interview guide, which I practised in a pilot interview with Beverley: acknowledge the distress, pause recording and offer water to give the participant a break, ask whether or not she wishes to continue the interview, offer a crisis number. When the first interviewee volunteered a reason for her therapy, I panicked that the disclosure might be triggering for her, and for me. So in the next question, I discouraged her from providing personal details. By reflecting on this in my research diary and discussing it with Beverley, who acted as a "clinical research supervisor" (Rolland et al., 2019, p. 287), I learned to recognise my own limitations and that it was acceptable to steer away from sensitive topics rather than contaminate the data. When a later interviewee disclosed her experience of domestic abuse, I was more able to tolerate emotionality. Although being "neutral" is typically advised of interviewers (Mann, 2016, p. 157), I held Nabeela's gaze for several, emotionally charged seconds, before quietly uttering "I'm sorry to hear that". This felt much more personal, but as Mann argues, interviews often involve dilemmas which require researchers to "[find] an appropriate point between two parameters" (ibid.), namely empathy and disclosure.

With sensitive topics, "The researcher, as the listener, can also be subject to (re) traumatisation" (Rolland et al., 2019, p. 286), which is why self-care is very important (Fawcett, 2003). Practitioners may feel better prepared than lay researchers, but key differences between a research interview and counselling (see Edge, 2020; Knox & Burkard, 2014) may make working with a "researcher hat" more challenging than expected.

Analysing the Interviews and Combining with the Survey

For each interview, analysis started practically immediately: I wrote down my first impressions and examined my own subjectivity (Roulston, 2010) in a reflexive diary, before typing a rough transcription of the audio-recording. I would then discuss the interview with Beverley. Next, I would refine the transcripts and carry out an inductive Thematic Analysis (Braun & Clarke, 2006, 2013), using NVivo to manage the volume of data.

I identified three over-arching themes, which matched the broad topics of the survey: "Language negotiation and use in therapy", "Impact of language practices" and "Perceptions of therapeutic empathy". In general, the interview data reinforced themes from the survey, providing more fine-grained detail. However, there were also new sub-themes. For example, interviewees' language preference(s) when relating to therapists appeared to be influenced by their acculturation strategies. Whilst those who preferred a relationship in English—a foreign language—held a discourse of assimilation towards life in the UK, those who valued multilingual relationships—anchored in a shared first language and the ability to switch between languages—held a discourse of integration (Rolland, 2019). This interpretation of why some migrant clients do not take up the option of code-switching when expressing themselves in psychotherapy was enabled by the more open-ended nature of interviews. Thus, examining how these helped to explain the results from the previous phase was a crucial part of the final interpretation stage.

Data analysis is a phase of intensive engagement with the data, which can also leave researchers vulnerable to (re)traumatisation (Rolland et al., 2019). Bager-Charleson et al. (2018) drew attention to the difficult feelings and physical symptoms reported by numerous therapists and highlighted coping strategies which they found helpful.

A Longitudinal Design

Another advantage of a sequential design is that it becomes a longitudinal study, with two datasets generated at different time points. Whilst the researcher can minimise the time between phases if need be, it can also be useful to have a period of reflection, for both the researcher and participants. In this case study, for example, one interviewee shared thoughts she had about the study topics since completing the survey. Engaging with the questions, Elena had asked herself why she did not wish to use any Italian—her first language—in her psychotherapy. She described how in the months between survey completion and our Skype interview, she had made the shift to introduce Italian into her therapy, in specific ways which she could tolerate (Rolland et al., 2021), without the need for her therapist to understand Italian. This had enabled her to feel connected to her childhood experiences and opened up a discussion with her therapist around language use and integrating her child and adult selves, particularly when visiting her home country. In her words, it allowed her to "reconnect with parts of myself that I didn't either explore, or I didn't want to explore" (op. cit.: 114). Thus, the time elapsed and opportunity to have a second say on the research topic revealed the impact which the first stage of the research had had on the participant. This example illustrates how the act of asking certain questions can empower research participants and clients to explore dilemmas for themselves and learn from this, at their own pace and with their own solutions. Elena's self-reflexivity may have been aided by her training as a psychotherapist, however the topic itself was new and not explored in her training.

A longitudinal element such as this model affords, then, can capture the client's journey of self-discovery and has the potential to be akin to action research, where the therapist-researcher's intervention has had a demonstrable impact. Ultimately, this study offers evidence, through a mixed methods design, that showing curiosity about language choices within therapy can lead the dyad to new places.

Conclusion

We quoted Ottolenghi in the introduction on what constitutes a well-made salad. According to him, it requires "a certain uniformity; it should make perfect sense for those ingredients to share a bowl". The same applies—by extension and with some metaphorical liberty—to a well-made mixed methods study. Our two "chefs", Sally and Louise, who came from different professional backgrounds but shared a passion about multilingualism in psychotherapy, used combinations of different methods, different types of data from different types of multilinguals in psychotherapy, to answer their own specific research questions on the role of languages in psychotherapy, taking into account participants' (known) level of vulnerability. In each case, they found that combining methods generated additional perspectives and allowed for a better understanding of the problem. Moreover, mixed methods may be particularly suited to researching with vulnerable participants since such designs can support relationship-building, be sequenced to allow for informed consent to each phase and create space for reflection, and include participatory approaches (e.g. Lenette, 2021). Thus, rather than being motivated by a desire to "mine" multiple types of data from participants, a sensitive approach to mixed methods offers opportunities to help participants to reach a new understanding of themselves through the research. In addition, both studies highlighted the need for appropriate supervision and self-care in order to protect researchers from traumatisation.

Our work also demonstrates the advantages of a cross-disciplinary perspective, where collaboration and supervision are the answer to no single person having all the expertise. Finally, the results point to a common finding, namely that code-switching and language preferences to discuss sensitive issues are very much linked to the participants' lived experiences and the embodiment of their various languages rather than just their proficiency in these languages.

Activities

(a) Can you think of an under-researched topic which would benefit from first quantifying (e.g. identifying the prevalence of a problem) before a qualitative phase to understand the experience under investigation?

(b) Can you think of other settings where ethnographic strategies would be an appropriate starting point for a follow-on qualitative study? What ethical questions would you need to consider, including around the shift in your role as a participant to researcher?

(c) What benefits and challenges could the longitudinal aspect of your chosen mixed methods design (qual-qual or quant-qual) bring to your exploration of your research topic or question?

(d) If you are multilingual and might share more than one language with some qualitative participants, consider the pros and cons of allowing

(*continued*)

(continued)
> them to choose the language(s) of communication. What additional resources and preparation might you need to carry out your chosen method(s) in more than one language?
>
> (e) Thinking about your research topic, which methods could you usefully combine and how (simultaneously or sequentially)?

Summary

The starting point of the present chapter is the fact that the languages of multilinguals have different amounts of emotional resonance. Languages acquired early in life are typically felt to be more powerful than languages acquired later. It means that multilingual clients in therapy may switch languages depending on their need to zoom in, or to distance themselves from the memories attached to words and allowing them to find the best channel for their emotions. The two studies presented in this chapter show different mixed methods approaches that allowed the researchers to uncover complex issues behind the language practices and attitudes of multilingual clients discussing sensitive issues with their therapist, and the role which using a later-learned language can play in the therapeutic journey of people who have experienced extreme trauma.

References

Bager-Charleson, S., Dewaele, J.-M., Costa, B., & Kasap, Z. (2017). A multilingual outlook: Can awareness-raising about multilingualism affect therapists' practice? A mixed-method evaluation. *Language and Psychoanalysis, 6*(2), 56–75.

Bager-Charleson, S., Du Plock, S., & McBeath, A. (2018). Therapists have a lot to add to the field of research, but many don't make it there: A narrative thematic inquiry into counsellors' and psychotherapists' embodied engagement with research. *Language and Psychoanalysis, 7*(1), 1–18.

Bager-Charleson, S., & Kasap, Z. (2017). Embodied situatedness and emotional entanglement in research – An autoethnographic hybrid inquiry into the experience of doing data analysis. *Counselling and Psychotherapy Research, 17*(3), 190–200.

Barton, J. (2020). Doing Qualitative Research with Interpretative Phenomenological Analysis. In S. Bager-Charleson and A. McBeath (Eds.), *Enjoying Research in Counselling and Psychotherapy* (pp. 51–69). Basingstoke: Palgrave Macmillan.

Barrett-Lennard, G. T. (1962). Dimension of therapist response as causal factors in therapeutic change. *Psychological Monographs, 76*, 1–36.

Bramley, N., & Eatough, V. (2005). The experience of living with Parkinson's disease: An interpretative phenomenological analysis case study. *Psychology and Health, 20*(2), 223–235.

Braun, V., & Clarke, V. (2013). *Successful qualitative research: A practical guide for beginners*. Sage.

Braun, V., & Clarke, V. (2006). Using thematic analysis in psychology. *Qualitative Research in Psychology, 3*(2), 77–101.

Burck, C. (2005). *Multilingual living: Explorations of language and subjectivity.* Palgrave Macmillan.

Burck, C. (2011). Living in several languages: Language, gender, and identities. *European Journal of Women's Studies, 18*(4), 361–378.

Byford, A. (2015). Lost and gained in translation: The impact of bilingual clients' choice of language in psychotherapy. *British Journal of Psychotherapy, 31*(3), 333–347.

Campbell, T. (2007). Psychological assessment, diagnosis, and treatment of torture survivors: A review. *Clinical Psychology Review, 27*, 628–641.

Connell, G., Macaskie, J., & Nolan, G. (2016). A third language in therapy: Deconstructing sameness and difference. *European Journal of Psychotherapy and Counselling, 18*(3), 209–227.

Cook, S. R. (2019) *Exploring the role of multilingualism in the therapeutic journey of survivors of torture and human trafficking.* Unpublished PhD thesis, Birkbeck, University of London.

Cook, S. R., & Dewaele, J.-M. (2022). 'The English language enables me to visit my pain'. Exploring experiences of using a later-learned language in the healing journey of survivors of sexuality persecution. *International Journal of Bilingualism, 26*(2), 125–139.

Costa, B., & Dewaele, J.-M. (2012) Psychotherapy across languages: beliefs, attitudes and practices of monolingual and multilingual therapists with their multilingual patients. *Language and Psychoanalysis, 1*, 18–40 (After winning the Equality and Diversity Research Award from the British Association for Counselling and Psychotherapy in 2013, it was revised and reprinted in *Counselling and Psychotherapy Research*, 2014, 14(3), 235–244.).

Costa, B., & Dewaele, J.-M. (2019). The talking cure – building the core skills and the confidence of counsellors and psychotherapists to work effectively with multilingual patients through training and supervision. *Counselling and Psychotherapy Research, 19*, 231–240.

Creswell, J. W., & Plano Clark, V. L. (2011). *Designing and conducting mixed methods research* (2nd ed.). Sage.

Cutcliffe, J. R. (2003). Reconsidering reflexivity: Introducing the case for intellectual entrepreneurship. *Qualitative Health Research, 13*(1), 136–148.

Dewaele, J.-M. (2013). *Emotions in multiple languages* (2nd ed.). Palgrave Macmillan.

Dewaele, J.-M. (2016). Emotions and Multicompetence. In V. J. Cook & L. Wei (Eds.), *The Cambridge handbook of linguistic multi-competence* (pp. 461–478). Cambridge University Press.

Dewaele, J.-M. (2019). The vital need for ontological, epistemological and methodological diversity in applied linguistics. In C. Wright, L. Harvey, & J. Simpson (Eds.), *Voices and practices in applied linguistics: Diversifying a discipline* (pp. 71–88). White Rose University Press.

Dewaele, J.-M. (2023). Research into multilingualism and emotions. In G. L. Schiewer, J. Altarriba, & B. Chin Ng (Eds.), *Language and emotion. An international handbook* (pp. 1217–1237). Mouton De Gruyter.

Dewaele, J.-M., & Costa, B. (2013). Multilingual clients' experience of psychotherapy. *Language and Psychoanalysis, 2*(2), 31–50.

Dewaele, J.-M., & Costa, B. (2014). A cross-disciplinary and multi-method approach of multilingualism in psychotherapy. In S. Bager-Charleson (Ed.), *A reflexive approach. Doing practice-based research in therapy* (pp. 28–37). London: Sage.

Dewaele, J.-M., Lorette, P., Rolland, L., & Mavrou, I. (2021). Differences in emotional reactions of Greek, Hungarian and British users of English when watching television in English. *International Journal of Applied Linguistics, 31*(3), 345–361.

Edge, J. (2020). *Continuing cooperative development.* University of Michigan Press.

Fawcett, J. (Ed.). (2003). *Stress and trauma handbook: Strategies for flourishing in demanding environments.* World Vision International.

Finlay, L. (2020). Ethical research? Examining knotty, moment-to-moment challenges throughout the research process. In S. Bager-Charleson & A. McBeath (Eds.), *Enjoying research in counselling and psychotherapy* (pp. 115–136). Palgrave Macmillan.

Frost, N., & Bailey-Rodriguez, D. (2020). Doing qualitatively driven mixed methods and pluralistic qualitative research. In S. Bager-Charleson & A. McBeath (Eds.), *Enjoying research in counselling and psychotherapy* (pp. 137–160). Palgrave Macmillan.

Hinchman, L. P., & Hinchman, S. (Eds.). (1997). *Memory, identity, community: The idea of narrative in the human sciences.* SUNY Press.

Jackson, S., Backett-Milburn, K., & Newall, E. (2013). Researching distressing topics: Emotional reflexivity and emotional labor in the secondary analysis of children and young people's narratives of abuse. *SAGE Open, 3*(2). https://doi.org/10.1177/2158244013490705

Josselson, R. (2013). *Interviewing for qualitative inquiry: A relational approach.* Guilford Press.

Kennard, D. (1998). *An introduction to therapeutic communities.* London: Jessica Kingsley.

Knox, S., & Burkard, A. W. (2014). Qualitative research interviews: An update. In W. Lutz & S. Knox (Eds.), *Quantitative and qualitative methods in psychotherapy research* (pp. 342–354). Routledge.

Langdridge, D. (2007). *Phenomenological psychology: Theory, research and method.* Pearson Education.

Leavy, P. (Ed.). (2014). *The Oxford handbook of qualitative research.* Oxford Library of Psychology.

Lenette, C. (2021). Health on the move: Walking interviews in health and wellbeing research. In D. Lupton & D. Leahy (Eds.), *Creative approaches to health education. New ways of thinking, making, doing, teaching and learning* (pp. 136–159). Routledge.

Maggs-Rapport, F. (2000). Combining methodological approaches in research: Ethnography and interpretive phenomenology. *Journal of Advanced Nursing, 31*(1), 219–225.

Mann, S. (2016). *The research interview: Reflective practice and reflexivity in research processes.* Palgrave Macmillan.

Marcos, L. R. (1976). Bilinguals in psychotherapy: Language as an emotional barrier. *American Journal of Psychotherapy, 36*(4), 347–354.

McBeath, A. (2020). Doing quantitative research with a survey. In S. Bager-Charleson & A. McBeath (Eds.), *Enjoying research in counselling and psychotherapy* (pp. 175–194). Palgrave Macmillan.

McBeath, A., & Bager-Charleson, S. (2020). Introduction: Considering qualitative, quantitative and mixed methods research. In S. Bager-Charleson & A. McBeath (Eds.), *Enjoying research in counselling and psychotherapy* (pp. 1–12). Palgrave Macmillan.

McGranahan, C. (2015). Anthropology as Theoretical Storytelling. In C. McGranahan (Ed.), *Writing Anthropology: Essays on Craft and Commitment* (pp. 73–77). New York, USA: Duke University Press.

Morse, J.-M. (2009). *Mixing qualitative methods.* Sage.

Morse, J. M. (2017). *Essentials of qualitatively-driven mixed-method designs.* Routledge.

Morse, J.-M., & Niehaus, L. (2009). *Mixed method design: Principles and procedures.* Coast Press.

Nightingale, D., & Cromby, J. (1999). *Social constructionist psychology: A critical analysis of theory and practice.* McGraw-Hill Education.

Ottolenghi, Y. (2012, March 9). Yotam Ottolenghi's end-of-winter salad recipes. *The Guardian.* https://www.theguardian.com/lifeandstyle/2012/mar/09/late-winter-salad-recipes-ottlenghi

Panicacci, A., & Dewaele, J.-M. (2017). 'A voice from elsewhere': Acculturation, personality and migrants' self-perceptions across languages and cultures. *International Journal of Multilingualism, 14*(4), 419–436.

Parker, I. (2007). *Revolution in psychology.* Pluto Press.

Pavlenko, A. (2005). *Emotions and multilingualism.* Cambridge University Press.

Pavlenko, A. (2012). Affective processing in bilingual speakers: Disembodied cognition? *International Journal of Psychology, 47*(6), 405–428.

Pérez-Rojas, A. E., Brown, R., Cervantes, A., Valente, T., & Pereira, S. R. (2019). "Alguien abrió la puerta": The phenomenology of bilingual Latinx clients' use of Spanish and English in psychotherapy. *Psychotherapy, 56*(2), 241–253.

Priest, A. (2020). Doing mixed methods research. Combining outcome measures with interviews. In S. Bager-Charleson & A. McBeath (Eds.), *Enjoying research in counselling and psychotherapy* (pp. 213–238). Palgrave Macmillan.

Rhodes, J., & Smith, J. A. (2010). "The top of my head came off": An interpretative phenomenological analysis of the experience of depression. *Counselling Psychology Quarterly, 23*(4), 399–409.

Rolland, L. (2019). *Multilingual selves in psychotherapy: A mixed methods study of multilingual clients' experiences in relation to language practices.* Unpublished PhD thesis, Birkbeck, University of London.

Rolland, L. (in prep.) "I'm sure at some point we'll be switching": Planning and enacting an interview language policy with multilingual participants.

Rolland, L., Costa, B., & Dewaele, J.-M. (2021). Negotiating the language(s) for psychotherapy talk: A mixed methods study from the perspective of multilingual clients. *Counselling and Psychotherapy Research, 21*, 107–117.

Rolland, L., Dewaele, J.-M., & Costa, B. (2017). Multilingualism and psychotherapy: Exploring multilingual clients' experiences of language practices in psychotherapy. *International Journal of Multilingualism, 14*(1), 69–85.

Rolland, L., Dewaele, J.-M., & Costa, B. (2019). Planning and conducting ethical interviews: Power, language and emotions. In J. McKinley & H. Rose (Eds.), *The Routledge handbook of research methods in applied linguistics* (pp. 279–289). Routledge.

Roulston, K. (2010). *Reflective interviewing.* Sage.

Silverman, D. (2003). *Doing qualitative research.* Sage.

Smith, J. A. (2017). Interpretative phenomenological analysis: Getting at lived experience. *The Journal of Positive Psychology, 12*(3), 303–304.

Smith, J., Flowers, P., & Larkin, M. (2009). *Interpretative phenomenological analysis: Theory, method and research.* Sage.

Yanow, D. (2006). Thinking interpretively: Philosophical presuppositions and the human sciences. *Interpretation and Method: Empirical Research Methods and the Interpretive Turn, 2*, 5–26.

Index